ANNALS OF
THE NEW YORK ACADEMY
OF SCIENCES

Volume 847

EDITORIAL STAFF

Executive Editor
BILL BOLAND

Managing Editor
JUSTINE CULLINAN

Associate Editor
MARION L. GARRY

The New York Academy of Sciences
2 East 63rd Street
New York, New York 10021

ULTRASOUND SCREENING FOR FETAL ANOMALIES: IS IT WORTH IT?

SCREENING REVISITED AFTER THE EUROFETUS DATA

ANNALS OF THE NEW YORK ACADEMY OF SCIENCES
Volume 847

ULTRASOUND SCREENING FOR FETAL ANOMALIES: IS IT WORTH IT?

SCREENING REVISITED AFTER THE EUROFETUS DATA

Edited by Salvator Levi and Frank A. Chervenak

The New York Academy of Sciences
New York, New York
1998

(SCI)
Q
11
.N5
Vol. 847

LOYOLA UNIVERSITY LIBRARY

∞ The paper used in this publication meets the minimum requirements of American National Standard for Information Sciences—Permanence of Paper for Printed Library Materials, ANSI Z39.48-1984.

Cover: A classic ultrasound representation of fetal ventriculomegaly. (Arrows point to the midline echo; LV, dilated lateral ventricle; CP, dangling choroid plexus; C, compressed cerebral cortex.)

Library of Congress Cataloging-in Publication Data

Ultrasound screening for fetal anomalies: Is it worth it? : screening revisited after the Eurofetus data / edited by Salvator Levi and Frank A. Chervenak.
    p.   cm.— (Annals of the New York Academy of Sciences, ISSN 0077-8923 : v. 847)
    Papers presented at a conference held in New York City on June 23-25, 1997.
    Includes bibliographical references and index.
    ISBN 1-57331-123-5 (cloth : alk. paper). — ISBN 1-57331-124-3 (paper : alk. paper)
    1. Fetus—Abnormalities—Ultrasonic imaging—Congresses. 2. Fetus—Diseases—Diagnosis—Congresses. 3. Ultrasonics in obstetrics—Congresses. 4. Prenatal diagnosis—Congresses. 5. Diagnosis, Ultrasonic—Congresses. I. Levi, Salvator, II. New York Academy of Sciences. III. Series.
    [DNLM: 1. Fetal Diseases—ultrasonography congresses. 2. Ultrasonography, Prenatal congresses. 3. Abnormalities—ultrasonography congresses. 4. Fetus—abnormalities congresses. W1 AN626YL v. 847 1998]
    Q11.N5 vol. 847
    [RG628.3.U58]
    618.3'207543—DC21
    DNLM/DLC
    for Library of Congress   98-17556
                                                                                 CIP

ComCom/RRD
Printed in the United States of America
ISBN 1-57331-123-5 (cloth)
ISBN 1-57331-124-3 (paper)
ISSN 0077-8923

ANNALS OF THE NEW YORK ACADEMY OF SCIENCES

Volume 847
June 18, 1998

ULTRASOUND SCREENING FOR FETAL ANOMALIES: IS IT WORTH IT?

SCREENING REVISITED AFTER THE EUROFETUS DATA[a]

Editors and Conference Organizers
SALVATOR LEVI AND FRANK A. CHERVENAK

CONTENTS

[a] This volume contains papers presented at a conference entitled Ultrasound Screening for Fetal Anomalies: Is It Worth It?, which was sponsored jointly by the New York Academy of Sciences and The Eurofetus Project and held in New York City on June 23–25, 1997.

Financial assistance was received from:

Supporter

- MARCH OF DIMES BIRTH DEFECTS FOUNDATION

Contributor

- ACUSON CORP.
- ALOKA CO. LTD.

Preface

SALVATOR LEVI[a] AND FRANK A. CHERVENAK[b]

[a]Ultrasound Laboratory, Department of Obstetrics and Gynecology, Centre Hospitalier
Universitaire Brugmann and Université Libre de Bruxelles, Brussels, Belgium
[b]Department of Obstetrics and Gynecology, The New York Hospital-Cornell Medical
Center, New York, New York, USA

One of the most important controversies in modern clinical medicine is the question,
"Ultrasound screening for fetal anomalies: Is it worth it?" The RADIUS study, the
largest randomized controlled clinical trial on this subject, suggests that routine screening is not efficacious or cost-effective. Although this conclusion has been supported by
the American College of Obstetricians and Gynecologists, most American obstetricians
disagree with the College. In contrast to this American study, a considerable body of
work has come forth from Europe supporting routine obstetric ultrasound. By far the
largest study on this subject is the Eurofetus database, in which 200,000 low-risk pregnant women in 60 hospitals had obstetric ultrasound examinations performed in centers proficient in prenatal diagnosis. The 61% overall detection rate of structural anomalies in the Eurofetus study contrasts sharply with the 35% overall detection rate in the
RADIUS study.

In order to address the conflicting data and conflicting opinions on this topic, a conference was held at The Rockefeller University in New York City, June 23–25, 1997,
sponsored by the New York Academy of Sciences. Over 150 scientists and clinicians
participated in the meeting, with highly informative presentations and lively discus-
sions. The purpose of this volume is to present the most important aspects of the conference.

Part I deals with the relevance of fetal anomalies in clinical practice. Dimensions of
this important topic are developed by an obstetrician-geneticist, a pediatrician, and a
mental health professional. There is a broad-based consensus that fetal anomalies do
indeed have an impact on medical care both before and after birth.

The question of whether the prenatal diagnosis of fetal anomalies affects perinatal outcome is presented in Part II. Anomalies of the central nervous system, cardiovascular system, gastrointestinal system, and the genitourinary system are reviewed
with an emphasis on the effect of prenatal diagnosis on outcome. The San Francisco
group that pioneered fetal surgery presents a comprehensive review of this important
topic.

Parts III and IV emphasize the methodology, results, and conclusions of the Eurofetus study. The importance of quality assurance in obstetric and gynecologic ultrasound is presented in the Hungarian model.

Parts V and VI cover the important topics of economic analysis, managed care,
ethics, law, education, psychology, biochemical screening, first trimester ultrasound,
and ultrasound screening for fetal anomalies in developing countries. Last, poster papers from the conference are presented.

In summary, at the conference and in this volume we have tried to put together
comprehensive state-of-the-art information on the routine obstetric ultrasound controversy. Our conclusion from this effort is that routine obstetric ultrasound is war-
ranted for all pregnancies, but only if it is performed in a quality manner. Although
there is still scientific and economic controversy about our conclusion, we would argue

that, at a minimum, there is an ethical obligation to present the option of an 18–22-week routine obstetric ultrasound examination in clinical centers in which quality ultrasound is available. We hope that our efforts will move public policy in this direction and encourage further discourse on this most important topic in contemporary obstetrics.

What Is an Anomaly?

MARK I. EVANS AND JENIFER LAMPINEN

*Departments of Obstetrics and Gynecology, Molecular Medicine & Genetics, and
Pathology, Wayne State University, Detroit, Michigan 48201, USA*

It has long been appreciated by geneticists, obstetricians, and pediatricians that the occurrence of babies born with congenital anomalies of a serious nature is between 2 and 4%, and that if one includes the minor anomalies, this number may approach 7–8%. This figure is far higher than most couples realize and may represent one of the reasons that obstetrics is particularly litigious, in that most couples feel they have an "inherent right" to a perfectly normal, healthy child. This conference attempts to investigate one particular approach to the identification of fetal anomalies—that of the use of ultrasound screening, which, at various times, has shown tremendous promise and expertise, and at other times has been highly ineffective.

As a starting point we must attempt to communicate in a language that is agreed upon by all. It has been commonplace throughout the literature that different terminologies have been used for the same event, thus making it particularly difficult to try to compare results from various centers around the world. This has led to confusion in many instances about the prognosis of particular conditions when they are given different names.

The purpose of this initial presentation is to bring together common usages of often misused terminologies, with the aim of arriving at a common ground for usage at this conference (TABLE 1). This overview is not intended to be a thorough discussion of each of these terms, which can be found in standard genetics and pathology textbooks, but merely to emphasize their proper usage.

TABLE 1. Glossary of Terms

• Anomaly	Deviation from the normal in regard to form, structure, or position
• Aplasia	Complete absence of cellular proliferation
• Hypoplasia	Results from insufficient or decreased cellular growth
• Hyperplasia	Results from excessive cellular growth
• Dysplasia	Abnormal growth or development of cells causing disorganized cellular structure
• Agenesis	Failure of a structure or organ to form
• Dysgenesis	Defective development resulting in some type of disorganization
• Atrophy	Degeneration of cells which results in wasting or a decreased size
• Hypotrophy	Undergrowth or the failure to reach the normal size
• Hypertrophy	Overgrowth of a structure or organ
• Genotype	Refers to an organism's genetic composition
• Phenotype	Outward physical appearance or genetic makeup of an individual; the direct result of the genotype and, in some cases, the environment

[Continued overleaf]

1

TABLE 1. Glossary of Terms *(Continued)*

• Congenital	Refers to conditions present at birth which may or may not be genetic
• Genetic	An inherited, but not always congenital, condition
• Malformation	A birth defect due to an intrinsic abnormality or incomplete development. Can be genetic, environmental or multifactorial, and typically occurs prior to 10 weeks of gestation. Cleft lip and/or cleft palate may be classified as malformations.
• Disruption	An interference with formation of an otherwise normal structure and a result from external forces such as amniotic bands or teratogens. May be the result of environmental agents or mechanical concerns
• Deformation	In contrast to a disruption, a deformation occurs *after* the normal formation of an organ or structure. It is the the result of compression, constriction, or immobility, e.g., club feet due to oliohydramnios. In some cases, it may have a genetic cause.
• Etiology	Underlying cause of an anomaly
• Pathogenesis	Specific mechanism by which an anomaly or disease occurs
• Syndrome, genetic	A group of features seen together with common, specific etiology
• Syndrome, complex	Composite of multiple features
• Spectrum	Considered complex, with considerable variation
• Association	Nonrandom occurrence of multiple features, with no known etiology, e.g., VACTRAL and CHARGE
• Sequence	Pattern of anomalies from a single anomaly or factor, e.g., Potter sequence vs. syndrome
• Teratogen	An environmental agent that causes a morphologic abnormality after fertilization, but prior to delivery
• Mendelian	Conditions, typically single gene, inherited in the manner conceived by Gregor Mendel
• Multifactorial	Caused by both genetic and environmental factors
• Sporadic	Occurring by chance, not hereditary
• Macrocephaly	Abnormal largeness of the head of uncertain origin
• Hydrocephaly	A large head due to ventriculomegaly; often colloquially referred to as "water" on the brain
• Ventriculomegaly	An increase in ventricle size, with or without a large head size

Fetal Anomalies and the Pediatrician

DOMINIQUE BIARENT

Pediatric and Neonatal Intensive Care Unit, Hôpital Universitaire des Enfants Reine Fabiola, Université Libre de Bruxelles, 15 avenue JJ Crocq, B-1020 Brussels, Belgium

ABSTRACT: The role of the pediatrician begins when the antenatal diagnosis of a congenital anomaly has been confirmed in a high-risk perinatal center. The pediatrician contributes in establishing the prognosis and to discuss the best therapeutic possibilities based upon his own experience and the literature. The pediatrician plays an important role in the informing of the parents, particularly when the malformation is correctable. He will provide them with a complete explanation about the care of the baby, possible complications, and the prognosis. The parents meet the medical staff, see the place where their child will be treated after birth, gain confidence, and prepare the best possible mother-infant and father-infant links. The delivery should be planned in a high-risk perinatal center to avoid the postnatal transportation of a sick newborn infant as well as the separation of the infant from the mother. A planned delivery is essential to permit the pediatrician to prepare and execute an early adapted-to-the-malformation resuscitation and prompt surgery in the hope of reducing mortality and morbidity. After birth, the pediatrician plays a role not only in the pre- and postoperative care, but also in supporting the parents and facilitating their investment in the sick baby. The antenatal diagnosis permits the pediatrician and the surgeon to prepare and optimize the care of the newborn and allows the parents to anticipate the mourning of the imagined infant, providing them time to accept the diagnosis and the sick baby before the birth.

The pediatrician (pediatrician must be understood as a team including neonatologist, pediatric intensivist, and pediatric surgeon) is increasingly concerned with congenital anomalies (CA) because they constitute a growing proportion among the causes of perinatal morbidity and mortality.[1-5] Moreover, the pediatrician's concern toward CA is changing because members of the pediatric team may be required to participate in the diagnosis and prognosis of the CA before the birth of their "patient-to-come." Their role in advising and preparing the parents is of utmost importance. Recently, the function of the pediatrician with respect to the fetus as a patient has changed. Instead of beginning with the care of the newborn in the delivery room—as was usually required by the obstetrician—it begins now largely before birth. This is explained by the antenatal diagnosis of a majority of CA depending on the screening efficiency for detecting anomalies.[2]

ANTENATAL DIAGNOSIS

When a malformation is suspected, examination at the tertiary level is required to confirm, correct, and complete the diagnosis using research of associated malformations or anomalies dramatically important to determine the prognosis.

Setting the Prognosis

The specially qualified pediatricians (neonatologists, intensivists, cardiologists, pediatric surgeons) are now usually invited to join a group of specialists involved in the care of CA: obstetric and perinatal specialists in high-risk pregnancy and in antenatal ultrasound, geneticists, radiologists, pathologists, nurses, and social workers. This "perinatal advisory group" (PAG) works in most of the tertiary centers involved in fetal and perinatal medicine that gathers information and knowledge about fetal disease and anomalies.

Indeed, the high number of various disorders that can be diagnosed nowadays by antenatal ultrasound do not allow one single group of care providers to counsel all cases.[2,5,6] The aim of the group is to discuss the accuracy of the diagnosis, the usefulness of analyses such as amniocentesis, cordocentesis, biochemical analysis and biochemical genetics, cytogenetics and molecular genetics—a recently growing field—and interpretation of the results and their implications for the pregnancy, birth management, and counseling for the parents.[5,7]

A PAG is active on our campus, including the obstetrics and gynecology department (Centre Hospitalier Brugmann) and the University Hospital for Children. During the last four years, the PAG has provided counseling in 138 cases at our institution. Fifty-four percent of the cases are referred by private obstetricians or other hospitals; 46% come from our own department of obstetrics and perinatology. In 123 out of 138 pregnancies (see TABLE 1), the diagnosis was confirmed at birth (87 live births) or at pathology after pregnancy termination (32) or spontaneous fetal death (4). Among the live births, 41 CA were treated by neonatal surgical correction, 23 CA were confirmed but did not require any neonatal surgery, 15 in both categories died in the follow-up, 23 had normalized ultrasound findings before birth and were confirmed as normal. In 6 other cases the ultrasound diagnosis was not confirmed at birth, but in none of those cases was the pregnancy terminated early. In 9 cases no follow-up was obtained. In 7 cases, the problem directly concerned the mother (maternal cardiopathy or phenylketonuria) or the vitality of the fetus (twin-to-twin transfusion syndrome).

The distribution of the frequencies of the discussed anomalies does not reflect the repartition of the fetal pathologies encountered in the sample of prenatal diagnoses managed by the ultrasound lab,[8] but corresponds only to the cases submitted to the

TABLE 1. Topics Discussed at the Perinatal Meetings (1993–1997, Brussels)

	Pregnancies (*n*)	Confirmed Diagnosis[a]		Diagnosis Not Confirmed[b]	
		Live Birth[c]	Stillbirth or Abortion[d]	by Follow-up[e]	No Follow-up[f]
Digestive malformations	35	30	3	1	1
Cardiac anomalies	23	17	4	1	1
Urologic malformations	18	9	3	2	4
Osseous and morphologic malformations	14	6	6	1	1
Chromosomal abnormalities	15	3	12		
Central nervous system defects	7	3	3	1	
Lung anomalies	4	3	1		
Metabolic disorders	9	5	2		2
Infectious diseases	5	3	2		
Maternal or fetal problems	8	8	0		
Total	138	87 (63%)	36 (26%)	6 (4.3%)	9 (6.5%)

[a]CA diagnosed by ultrasound or absence of CA after referral by private obstetrician or other hospital. Both diagnoses made by the PAG and confirmed at birth[c] or at pathology in the case of stillbirth or fetal death.[d]

[b]CA diagnosed by ultrasound but not confirmed at birth[e] or lost from the follow-up.[f]

PAG and reflects the need to confront an expert multidisciplinary team with a series of anomalies to help the obstetrician make the right decision.

The PAG handles severe as well as more moderate cases of CA. Advice about lethal or noncurable and severe CA usually end up with a unanimous and clear decision as to their management and counseling for the parents. In most of the cases, the issue should be termination of the pregnancy with the agreement of the parents.[9] For all the other types of abnormalities, the question should be whether or not to continue the pregnancy.

The Obstetrician–Pediatrician Relationship

The pediatrician brings to the PAG his knowledge of the best therapeutic possibilities and their application for each kind of anomaly, the relative risk of complications, the prognosis for each modality of treatment, the timing of appearance of the symptomatology, the eventuality of resuscitation in the delivery room, the preoperative care to apply, and the expected duration of the hospitalization. The members of the pediatric team also know the results for each pathology and the related literature.

The presence of a fetal anomaly indicates that the pregnancy should be evaluated in a high-risk perinatal center to gather complete information; it also indicates that the delivery should ideally be planned in a high-risk perinatal center to avoid the postnatal transportation of a sick newborn infant as well as the separation of the infant from the mother.[10] This situation is highly desired by the pediatric team because it guarantees the presence of a specialized team at birth allowing early resuscitation adapted to the malformation and prompt surgery if needed. Even with an inaccurate diagnosis, the presence of a specialized team will permit a rapid diagnosis and the adaptation of the treatment to the reality. The common goal must be to define an obstetric-pediatric consensus for an optimal and definitive therapeutic approach for the benefit of the parents and their baby-to-come.

Announcement to the Parents

The antenatal diagnosis and announcement of a fetal anomaly highly modify the perception of a wanted pregnancy. From a joyfully anticipated event, the pregnancy becomes stressful and full of questions for the couple.[11] The baby as it is imagined is modified by the ultrasound findings. It is the team's responsibility to provide sufficient information to permit the future parents to make an informed decision, that is to say:[5,12]

- To help them understand the malformation.
- To give them correct and complete information about the treatment
- To give them information about the prognosis of morbidity, mortality, and disability of the newborn
- To provide them with genetic counseling, if possible
- To enable them to decide whether they want to continue the pregnancy and support them in their decision.[7]

The main concern of the team must be to respect and protect parental autonomy.[12]

Parents–Pediatrician Relationship: Prenatal Meeting

The counseling of the parents is done individually by one or several members of the PAG or any other specialist according to the recommendations of the PAG. In the case of a correctable malformation, a meeting between the parents, pediatrician, and pediatric surgeon should be organized by the obstetrician. The pediatric surgeon explains the risks and benefits of proposed surgical correction and those of alternative treatments as well as of no treatment. Description of the intervention should be clear: resection and end-to-end anastomosis or stoma in gut atresia, for example, or the eventuality of palliation if the immediate and complete correction is not possible during the neonatal period (as in some congenital cardiopathies or in the case of esophageal agenesis). The surgeon and pediatrician will show the parents the neonatal intensive care unit where the child will be treated, making them comfortable with the future care of the baby. The pediatrician explains the general technical care the baby will need before and after the operation such as artificial ventilation, thoracic drainage, central lines or parenteral nutrition. Specific techniques like silo in giant exomphalos or extracorporeal circulation in diaphragmatic hernia should also be shown or explained. Expected duration of care is also stated. The pediatrician assures the parents that the goal of the pediatric team is that a relatively normal child is born. He tries to show them that even with extensive care, the parents play an important role in the nurturing of the baby and that loving care[13] is as important as medical care. Parents are strongly encouraged to stay close to their child and provide some of the care themselves, to breast-feed and kangaroo-carry their child. Brothers and sisters are allowed to come and visit the baby. To see where the child will be after birth and to meet the medical staff fosters confidence in the parents.[9]

Details are given not to emphasize the stress of the future parents, but to make them familiar with the management of the baby. Hesitation and conflicting advice from the members of the team reflect some incompetence on the part of the medical team and are more likely to increase the stress of the parents than are simple but precise and competent explanations about the future. However, it is extremely important to underline the probabilistic nature of medicine, neonatalogy, and neonatal surgery.[12] Treatments vary in their efficacy and the risks are not always predictable. The published results of follow-up studies are always given in terms of group statistical measures and therefore are not necessarily applicable individually in a simple way.[14]

POSTNATAL CARE

Enormous enthusiasm has been expressed in past years for the antenatal ultrasound diagnosis of major fetal malformations. Antenatal detection of surgically correctable malformations would ideally reduce mortality and morbidity.[15,16] It is difficult to evaluate the true benefit offered by the antenatal diagnosis to a baby with a CA.

Of 127 newborns admitted in our neonatal and pediatric intensive care unit for surgical correction of a digestive anomaly, 84 had gastrointestinal atresia (10 duodenal, 29 esophageal, 22 anal, 23 gut atresia or obstructions), 19 had wall defects, and 24 had diaphragmatic hernias. Forty-one newborns had been diagnosed antenatally (32%). Eighty-six babies were diagnosed postnatally (68%). Only 44% of the babies with an antenatal diagnosis were transferred *in utero* and, in fact, only diaphragmatic hernias and wall defects were systematically transferred *in utero* when diagnosis was made before birth, because Belgium unfortunately has no regional policies concerning this issue. Moreover, despite antenatal diagnosis, the newborns not transferred antenatally were transferred in a tertiary level center for surgery only at a mean age of 15 hours. Infants in whom the CA was diagnosed postnatally were transferred at a mean age of 30 hours. Some obstetricians do not seem to consider anomalies other than diaphragmatic hernias and wall defects at risk during and immediately after delivery and continue to prefer to transfer the baby postnatally.

Contrary to this opinion, in this series, babies with antenatal detected CA (group A) were sicker than babies with postnatal detected CA (group P). The mortality was 32% in group A and 16% in group P despite the fact that group A babies had fewer associated malformations. Twenty-nine percent of the group A babies had one or more malformations associated with the digestive CA. Fifty percent of the associated malformations are considered as major (with a vital risk such as cardiopathy, and other severe digestive, neurologic or renal malformation). As expected, none of them had chromosomal anomalies. Group P newborns had other malformations in 54% of the cases with 54% of major malformations and 7% of chromosomal anomalies. With respect to those results, one can assume that the severity of the illness is related to the digestive disease itself as well as to the associated malformations.

In another study made in our hospital, Viart et al.[17] showed that 24.5% of 139 ductus-dependent congenital heart diseases (CHD) were diagnosed during fetal life. The severe duct-dependent CHD were more frequently detected antenatally than the less severe left-heart obstructions, Fallot tetralogy and pulmonary stenosis (31 vs. 16%). In the same way, detected duct-dependent CDH had a worse prognosis than the undetected (mortality rate of 42 vs. 14%).[18] In the literature, other studies have also shown no difference[15,16,19,20,21] or a worse prognosis[22,23] in antenatal diagnosis of congenital malformations when compared with postnatal diagnosis.

We cannot exclude a "hidden mortality" of the most severe cases of infants with undiagnosed CA, who were not adequately resuscitated and who died in the delivery room before transfer or later. This hidden mortality had been demonstrated in the case of diaphragmatic hernia by Harrison and co-workers.[24] Nevertheless, antenatal diagnosis seems to detect more serious diseases, and this emphasizes the need for *in utero* transportation to optimize the care to those seriously ill newborns.

Mother–Infant and Father–Infant Relationship

In the case of congenital malformation, parental feelings of love, concern, and hope for their baby's well-being mix with feelings of guilt, fear, and grief. The parents are frequently disappointed by the loss of the fantasized baby as can also happen in a normal pregnancy. However, they also feel guilty not to have produced a healthy baby and to be incapable of protecting him from harm after birth. They are afraid of losing the baby, but are anxious about the impact of their baby's illness on their well-being and that of their family.[12] The pediatrician should recognize and verbalize those feelings to help the parents to cope with the baby's anomaly. All those stages—loss of the fantasized baby, recognition of the anomaly, feeling of guilty, understanding of the medical implication, acceptance and rebuilding of a different imagined baby, coping with the malformation—will begin before birth in the case of antenatal diagnosis, but only after birth in the case of postnatal diagnosis.[12]

Prenatal knowledge of an anomaly could increase parental anxiety during the remainder of the pregnancy, but is always seen as beneficial in allowing time to prepare for the arrival of a sick baby and the medical and surgical interventions required. In the absence of ultrasound diagnosis in diagnosticable malformations, parents always feel frustrated. They regret they did not have the time to prepare the birth and the opportunity to decide or not to continue the pregnancy.

Collaboration between obstetricians and pediatricians has changed since the development of the ultrasound screening of pregnancies. Nowadays, the pediatrician has a role to play in the care of the fetus.

A perinatal advisory group is required in case of CA to complete the diagnosis, make a prognosis, guide the care of the mother and the fetus, and encourage the *in utero* transfer. Prenatal diagnosis has a psychological benefit for the parents by improving their ability to cope with the anomaly of their child.

REFERENCES

1. FEKETE, C.N. 1984. Attitudes du chirurgien face au diagnostic antenatal d'une malformation. J. Génét. Hum. **32:** 15–22.
2. LEVI, S., Y. HYJAZI, J.P. SCHAAPS, P. DEFOORT, R. COULON & P. BUEKENS. 1991. Sensitivity and specificity of routine antenatal screening for congenital anomalies by ultrasound: The Belgian Multicentric Study. Ultrasound Obstet. Gynecol. **1:** 102–110.
3. SAARI-KEMPPAINEN, A., O. KARJALAINEN, P. YLOSTALO & O.P. HEINONEN. 1990. Ultrasound screening and perinatal mortality: Controlled trial of one-stage screening of pregnancy. The Helsinki ultrasound trial. Lancet **336:** 387–391.
4. VINTZILEOS, A.M., W.A. CAMPBELL, D.J. NOCHIMSON & P.J. WEINBAUM. 1987. Antenatal evaluation and management of ultrasonically detected fetal anomaly. Obstet. Gynecol. **69:** 640–660.
5. WILCOX, D.T., H.L. KARAMANOUKIAN & P.H. GLICK. 1993. Antenatal diagnosis of pediatric surgical anomalies. Counseling the family. Pediatr. Clin. North Am. **40:** 1273–1287.
6. STEPHENSON, S.R. & D.D. WEAVER. 1981. Prenatal diagnosis. A compilation of diagnosed conditions. Am. J. Obstet. Gynecol. **141:** 319–343.
7. VAMOS, E., K. VANDENBERGHE & J.J. CASSIMAN. 1997. Prenatal diagnosis in Belgium. Eur. J. Hum. Genet. **5(Suppl. 1):** 7–13.
8. LEVI, S., J.P. SCHAAPS, P. DE HAVAY, R. COULON & P. DEFOORT. 1995. End-result of routine ultrasound screening for congenital anomalies: The Belgian multicentric study 1984–92. Ultrasound Obstet. Gynecol. **5:** 366–371.
9. DUMEZ, Y. 1993. Prise en charge obstétricale des malformations foetales chirurgicalement curables. Pédiatrie **48:** 99–107.
10. SARDA, P., H. BARD, F. TEASDALE & A. GRIGNON. 1983. The importance of an antenatal ultrasonographic diagnosis of correctable fetal malformations. Am. J. Obstet. Gynecol. **147:** 443–445.
11. WHITE-VAN MOURIK, M.C., J.M. CONNOR & M.A. FERGUSON-SMITH. 1992. The psychosocial sequelae of a second trimester termination of pregnancy for fetal abnormality over a two year period. Birth Defects **28:** 61–74.
12. ROSTAIN, A.L. & V.K. BHUTANI. 1989. Ethical dilemmas of neonatal-perinatal surgery. Clin. Perinatol. **16:** 275–302.
13. ALS, H., G. LAWHON, F.H. DUFFY, G.B. MCANULTY, R. GIBES-GROSSMAN & J.G. BLICKMAN. 1994. Individualized developmental care for the very low-birth-weight preterm infant. Medical and neurofunctional effects. JAMA **272:** 853–858.
14. KINLAW, K. 1996. The changing nature of neonatal ethics in practice. Clin. Perinatol. **23:** 417–428.
15. HANCOCK, B.J. & N.E. WISEMAN. 1989. Congenital duodenal obstruction: The impact of an antenatal diagnosis. J. Pediatr. Surg. **24:** 1027–1031.
16. QUIRK, J.G., H. FORTNEY JOHN, BRECKENRIDGE COLLINS II, J. WEST, SJ. HASSAD & C. WAGNER. 1996. Outcomes of newborns with gastroschisis: The effects of mode of delivery, site of delivery, and interval from birth to surgery. Am. J. Obstet. Gynecol. **174:** 1134–1140.
17. VIART, P., G. RONDIA, H. DESSY, A. GALLEZ, F.E. DEUVAERT, D. BLUM, P. HEIMANN & E. VAMOS. 1993. Cardiologie foetale: le diagnostic anténatal des malformations cardiaques. Rev. Med. Brux. **14:** 252–257.
18. LEVI, S., D. BIARENT & P. VIART. 1993. Routine ultrasound screening for fetal malformations: Genuine utility or intellectual pastime? (abstract). *In* Clinical Basis and Research, Fetal Diagnosis and Therapy **5:** 8 S2.
19. NICHOLLS, G., V. UPADHYAYA, P. GORNAMLL, R.G. BUICK & J.J. CORKERY. 1993. Is specialist centre delivery of gastroschisis beneficial? Arch. Dis. Child. **69:** 71–73.
20. ROBERTS, J. P. & D.M. BURGE. 1990. Antenatal diagnosis of abdominal wall defects: A missed opportunity? Arch. Dis. Child. **657:** 687–689.
21. WILSON, J. M., D.O. FAUZA, D.P. LUND, B. R. BENACERRAF & W. H. HENDREN. 1994. An-

tenatal diagnosis of isolated congenital diaphragmatic hernia is not an indicator of outcome. J. Pediatr. Surg. **29:** 815–819.

22. DOMMERGUES, M., C.L. SYLVESTRE, L. MANDELBROT, J.F. OURY, M. HERLICOVIEZ, G. BODY, M. GAMERRE & Y. DUMEZ. 1996. Congenital diaphragmatic hernia: Can prenatal ultrasonography predict outcome? Am. J. Obstet. Gynecol. **174:** 1377–1381.

23. FAUZA, D.O. & J. M. WILSON. 1994. Congenital diaphragmatic hernia and associated anomalies: Their incidence, identification, and impact on prognosis. J. Pediatr. Surg. **29:** 1113–1117.

24. HARRISON, M.R., R.I. BJORDAL, F. LANGMARK & O. KNUTRUD. 1978. Congenital diaphragmatic hernia: The hidden mortality. J. Pediatr. Surg. **13:** 227–230.

Anomalies and the Mental Health Professional

THOMAS F. McNEIL[a,b] AND GUN TORSTENSSON NIMBY[c]

Departments of Epidemiology/Community Medicine[a] and Psychiatry[c]
Lund University, University Hospital UMAS, S-205 02 Malmö, Sweden

ABSTRACT: Parental attitudes and reactions to the identification of fetal anomalies generally represent well-documented, normally occurring phenomena. The appropriate clinical management of such emotional reactions is an important responsibility of the medical units delivering care and services to the parents. Medical policy decisions about whether and when to screen for offspring anomalies is a considerably more complex and controversial topic. Attitudes, feelings, and reactions both of parents and professionals to the identification of fetal abnormality and fetal normality have come to play an increasingly important role in such policy decisions. Adequate evaluation of the topic requires scientifically based knowledge of the psychological and psychosocial effects of screening of normal-risk and high-risk cases, as well as the short-term and long-term consequences of true positive, true negative, false negative, and false positive identifications of offspring abnormality. Only partial answers to these questions are available to date, and further empirical work is needed.

INTRODUCTION

Advances in the field of fetal screening and diagnosis have consistently presented new opportunities for identifying—and consequently for selecting and eliminating—offspring with various characteristics or the characteristics themselves. These opportunities have sharpened the focus of the naturally occurring questions about whether, when, and how to identify physical abnormality in offspring, and what to do when it is identified.

Parental feelings, attitudes, and reactions associated with the very early identification of *offspring normality and abnormality* have come to play an increasingly important role in medical policy decisions about these central questions.[e.g. 1–5] In many parts of the world, prospective parents have come to expect prenatal evaluation of the fetus as a natural part of the reproductive sequence, but questions have been raised concerning the relative "costs and benefits" of both existing screening/diagnosis and new possibilities for identifying and treating offspring abnormality. The identification of serious fetal abnormality during pregnancy permits selective abortion, but, in cases where the pregnancy is to be continued, requires the parents to live with the awareness of the fetus's abnormality for the duration of the pregnancy. Adequate answers are needed as to whether this knowledge represents an unnecessary psychological burden for the parents, with short- and/or long-term negative consequences, or instead whether it gives the parents the opportunity to become accustomed and adapt psychologically to the abnormality prior to the birth of the offspring. Furthermore, a substantial proportion of abnormality in fetuses is not identified through prenatal screening,[5] and the question may be raised about the psychological effects on the parents resulting from the failure of the medical system to detect fetal abnormality during pregnancy—for example, having informed parents that the fetus appears to be normal and then later finding the off-

[b] Corresponding author; e-mail: Thomas.McNeil@smi.mas.lu.se

spring to be abnormal after birth. In the case of somatically meaningful fetal abnormality which will be identified sooner or later, a central question concerns whether it is best for the prospective parents to experience the resultant mental trauma early or late in the reproductive process?

Concern has also been expressed that prenatal screening for fetal anomalies can cause totally unnecessary psychological trauma to parents by (1) identifying completely benign malformations that otherwise would be missed in postnatal examinations,[6] (2) identifying temporary abnormality which the fetus later outgrows (a "temporary true positive finding")[7] or (3) identifying false positive abnormality in a truly normal fetus.[8-11]

Professionals in the medical services associated with this process have their own feelings and attitudes toward these questions—partly as providers of medical service, and partly as human beings and often parents in their own right. Opinions on the topic abound, and the professional literature seems to us to be characterized by an unusually high proportion of "opinions to the editor" espousing views, warnings, and personal experiences, rather than scientific studies based on systematic empirical investigations of carefully selected samples. In such an emotionally loaded field, valuable opinions provide no substitute for well-designed, impartial scientific studies. Fortunately, many scientists are in the process of attempting to provide empirically based, informative answers to these most poignant questions.

The process of identifying fetal normality and abnormality has reached such an advanced stage of development and implementation that an adequate empirical evaluation of the psychological aspects of these phenomena necessarily includes all four types of situations that occur in screening or diagnosis of early offspring anomalies, i.e., "true negative," "true positive," "false negative," and "false positive" findings of abnormality. We make an attempt below to explore briefly each of these situations, and thereafter discuss psychic crisis reactions associated with offspring abnormality and appropriate clinical management of these reactions. Selected literature is reviewed, and we present results from several studies done in Malmö.

IDENTIFICATION OF NORMALITY IN OFFSPRING: "TRUE NEGATIVE" FINDINGS DURING PREGNANCY

Prenatal screening for fetal abnormality is a routine part of prenatal care in many countries, and a vast majority of normal-risk offspring who are screened by ultrasound will be defined as physically normal.[5] An increasing number of publications in medical and other scientific journals have explored parental expectations and experiences associated with ultrasound examinations per se and the effect of normal findings on parents' anxiety, attitudes, and feelings concerning the pregnancy, health behaviors, and feelings toward the offspring (bonding).

Pregnant women, and especially primigravidas, generally have very positive expectations for routine ultrasound, especially at the first examination during pregnancy.[4,12] The reality of ultrasound, and notably the visual image of the fetus, leaves some women somewhat disappointed,[12] but little support has been obtained for some authors' fears that confrontation with the image of the real fetus (rather than the fantasy fetus) would be psychically traumatic and lead to high anxiety in the pregnant woman.[12] Instead, most studies suggest that ultrasound identifying fetal normality leads to reduced maternal[1,4,13-15] (and paternal[13]) anxiety, especially when conditions had indicated increased risk for pathology.[13,16]

A series of studies has provided evidence for the psychological and behavioral benefits for parents resulting from receiving increased levels of feedback about the ultrasound procedure and image.[4,13,14,17] For example, a comparison of high feedback conditions (i.e., full view of the monitor and description of fetal anatomy, size, and movements) versus low feedback (i.e., only summary results of the exam) indicated the former condition to lead to less maternal anxiety, more sleep per night, and less food aversion late in pregnancy, as well as less fetal movement. Primiparous women receiving high feedback also had significantly improved reproductive outcomes, with fewer obstetric complications and more positive offspring characteristics concerning birth weight, habituation, motor behavior, irritability tendency, and activity level.[17] These positive benefits of ultrasound were observed under what represented unusually "high" feedback conditions in the 1980s,[14] but some of this high feedback may have become implemented as routine procedure in ultrasound examinations since then.

The effect of ultrasound on prospective parents' feelings toward the pregnancy and offspring has been a topic of considerable interest, and observations show positive effects in both somatic high-risk and low-risk groups.[16] Ultrasound performed prior to quickening is found to increase the experience of the reality of the pregnancy for both the woman and her partner,[3,14] increase maternal awareness of the fetus as an individual[12] and increase compliance with smoking, alcohol consumption, and dental care recommendations in most, but not all,[5] studies.[18,19] Early reports indicated that ultrasound experience prior to quickening promoted early maternal bonding to the fetus.[14] Although early bonding would be conducive to early compliance with health behaviors and would thus speak in favor of early ultrasound, the positive effect on bonding may only be temporary. Bonding occurs even more strongly as a consequence of quickening,[12] and ultrasound during pregnancy bears no relationship to bonding measured after delivery.[14] Early bonding through ultrasound may also have negative consequences for the few cases who will experience subsequent fetal loss.[4] Black[3] found that increased awareness of the fetus had made subsequent fetal loss harder for 44% and easier for 9% of cases followed up 1–6 months later. No information appears to be available concerning the effects of ultrasound on *long-term* adjustment to subsequent fetal loss, and a lack of long-term follow-up results is generally descriptive of this total field of research.

Parents typically have very positive attitudes and expectations toward routine ultrasound examinations, and some authors have expressed concern that parents conceive of ultrasound only as an interesting confirmation of the pregnancy and of the normality of the fetus rather than as representing screening for fetal abnormality.[1,2] For example, a prospective Swedish study of 40 randomly chosen nulliparae undergoing ultrasound examinations (Bjarnevik and Fahl, unpublished data) showed that one-half of the sample had given little contemplation to the rountine examination, whereas the other half had positive expectations for its results. The women reported feeling less anxiety prior to ultrasound than they usually felt when going to other medical examinations, and almost none of these randomly chosen women felt any reason for concern. Although this positive parental attitude could be gratifying for proponents of ultrasound examinations, pregnant women with such a conceptualization of ultrasound may be poorly prepared for the identification of fetal abnormality. This may be so problematic in cases with abnormality that some authors have suggested requiring compulsory presentation of routine ultrasound as prenatal screening for malformations, with informed consent given by parents.[1,2] Parents undergoing ultrasound screening because of high-risk conditions generally have other expectations for fetal abnormality, but its identification is not necessarily more psychologically benign (see below). The confirmation of fetal normality versus abnormality is naturally more important than any other factor (including level of feedback) for the parents' emotional experience of ultrasound and other diagnostic procedures.[12]

IDENTIFICATION OF ABNORMALITY IN OFFSPRING: "TRUE POSITIVE" FINDINGS DURING PREGNANCY

Effective empirical assessment of the psychological effects of identifying fetal anomalies during pregnancy is complicated, because the research design must also take into account the psychological effects of (1) the offspring having abnormality per se (regardless of when it is identified), as well as of (2) possible antecedent psychosocial conditions related to the development of the abnormality. Our prospective study of psychosocial background factors for congenital malformations indicated that pregnant women with malformed fetuses already have increased rates of psychosocial difficulties prior to the identification of the malformation,[20] and such antecedents could easily be incorrectly interpreted as consequences of the malformations. We thus use a research design that includes all four combinations of outcomes in the very same study, comparing true positive, false negative, false positive, and true negative cases with each other on both hypothetical consequences and antecedents of offspring abnormality. Furthermore, the importance of parental preparedness for fetal abnormality is evaluated by investigating the psychological effects in both general screening of normal-risk cases and in fetal diagnosis performed on high-risk cases. Research findings from our group are presented to illustrate both types of situations.

A new study by Torstensson Nimby *et al.* (unpublished data) has investigated a true positive group consisting of 84 pregnancies in which the fetuses were identified as malformed in ultrasound exams typically in gestational week 17 or 33. The malformations concerned the kidney/abdomen (one-third), brain (one-quarter), heart (one-sixth), and chromosome disorders (one-sixth), and resulted in severe offspring disorder or death in almost 80% of the cases. A major subset of the cases was followed up and interviewed in their homes on the average of about six years after the reproduction in question, to determine long-term consequences of the events.

The women's initial reactions to the identification of the malformation during pregnancy were "strong" or "very strong" in most cases, three-quarters of the group showing a maximal strength of reaction. The emotional reactions were clearly similar to those in psychic crisis reactions (see below), and represented psychological shock, desperation, worry, crying, anxiety, sadness, depression, etc. For almost all cases, these reactions began immediately upon identification of the fetal abnormality at the ultrasound examination, and lasted a year or longer in about half the sample.

In about one-quarter of the cases, some condition (objective or subjective) had led the women to expect that fetal abnormality might be identified by the ultrasound, and these women were compared with the remaining cases to determine whether mental preparedness influenced the woman's initial reaction to the identification of fetal abnormality. The results of the comparison showed that women who were mentally prepared for finding fetal abnormality reacted as strongly or even stronger than the remaining cases (80 vs. 75% maximal strength, respectively), with reactions lasting more than a year in more than 60% of the former cases (vs. 40% of the remaining cases). Mental preparedness for identifying fetal abnormality did not appear to reduce the psychological trauma of actually identifying abnormality.

The results obtained thus far from the follow-up interview about six years later suggest no negative long-term effects of prenatal identification of malformations on the women's mental or physical health (as compared with demographically similar control women); these results contrast clearly with the findings for women whose fetus's malformations were missed by ultrasound but identified at or after birth (see false negatives below). If these results are confirmed in the project's remaining data sets, then this would represent evidence for the psychological benefits of identifying fetal abnormality during pregnancy, as compared with after birth.

The psychological and psychosocial effects of prenatal diagnosis (PND) of hemophilia in offspring of pregnant carriers have been investigated by our group in two separate series of patients,[21-23] each reflecting the state of development of diagnostic methods at a particular time. Before PND became available, gene carriers frequently abstained from having children at all. With the advent of amniocentesis, fetal sex could be determined, permitting selective abortion of male offspring, only 50% of whom actually had hemophilia.[21,22] Further advances in the 1970s allowed PND through fetal blood sampling (FBS) in the second trimester, permitting selective abortion of only the hemophilic offspring at that stage of gestation.[24,25] Sex determination in gestational weeks 15–16 took about two weeks, whereas the results of FBS in weeks 18–20 were available within about two days.

Tedgård and co-workers have investigated the psychological and psychosocial consequences of this second-trimester PND, interviewing 29 Swedish and Danish women 1–4 years after the occurrence of the PND.[21,22] Most of the women felt that all female carriers of hemophilia should be made aware of the possibility for PND and that genetic counseling should be performed prior to pregnancies. All of the women had experienced notable psychological distress associated with one or more of the various aspects of the PND (i.e., the procedure itself, awaiting sex-determination results, awaiting the FBS—the procedure itself and its potential threat to the fetus's health, awaiting results of the FBS).[22] The periods waiting for the results of the tests were especially problematic for the women and were frequently described as the worst time in their lives.

Half of the group had experienced most of these aspects of the PND as psychologically problematic, and the group of "strong reactors" evidenced frequent psychosomatic and psychological symptoms (sleep problems, anxiety, headache, gastritis) during the six months that followed the PND. These strong-reacting women also had significantly more often than the other women a generally negative view of themselves and of being a gene carrier, had planned the pregnancy, had a higher education and a good general knowledge of hemophilia, and also espoused a guiding philosophy or religious view of life.[23] Having received misleading or insufficient information about the PND did not influence women's reactions. The results question whether giving increased information and encouraging knowledge about hemophilia will lead per se to better psychological coping with PND, and we suggested that giving psychosocial support before the PND may promote better adaptation.[23]

The psychological effects of the PND were only partially dependent upon its somatic outcome. Although women with healthy fetuses experienced joy and relief, a majority of the Swedish women with healthy fetusues nevertheless experienced notable psychological distress during the remaining pregnancy period. The psychological reactions of the nine women with hemophilic offspring were even stronger, with eight of them experiencing emotional breakdowns, sorrow, or disgust at the thought of having to have an abortion. The 12 women with subsequent abortions (9 therapeutic, 3 spontaneous) experienced very strong, negative emotions during the following half year, many reporting psychosomatic and somatic symptoms. Nevertheless, about half of the total group (58%) said they would again choose to use second-trimester PND in a new pregnancy.

Other research has shown that the later in pregnancy the diagnosis is carried out, the greater the distress experienced by the prospective parents.[26,27] PND in the first trimester was thus thought possibly to yield less psychic trauma for the parents.[28] PND of hemophilia later became available in the first trimester through chorionic villi sampling (CVS), and systematic follow-up and interview was done with 29 carriers of hemophilia and 23 of their partners a median of 3.5 years after they had undergone their first CVS (Tedgård *et al.*, manuscript submitted). Three-quarters of these couples had chosen to become pregnant because of the possibility of obtaining PND by CVS, and most had obtained genetic counseling both before and during the pregnancy. In spite of this, almost one-third of the cases expressed dissatisfaction with the information about CVS, irrespective of who had provided this information. One-third had experienced the CVS as more psychologically complicated than they had expected, registering unexpected pain and discomfort at the necessity of having to repeat the testing. Although few women expressed concern about hazards of CVS to their own health, almost all were worried about the potentially negative effect on the fetus.

The two-week period while awaiting the results of the PND was experienced as very emotionally trying by two-thirds of the women and one-half of the men, the women having significantly more psychiatric or psychosomatic symptoms (anxiety, depression, gastritis, etc) than did their partners. Almost 80% of the women had a priori decided to abort a hemophilic fetus; women with a basically negative attitude toward abortion experienced the waiting period in an especially negative manner. Eight couples chose termination of the pregnancy because of hemophilia in the offspring. In spite of total agreement about the decision, the couples experienced the subsequent six months as very emotionally difficult. These eight women showed significantly more signs of depressive mood than did other women when followed up three years later, and two of the eight couples had divorced since the CVS (as compared with none of the remaining 21 couples). All but one of the cases who continued pregnancies with normal fetuses experienced the remainder of pregnancy as a psychologically benign period.

The notable problems associated with both the CVS itself and first-trimester abortions of hemophilic fetuses did not fulfill hopes that trimester-1 procedures would lead to fewer mental and psychosocial difficulties than was the case for trimester-2 PND and abortion. Nevertheless, about 80% of the women and all of their partners said they would choose PND by CVS in a new pregnancy, this being more positive than attitudes regarding second trimester PND.[22]

These parents actively chose the PND, were highly prepared for identifying fetal abnormality, and were prepared for acting upon it—but they still suffered notable psychological distress when the CVS identified fetal abnormality. A basic conclusion seems to be that, regardless of when and how PND is done, the health of the fetus is of utmost importance for the parents' experiences and psychological well-being in association with prenatal screening. However, even findings of fetal normality provide no guarantee of psychological well-being during the remainder of the pregnancy after prenatal screening or diagnosis.

IDENTIFICATION OF NORMALITY IN ABNORMAL OFFSPRING: "FALSE NEGATIVE" FINDINGS

Many malformations are not identified during pregnancy but become apparent at birth or later during neonatal or childhood periods.[5] Our new study of the psychological consequences of identifying malformations during pregnancy included a comparison group of 77 women whose fetuses were not identified as malformed at two ultrasound examinations during pregnancy, but whose offspring showed malformations within one year after birth (half within 24 h of birth, and one-sixth within the following three weeks). The malformations were similar in nature and severity to those in the true positive group described above.

This false negative group evidenced more negative psychological characteristics at follow-up than did the true positive cases: First, the false negative cases were twice as reluctant as any other subject group to participate in the follow-up interview about ultrasound and its consequences, and about one-third of the group that did participate expressed bitterness or skepticism about the ultrasound having missed the malformation. Second, the false negative group clearly reported poorer mental health at the time of follow-up than that for both normal control and true positive cases, as blindly assessed by a psychiatrist. If these results hold up in remaining data analyses, then identifying fetal abnormality after birth would appear to be clearly more psychologically problematic for the parent in the long run than is the identification of malformations during pregnancy.

Are Mothers of Malformed Fetuses Different?

The cases of malformed offspring in our new study (true positive and false negative cases combined) were found not to differ from reproducing control cases with respect to the demographic characteristics of age, marital or cohabitation status, social class or parity, but women with malformed offspring at the index reproduction significantly more often had a history of two or more previous offspring deaths (i.e., spontaneous or legal abortion, extrauterine pregnancy, stillbirth or postnatal offspring death up to one year of age) (Torstensson Nimby *et al.*, unpublished data). The women with malformed offspring also reported significantly more often having experienced stress at the time of the index pregnancy prior to identification of the offspring abnormality, with trends toward less appropriate timing of the pregnancy and a poorer life situation. These apparent antecedent conditions need to be taken into account when evaluating effects of the identification of offspring abnormality.

IDENTIFICATION OF ABNORMALITY IN NORMAL OFFSPRING: "FALSE POSITIVE" FINDINGS

Professionals have been especially interested in both the frequency and consequences of false positive diagnoses. One of the nightmares associated with prenatal screening is the possibility that incorrect identification of fetal abnormality could lead to dire somatic consequences (e.g., abortion) or to completely unnecessary psychological damage to the parents. An important issue is whether these false positive identifications leave lasting traces of psychological trauma on the parents or instead reflect a benign "all's well that ends well" phenomenon. This question was assessed in our new study, which included 11 women whose fetuses were found to be malformed during pregnancy (10 kidney abnormalities and one esophageal atresia) but were normal at birth. As might be expected, these women reacted immediately (as did "true positive" cases) with anxiety and worry upon identification of the fetal abnormality. However, at follow-up six years later they were clearly positive toward sharing their views in interviews regarding ultrasound, expressed entirely positive attitudes toward ultrasound examinations (all 11 cases), and generally lacked bitterness about the false finding (10 of 11 cases). The women were also indistinguishable from control mothers with normal offspring concerning their own reported mental and physical health. These results yield no evidence of long-term negative psychological effects of false positive findings.

In contrast, other systematic studies of psychological effects of false positive identifications in screening for metabolic disorders have shown some negative psychological consequences. Interestingly, these studies concerned screening in which the false positive rate was moderately (e.g., 50%[10]) to extremely (e.g., 95%[8]) high. For example, Bodegård *et al.*[8] studied 102 families of newborns with a false positive finding of congenital hypothyroidism, and found evidence of very strong emotional reactions to the initial news of the abnormality. Although the falseness of the diagnosis was revealed one week later, almost one-fifth of the families showed remaining insecurity about the child's health at 6–12 months of age. When the children were 4 years old, 60% of the families were judged not to have fully integrated this threat emotionally, as defined according to Bodegard et al.'s psychoanalytic theory model. A subsequent study of 11 false positive cases from screening for hypothyroidism (with 50% false positives[10]) found that only two of the 11 families showed a complete emotional integration of the events 1–4 years later.

In our view, serious questions may be raised as to the value of the operational definition of psychological damage in these important studies.[8,10] The researchers counted such things as vague parental memories of events or not having an entirely "rational view" of the screening as evidence of a lack of emotional integration; parental worry about the child or something else was counted as a sign of "displaced anxiety," and disturbed behavior (e.g., shyness) in the children during standardized testing was taken as signs of a negative effect of the false positive identification. However, the somatic follow-up program was fraught with seemingly inappropriate contacts and after-care[9,11] (which could justifiably make parents "irrational"), no objective criteria or interjudge agreement was used to define the damage, and no control group was available for comparison of "disturbed" behavior in the offspring. In our opinion, the interpretation of these phenomena as evidence of damage due to false positive identification remains very questionable.

Sorensen et al.[11] also conducted a follow-up of 60 parents whose newborns were being retested because of equivocal test results for metabolic disorders such as galactosemia and phenylketonuria. All subsequent test results were normal (as had been expected), but the request to the parent to bring the newborn in for renewed testing represented a "false positive" event. Parents showed a significant reduction in anxiety and depression levels after the normalizing results were obtained, but about one-third of the parents were still worried about the neonate's health when followed up within two weeks after receiving the final test results. Tymstra[29] presented similar research findings showing that some parents remained concerned about the health of offspring found to be healthy after false positive findings of thyroid deficiency.

In total, false positive findings of early abnormality in offspring appear to have at least initially negative psychological consequences for the parents, as well should be the case, but the long-term consequences after the child is pronounced to be normal are less well determined. More research of high scientific quality is needed in this particular area.

PSYCHIC CRISIS REACTIONS: CHARACTERISTICS AND CLINICAL MANAGEMENT

Prospective parents (especially mothers) are generally considered to be unusually psychologically sensitive during the prenatal, perinatal, and early infancy/parenthood periods. Parents very frequently react with a classical psychic crisis reaction (CR) at the identification of suspected or manifest abnormality in the unborn or newly born offspring. In our opinion, the proper identification and clinical management of an acute or prolonged CR is an important responsibility of the clinical services that identify the offspring abnormality. A description of CRs and strategies for appropriate clinical management may be helpful to professionals coming in contact with these important phenomena.

CRs have four phases (shock, reaction, reparation, new orientation), the first two of which represent CRs' acute phase and which are often intertwined with each other chronologically.[30] Psychological defense mechanisms such as denial ("it didn't happen") and isolation ("it happened, but it's not important to me") dominate the shock phase, and have the function of keeping the unbearable facts out of the person's emotional consciousness. The person in a CR following an offspring's death may evidence denial, for example, by discussing what he/she will do when the baby comes home from the hospital, while a person showing signs of isolation may, for instance, discuss the baby's death and disease in a clear intellectual manner, but without showing any evidence of feelings associated with the event.

Professional care and contact need to be optimized during the acute stage of CRs. CRs have a number of practical clinical implications: First, the most important assistance the person can receive in the acute phase is to have her/his basic biological and psychological needs attended to, that is, to receive physical warmth and have the presence and support from another person. A person in an acute CR must not be left alone even for a short time. Women who have been left alone in the examination room, even for extremely short intervals, have experienced their aloneness in a very negative manner, and developed catastrophic feelings and ideas about the fetus which are often incorrect. Medical personnel who remain in the room with the woman can be there to answer questions and receive emotional expressions which occur.

Second, a person in the shock phase has difficulty comprehending and incorporating new information, and any information that is given can be easily misinterpreted. While many people in acute CRs appear to actively seek information, their capacity for taking it in is frequently quite limited at that time. The professional who gives information about results of examinations, outcome for the offspring, etc., thus needs to take plenty of time, speak in a simple and calm manner, repeating information as needed, and possibly also sit down close to the person so that body contact can be established when and if appropriate. The suggestion to offer the person a "nice cup of tea" symbolizes the creation of an atmosphere which would allow the person to take in the information at an appropriate pace and in a warm personal setting.

In the subsequent reaction phase of the crisis, the person reacts not only with intellectual understanding but also with the emotions associated with the traumatic event. Many different types of feelings may be evident, including those which appear frightening, distasteful or unfitting to other persons. For example, the person in a CR may behave unjustifiably aggressively toward other persons, including the damaged/dead offspring, the medical personnel who have informed the parent about the traumatic condition or tried to help afterwards, or their relatives. If this occurs, the caregivers and relatives must recognize their own possible negative reactions to the person's behavior, and in no case act negatively or retaliate. The caregiver can often make an important contribution to the resolution of the CR by "labeling" the person's feelings for them (e.g., "I don't blame you for being angry or shocked"), thus giving the person a chance to recognize and express their feelings directly. The caregiver should also clearly give the impression that all of the person's feelings are important and normal in such circumstances.

We recommend that renewed contact with the parent or family be made as soon as possible, e.g., the day following the trauma/first information, and that the caregiver or another informed person should be available by telephone in the meantime. On renewed contact, the medical personnel should be open to the parents' emotional reactions, contemplations, and speculations, and the parents should be encouraged to ask questions and to describe how they experienced the information/results. Giving advice to the parent (especially to "have another baby") is contraindicated, as it may hinder mourning and lead to psychological problems at the next reproduction.

In time, the normal CR will progress to reparation and new orientation phases in which the traumatic event and its consequences will be let into the person's consciousness and integrated into the new reality of the person's life. CRs to traumatic events are natural and normal phenomena, but can at times become abnormally exaggerated in strength, form or duration, and the question is sometimes raised as to whether a particular CR exceeds the limits for normality. Exact limits are difficult to define, but should the reactive phase be prolonged (e.g., exceed one month) or increase notably in strength, for example, with great anxiety and sleep difficulties, or change in form (show the development of notable depression, hallucinations or bizarre behavior), then further help may be needed. In milder cases, contact might be sought perhaps with a social worker within the obstetric or pediatric clinical system. Our own preference is that, if possible, all medical care including crisis intervention be kept within the realm of the obstetric/pediatric services, where expertise also exists concerning the offspring. In contrast, referral to psychiatric or other mental health services would tend to indicate to the parent that the parent's reaction is psychically abnormal and/or that the obstetric/pediatric services do not have the capability or desire to help them. Referral to psychiatry should, in our opinion, be reserved for the unusual cases in which a CR develops into a true depressive or (borderline) psychotic condition. Psychiatric services may nevertheless be helpful as consultants to the obstetric/pediatric personnel who provide the primary care and contact for the parent.

REFERENCES

1. THORPE, K., L. HARKER, A. PIKE & N. MARLOW. 1993. A comparison of women's experiences of antenatal ultrasound screening with cerebral ultrasound of their newborn infant. Soc. Sci. Med. **36:** 311–315.
2. BUCHER, H.C. & J.G. SCHMIDT. 1993. Does routine ultrasound scanning improve outcome in pregnancy? Meta-analysis of various outcome measures. Br. Med. J. **307:** 13–17.
3. BLACK, R. 1992. Seeing the baby: The impact of ultrasound technology. J. Genet. Counseling **1:** 45–54.
4. PERSUTTE, W.H. 1995. Failure to address the psychosocial benefit of prenatal sonography: Another failing of the RADIUS study. J. Ultrasound Med. **14:** 795–796.
5. SAARI-KEMPPAINEN, A., O. KARJALAINEN, P. YLÖSTALO & O.P. HEINONEN. 1990. Ultrasound screening and perinatal mortality: Controlled trial of systematic one-stage screening in pregnancy. Lancet **336:** 387–391.
6. GRIFFINS, D.M. & M.H. GOUGH. 1985. Dilemmas after ultrasonic diagnosis of fetal abnormality. Lancet **1:** 623–624.
7. CHITTY, L.S., G.H. HUNT, J. MOORE & M.O. LOBB. 1991. Effectiveness of routine ultrasonography in detecting fetal structural abnormalities in a low risk population. Br. Med. J. **303:** 1165–1169.
8. BODEGÅRD, G., K. FYRÖ & A. LARSSON. 1983. Psychological reactions in 102 families with a newborn who has a falsely positive screening test for congenital hypothyroidism. Acta Paediatr. Scand. Suppl. **304:** 1–21.
9. FYRÖ, K. & G. BODEGÅRD. 1987. Four-year follow-up of psychological reactions to false positive screening tests for congenital hypothyroidism. Acta Paediatr. Scand. **76:** 107–114.
10. FYRÖ, K. & G. BODEGÅRD. 1988. Difficulties in psychological adjustment to a new neonatal screening programme. Acta Paediatr. Scand. **77:** 226–231.
11. SORENSON, J.R., H.L. LEVY, T.W. MANGIONE & S.J. SEPE. 1984. Parental response to repeat testing of infants with "false-positive" results in a newborn screening program. Pediatrics **73:** 183–187.
12. VILLENEUVE, C., C. LAROCHE, A. LIPPMAN & M. MARRACHE. 1988. Psychological aspects of ultrasound imaging during pregnancy. Can. J. Psychiatry **33:** 530–536.
13. COX, D.N., B.K. WITTMANN, M. HESS, A.G. ROSS, J. LIND & S. LINDAHL. 1987. The psychological impact of diagnostic ultrasound. Obstet. Gynecol. **70:** 673–676.
14. LUMLEY, J. 1990. Through a glass darkly: Ultrasound and prenatal bonding. Birth **17:** 214–217.
15. SPARLING, J.W., J.W. SEEDS & D.C. FARRAN. 1988. The relationship of obstetric ultrasound to parent and infant behavior. Obstet. Gynecol. **72:** 902–907.
16. TSOI, M.M., M. HUNTER, M. PEARCE, P. CHUDLEIGH & S. CAMPBELL. 1987. Ultrasound

scanning in women with raised serum alpha fetoprotein: Short-term psychological effect. J. Psychosom. Res. **31:** 35–39.

17. FIELD, T., D. SANDBERG, T.A. QUETEL, R. GARCIA & M. ROSARIO. 1985. Effects of ultrasound feedback on pregnancy anxiety, fetal activity, and neonatal outcome. Obstet. Gynecol. **66:** 525–528.

18. READING, A.E., S. CAMPBELL, D.N. COX & C.M. SLEDMERE. 1982. Health beliefs and health care behavior in pregnancy. Psychol. Med. **12:** 379–382.

19. WALDENSTRÖM, U., S. NILSSON, O. FALL, O. AXELSSON, G. EKLUND, S. LINDEBERG & Y. SJÖDIN. 1988. Effects of routine one-stage ultrasound screening in pregnancy: A randomised controlled trial. Lancet **2:** 585–588.

20. MCNEIL, T.F., G. BLENNOW & L. LUNDBERG. 1988. A prospective study of psychosocial background factors associated with congenital malformations. Acta Psychiatr. Scand. **78:** 643–651.

21. LJUNG, R., U. TEDGÅRD, T. MCNEIL & E. TEDGÅRD. 1987. How do carriers of hemophilia experience prenatal diagnosis by fetal blood sampling? Clin. Genet. **31:** 297–302.

22. TEDGÅRD, U., R. LJUNG, T. MCNEIL, E. TEDGÅRD & M. SCHWARTZ. 1989. How do carriers of hemophilia experience prenatal diagnosis (PND)? Acta Paediatr. Scand. **78:** 692–700.

23. TEDGÅRD, U., R. LJUNG, T.F. MCNEIL & E. TEDGÅRD. 1997. Identifying carriers at high risk for negative reactions when performing prenatal diagnosis of haemophilia. Hemophilia **3:** 123–130.

24. RODECK, C.H. & S. CAMPELL. 1979. Umbilical-cord insertion as a source of pure fetal blood for prenatal diagnosis. Lancet **1:** 1244–1245.

25. GUSTAVII, B., E. CORDESIUS, L. LÖFBERG & P. STRÖMBERG. 1979. Fetoscopy. Acta Obstet. Gynecol. Scand. **58:** 409–410.

26. SPENCER, J.W. & D.N. COX. 1987. Emotional responses of pregnant women to chorionic villi sampling or amniocentesis. Am. J. Obstet. Gynecol. **157:** 1155–1160.

27. SJÖGREN, B. & N. UDDENBERG. 1989. Prenatal diagnosis and psychological distress: Amniocentesis or chorionic villus biopsy? Prenatal Diagn. **9:** 477–487.

28. BURKE, B.M. & A. KOLKER. 1993. Clients undergoing chorionic villus sampling versus amniocentesis: Contrasting attitudes toward pregnancy. Health Care Women Int. **14:** 193–200.

29. TYMSTRA, T. 1986. False positive results in screening tests: Experiences of parents of children screened for congenital hypothyroidism. Fam. Pract. **3:** 92–96.

30. OTTOSSON, J.-O. 1995. Psykiatri (Psychiatry). Almqvist & Wiksell. Stockholm.

Central Nervous System Anomalies

LÁSZLÓ CSABAY,[a] ISTVÁN SZABÓ, CSABA PAPP, ERNŐ TÓTH-PÁL, AND ZOLTÁN PAPP

I. Department of Obstetrics and Gynecology, Semmelweis University Medical School, Budapest, Hungary

ABSTRACT: The authors review the most common congenital anomalies of the central nervous system (CNS): neural tube defects (NTDs), ventriculomegaly/holoprosencephaly, hydranencephaly, holoprosencephaly sequence, iniencephaly, and microcephaly. They emphasize the importance of the diagnostic tools (biochemical markers of the maternal serum, ultrasound screening, invasive techniques), methods which are complementary to each other.

NEURAL TUBE DEFECTS

Neural tube defects (NTDs) constitute the most frequently encountered group of severe congenital anomalies of the central nervous system. In very early embryogenesis the neural plate develops into a tube-like structure, and disturbed development at that stage results in persistently open structures derived from that tube. Three major types of malformation result: anencephaly/exencephaly, spina bifida, and encephalocele. The first two account for 95% of all NTDs, and encephalocele for 5%.

Anencephaly/Exencephaly. Apparent failure of closure at the cranial pole results in anencephaly, a gross malformation incompatible with survival postnatally. The calvaria is largely or totally absent, the frontal, parietal and occipital bones being present only in a rudimentary form. The bony orbits are shallow, with associated exophthalmos. The neural tube lesion is covered by an abundantly vascularized spongy connective tissue, the area cerebrovasculosa, containing some glial cells, and a disordered choroid plexus.[1] Primordial remnants of the brain stem and basal ganglia can be recognized beneath this transparent membrane (Figs. 1 and 2).

The cranial defect may continue downward as a cleft involving the whole length of the spinal column (craniorachischisis) or, more frequently, be accompanied by a separate lumbosacral spina bifida. In some cases the skull vault is entirely absent (acrania).

Defective closure of the neural tube (encephaloschisis) is the primary factor leading to anencephaly, subsequent extroversion of the brain is a secondary factor, and gradual degeneration of the exposed tissues a tertiary one. Ultrasound in the first half of pregnancy will rather consistently show some exposed cerebral tissue (exencephaly) (Fig. 3).

On serial ultrasound this initially extruded mass becomes smaller, a regression

[a] Address correspondence to László Csabay, M.D., I. Department of Obstetrics and Gynecology, Semmelweis University Medical School, Budapest, Baross utca 27, Hungary, H-1088.

brought about by the large number of macrophages present in the fetal circulation and the amniotic fluid ("scavenger function"). This cellular reaction can be identified in the amniotic fluid and is useful in prenatal diagnosis.[2-6]

"Classical" anencephaly is seen mainly in the second half of gestation; before week 20 one finds exencephaly more frequently. To differentiate the two is important only at the time of diagnosis; in statistics on malformation both forms are registered as anencephaly. Anencephaly is found more frequently in female fetuses. Many die *in utero,* and the remainder within a few hours of birth.

Spina Bifida. Spina bifida results from defective neural tube closure along some or the entire length of the vertebral column.[7,8] When no tissue is extruded through the defect, and it is covered by normal skin, it is termed spina bifida occulta. When the defect forms a protruding sac, the term spina bifida cystica is used. The simple designation "spina bifida" usually refers to this latter term. This group can be subdivided into "closed" defects—the sac is covered by intact skin or thick opaque membrane (not to be confused with spina bifida occulta), and "open" defects, which are covered by a reddish semitransparent oozing membrane, the area medullo-vasculosa, which at its edges merges into the more normal surrounding skin. This represents a primary tissue defect and contains remnants of the original protecting

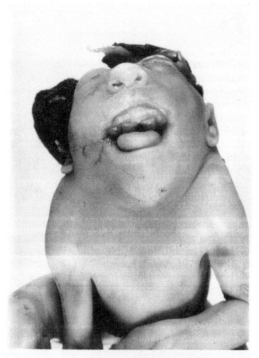

FIGURE 1. Anterior view of an anencephalic fetus. Note the protruded eyes (frog-like face).

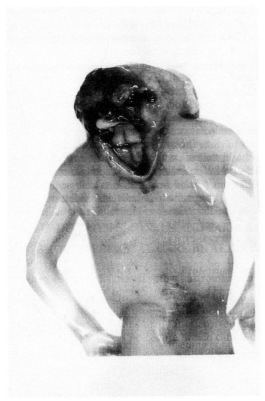

FIGURE 2. Posterior view of a fetus with anencephaly and open cervical and upper thoracic spina bifida. The brain stem and cervical part of the spinal cord remain uncovered.

membrane: both this membrane and the neighboring intact skin are very easily injured (FIGS. 4–6).

When the saccular formation contains cerebrospinal fluid (CSF) and extruded meningeal tissue, but no neural elements, it is called a meningocele. When spinal cord tissue and/or nerves are present, it is termed a myelomeningocele. Occasionally no protective membrane is present, and the neural tube is completely open, like a book, not covered by skin, vertebral arch or meninges, the defect exposing the central canal of the cord (myeloschisis, rachischisis). All of the above are frequently associated with malformations of the fourth ventricle and medulla (Arnold-Chiari malformation) and with hydrocephalus.

Myelocystocele (hydromelia) should be clearly distinguished from spina bifida; it results from cystic dilatation of the central canal of the cord, and is often associated with bladder exstrophy or with persistent cloaca.

Pilonidal sinus, a blind soft-tissue dimple at the level of the sacrum, is not a form of spina bifida. However, dermal sinuses may represent a mild form of closure defect, because they do connect with the spinal canal. On the skin surface a lipoma or a dermoid cyst, or sometimes a dimple, may draw attention to the opening of the sinus; spinal fluid leakage may occur.

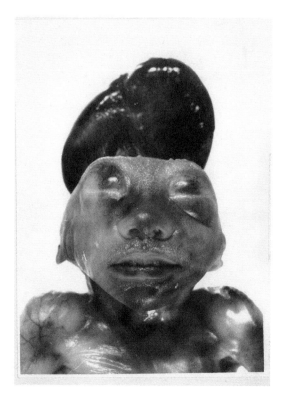

FIGURE 3. Anterior view of a fetus with exencephaly.

Spina bifida cystica is a severe malformation often leading to death in the neonatal period. Surgical treatment includes direct closure of the defect (skin grafting), insertion of shunts to relieve hydrocephalus, and operations to relieve urinary and intestinal obstruction. Nonetheless, many of the survivors suffer paralysis of the lower limbs, urinary and fecal incontinence, and some form of mental retardation, focal neurological damage, and unrelieved hydrocephalus.

Criteria for selective surgery have been introduced, taking into account the severity, extent and location of the neural tube lesion, the presence or absence of associated malformations, the general condition of the newborn baby, and the attitudes of the parents. Only one-third of liveborn babies with open spina bifida reaches five years of age, and among these survivors 80% suffer from severe handicaps; only 5–10% are able to lead a completely normal life. For babies with closed spina bifida lesions detected at birth, the prognosis is better, but 60–70% of them have a persisting handicap.[9]

Encephalocele. An encephalocele is a hernia-like protrusion of meninges and/or brain tissue through an opening in the cranium. The occipital bone is most frequently involved (FIG. 7). Sphenopharyngeal, sphenoorbital, and frontoethmoidal forms sometimes occur, the latter being the most common form of NTD in Thailand. Many

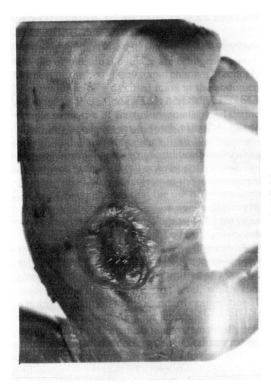

FIGURE 4. Large thoracolumbar spina bifida cystica. The opened book-like spinal cord can be seen on the bottom.

affected infants die, despite surgical treatment, and survivors usually exhibit serious neurological handicaps.

Genetics

Excluding cases presenting as part of multiple congenital anomalies (e.g., chromosome aberrations, Meckel's syndrome, Robert's syndrome), NTDs are multifactorially determined. Within a family, recurrence risks are based on survey data. For a healthy couple who have had one child with NTD, for subsequent children the risk may rise to 3%; the same risk applies to children born to a parent with NTD (spina bifida). For parents who already have had two or three children with NTD, risks for a further child may rise to 10–20%. Anencephaly, spina bifida, and encephalocele can appear within the same family.[10,11]

Prenatal Ultrasound Diagnosis

All anencephalic babies die early, at about or shortly after the time of birth. Some spina bifida babies also die very early, but others survive for varying periods, often with

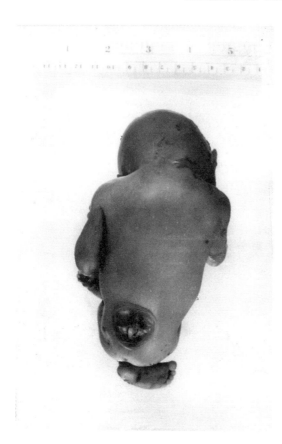

FIGURE 5. Midtrimester fetus with lumbosacral spina bifida.

a high degree of handicap, involving a heavy burden for their families and for society. Many couples with a previous spina bifida baby, or at high risk for an NTD pregnancy (identified on screening), request prenatal diagnosis.

Polyhydramnios is easily demonstrated with ultrasound. In anencephaly, absence of the calvaria results in an open bowl-like or flower-like echo, and exophthalmos is obvious. In exencephaly and encephalocele, the extracranial tissue is usually easily seen, and lack of continuity of the vault bones can be demonstrated. In spina bifida, the two posterior lines of the vertebral column diverge at the level of the defect; in transverse section a "U" or "V" pattern is seen instead of a circular one. Because of the sharp outline of the excess tissue, closed forms are easier to recognize than open spina bifida. With spina bifida, dilated or abnormally shaped cerebral ventricles can often be demonstrated. The recent identification of easily recognizable cranial and cerebellar signs by Campbell will facilitate the detection rate of spina bifida at the routine booking scan. (Lemon sign: scalloping of the frontal bones; banana sign: anterior curvature of the cerebellar hemispheres)[12–21] (FIGS. 8–16).

In most prenatal diagnosis centers, women with a previous history of NTD will be offered amniocentesis at 16 to 18 weeks of gestation, and the diagnosis of NTD is

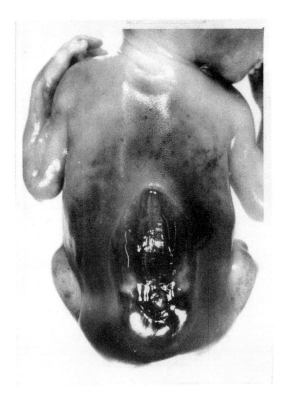

FIGURE 6. Midtrimester fetus with extensive open thoracolumbar spina bifida.

based on the amniotic fluid AFP. The amniocentesis seems not to be necessary, the diagnosis can be made by ultrasound instead of amniotic fluid analysis.[22]

Prenatal Screening

In certain families there is a greatly elevated risk of bearing a child with NTD. However, 95% of the children with NTD are born to low-risk couples. Screening tests in pregnancy are available and practicable. Many consider the advantages and benefits of screening programs to outweigh their initial costs and their few other disadvantages[22-33] (TABLES 1 and 2).

Before the introduction of prenatal screening, the birth prevalence of NTD was 3 per 1000. As a result of screening and also apparently of improvements in general health, the prevalence has fallen in some populations by 60–80%.[1,34-43]

VENTRICULOMEGALY/HYDROCEPHALUS

Megalencephaly resulting from a pathologic increase in the volume of CSF is called hydrocephalus. The excess CSF is most frequently present within the cerebral ventricles.

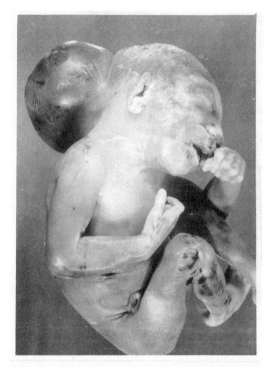

FIGURE 7. Lateral view of a fetus with large occipital meningoencephalocele, partly covered by normal skin.

Ventricular dilatation, due to increased CSF pressure, usually precedes the appearance of other signs, for example, cranial enlargement, and the term ventricular dilatation (ventriculomegaly) is also used, in prenatal diagnosis, independently of the idea of hydrocephalus. Birth prevalence of hydrocephalus is 2 per 1000.

The CSF is mainly produced in the choroid plexuses of the lateral ventricles, reaches the third ventricle through the foramen of Monro, and then the fourth ventricle through the aqueduct of Sylvius. It then passes into the subarachnoid space through the foramina of Luschka and Magendie. Ninety percent of the CSF is reabsorbed into the superior sagittal sinus, and any obstacle to the free outward flow of fluid leads to its accumulation.

When the obstruction is within the ventricular system, that is, between the foramen of Monro and the foramina of Luschka and Magendie, the consequent hydrocephalus is called intraventricular obstructive, or noncommunicating. When the block is between the basal cisterns and the subarachnoid space, the designation is extraventricular obstructive, or communicating, hydrocephalus (FIGS. 17 and 18).

Ninety percent of hydrocephalus seen at birth is secondary to some other pathology, either (1) defective closure or other abnormality of the neural tube, (2) intrauterine infection (toxoplasmosis, CMV, listeriosis), (3) intracranial hemorrhage or (4) choroid plexus papilloma. This secondary hydrocephalus may be communicating or noncommunicating, depending on the primary pathologic process.[1,2,41]

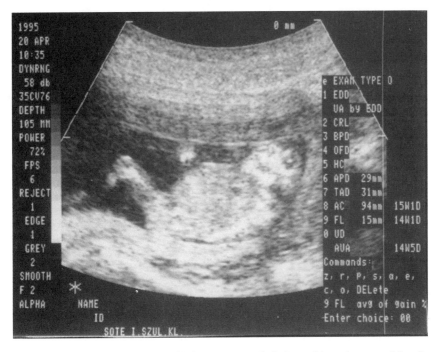

FIGURE 8. Longitudinal scan of a midtrimester anencephalic fetus with an absent cranial vault.

Isolated Forms. In 10% of cases the primary defect is agenesis, hypoplasia or malformation of one of the openings within the ventricular system. These are noncommunicating forms and are always isolated. Inheritance is monogenic in one-third or less of the cases, and multifactorial in the remainder. In most of the monogenic cases there is a primary block within the aqueduct. It may sometimes be difficult to demonstrate this block even in cases diagnosed prenatally. A low-set abnormally flexed thumb may be associated with the X-linked recessive form.

Dandy-Walker Sequence. This anomaly is characterized by hypoplasia or agenesis of the cerebellar vermis and a cystic dilatation of the scala posterior. The degree of anatomical abnormality is highly variable. Hydrocephalus is caused by atresia or obliteration of the foramina of Magendie and Luschka; the fourth ventricle is enormously dilated, resulting in the dilatation of the third and lateral ventricles, while the basal cisterns are obliterated (FIG. 19). The etiology is unknown. Autosomal recessive inheritance has sometimes been observed. It may be part of a syndrome, i.e., hydrolethalus.

Arnold-Chiari Malformation. A downward displacement of the cerebellum and the medulla oblongata into the spinal canal leads to a communicating obstructive

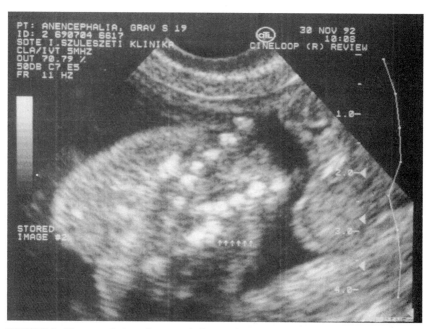

FIGURE 9. Ultrasound view of anencephaly, together with open cervical and upper thoracic spina bifida.

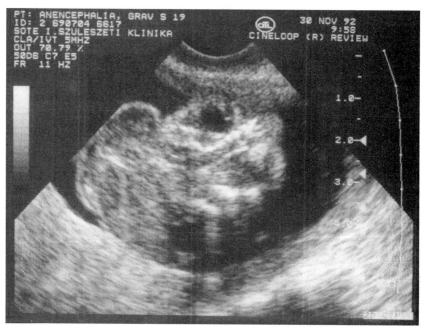

FIGURE 10. Transverse scan of an anencephalic fetus.

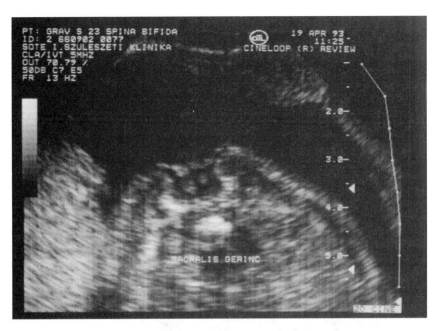

FIGURE 11. Transverse ultrasound scan of a 23-week-old fetus with sacral spina bifida.

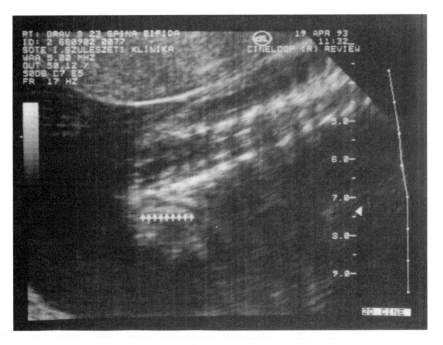

FIGURE 12. Longitudinal scan of the spina bifida.

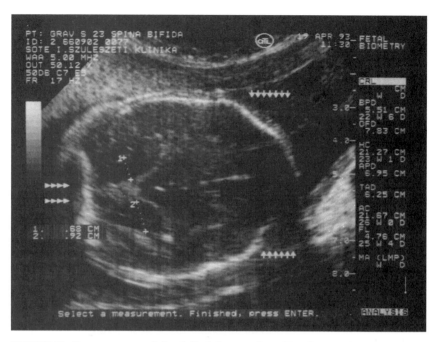

FIGURE 13. Transverse scan of the skull of the same fetus. The distances between the small crosses demonstrate the ventriculomegaly. The horizontal arrows show the banana-sign, the vertical ones the lemon-sign.

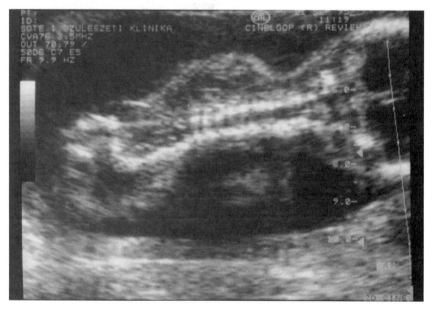

FIGURE 14. Longitudinal sonogram of a fetus with large lumbosacral spina bifida.

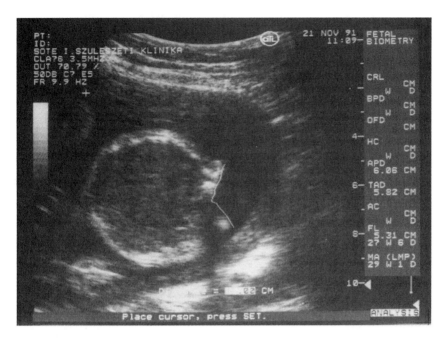

FIGURE 15. Transverse scan showing a wide, open spinal tube in a 29-week-old fetus.

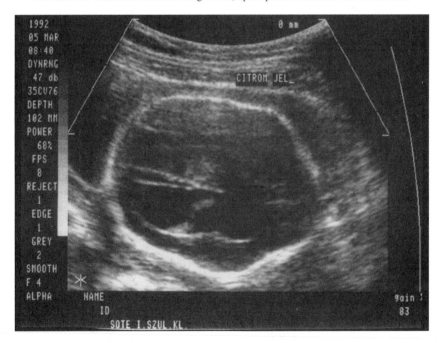

FIGURE 16. Typical lemon-sign of the skull and ventriculomegaly in a fetus with spina bifida.

TABLE 1. Impact of the Prenatal Midtrimester Screening on the Prevalence of Severe Major Fetal Anomalies

Anomaly	Detected/ Searched for	Not Screened	Total	Midtrimester Prevalence (per 1000)	Selective Termination	Birth Prevalence (per 1000)	Prevalence at 1 Year (per 1000)
Anencephaly/exencephaly without spina bifida	27/27	0	27	0.42	27	0	0
Anencephaly/exencephaly with spina bifida	17/17	0	17	0.26	17	0	0
Spina bifida, isolated	12/16	4	20	0.31	12	0.13	0.11
Spina bifida with hydrocephalus	28/28	0	28	0.43	28	0	0
Iniencephaly	5/5	0	5	0.08	5	0	0
Encephalocele, occipital	6/7	2	9	0.14	6	0.05	0.02
Encephalocele, nonoccipital	1/2	1	3	0.05	1	0.03	0.02
Hydrocephalus, isolated	46/50	9	59	0.91	46	0.21	0.08
Holoprosencephaly sequence	8/8	0	8	0.12	8	0	0
Hydranencephaly	—	1	1	0.02	0	0.01	0
Dandy-Walker malformation	1/1	0	1	0.02	1	0	0
Agenesis/dysgenesis of corpus callosum	2/4	1	5	0.08	2	0.05	0.03
Microcephaly	1/2	5	7	0.11	1	0.09	0.10
Total	154/167	23	190	2.94	154	0.57	0.36

TABLE 2. Detection Rates of Maternal Serum Alpha-Fetoprotein and Ultrasound Screening in Cases of Screened Fetal Abnormalities[33]

Anomaly	MSAFP[a] > 2.5	MoMs	Ultrasound	
	n	%	n	%
Anencephaly/exencephaly without spina bifida	19/20	95.0	27/27	100.0
Anencephaly/exencephaly with spina bifida	12/12	92.3	17/17	100.0
Spina bifida, isolated	11/16	68.8	12/16	75.0
Spina bifida with hydrocephalus	14/20	70.0	28/28	100.0
Iniencephaly	1/2	50.5	5/5	100.0
Encephalocele, occipital	3/4	75.0	6/7	85.7
Encephalocele, nonoccipital	—	—	1/2	50.0
Hydrocephalus, isolated	5/39	12.8	46/50	92.0
Holoprosencephaly sequence	2/8	25.0	8/8	100.0
Hydranencephaly	0/1	0.0	—	—
Dandy-Walker malformation	—	—	1/1	100.0
Agenesis/dysgenesis of corpus callosum	0/2	0.0	2.4	50.0
Microcephaly	—	—	1/2	50.0
Total	67/125	53.6	154/167	92.2

[a]MSAFP, maternal serum alpha-fetoprotein; MoMs, multiples of median.

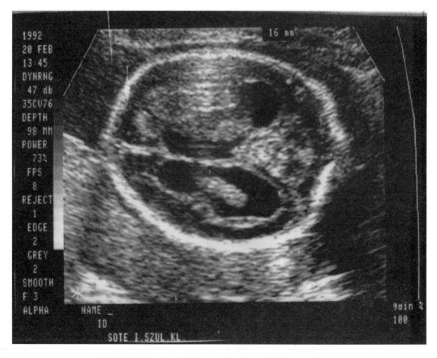

FIGURE 17. Ventriculomegaly of a midtrimester fetus.

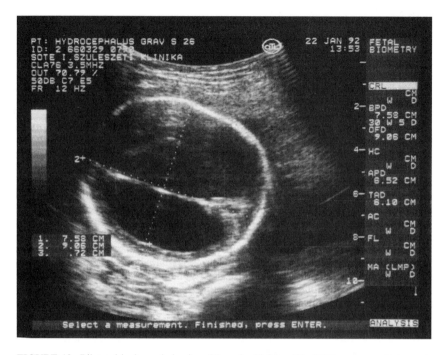

FIGURE 18. Bilateral hydrocephalus in a 26-week-old fetus. The BPD corresponds to week 30–31 of gestation.

hydrocephalus. Sometimes only the cerebellar tonsils lie below the level of the foramen magnum, sometimes the entire cerebellum, sometimes the caudal part of the medulla oblongata, and sometimes the medulla with the entire fourth ventricle. It is always accompanied by cervical spina bifida. It is unknown which change is the primary one (a slight herniation is always demonstrable with spina bifida). The etiology is unknown; autosomal recessive inheritance has sometimes been observed.

Brain Cysts. Choroid plexus cysts (FIG. 20), which are commonly bilateral and within the lateral ventricles, resolve spontaneously before the third trimester of pregnancy and are of no pathologic importance. However, if the cysts are associated with other malformations, they may indicate the presence of an underlying chromosomal abnormality. Large cystic spaces within the substance of the brain represent porencephalic cysts that are often associated with ventriculomegaly and are thought to result from intracranial hemorrhage.

Prenatal Ultrasound Diagnosis

Prenatal diagnosis of hydrocephalus can be made with ultrasound. The process begins *in utero* with dilatation of the ventricles and is then followed by enlargement of the skull. In prenatal diagnostic practice ventricular dilatation and hydrocephalus should

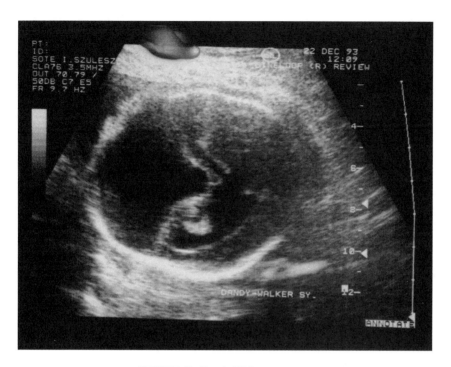

FIGURE 19. Dandy-Walker sequence.

be clearly distinguished. Hydrocephalus includes megalencephaly, that is, an excessive growth of the biparietal diameter (BPD), additional to a dilatation of the ventricular system.

By 14 weeks of gestation the lateral ventricles, filled with choroid plexus, can be seen on the ultrasound screen. The diagnosis of ventricular dilatation can be established by 18–20 weeks. Obstructive ventricular dilatation is easier to diagnose in the third trimester, at which time gestation and also hydrocephalus, if present, can be diagnosed (BPD > 90th percentile).

One should remember that a dilated monoventricle may be associated with the alobar type of holoprosencephaly. Ventricular dilatation may also result from *in utero* infection. In such cases the process is not progressive and may even be reversible.

For the diagnosis of cerebral ventricular dilatation the lateral ventricle/hemisphere ratio is a useful index. The numerator of the fraction derives from the distance between the midline and the lateral wall of the lateral ventricle; the denominator denotes the distance between the midline and the internal bony wall of the cranium. A quotient exceeding 0.5, in 17 weeks of gestation or later, suggests the ventricular system is probably dilated. However, dilatation commences in the occipital horns of the lateral ventricles, and the medial wall of the lateral ventricle is at first pressed toward the midline by the increasing volume of CSF, so a normal quotient may not necessarily indicate that dilatation has not already begun.

When the ventricles are dilated the falx cerebri may appear to float or flap, moving with movements of the scanning head. The presence of associated malformations, for

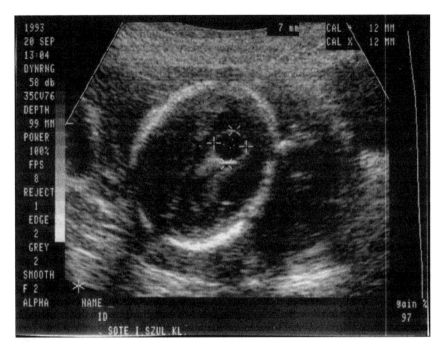

FIGURE 20. Unilateral choroid plexus cyst with diameter of 12 mm in a midtrimester fetus.

example, spina bifida or encephalocele, may help the recognition of ventricular dilatation; it may be seen together with the sonographic signs of Dandy-Walker sequence or Arnold-Chiari malformation.

In spina bifida, the biparietal diameter is often below the 10th percentile by or before week 20 of gestation. Ventricular dilatation is then usually demonstrable, and is very often seen in cases diagnosed earlier. Isolated spina bifida, without ventricular dilatation, is rare.

Once ventricular dilatation has been diagnosed convincingly, most couples insist on termination of the pregnancy. One must remember that nearly two-thirds of all fetuses with a pregnancy diagnosis of hydrocephalus are born dead or die within a few days of birth. Fifty percent of children who are operated on die before 5 years old, and only one-third of all survivors are of more or less normal intelligence.

An intrauterine shunting procedure can be considered as a possible alternative to termination of pregnancy, but only a small proportion of cases diagnosed before 24 weeks is suitable for this procedure; in later pregnancy the cortical mantle is thinned to a degree that implies permanent damage.

HYDRANENCEPHALY

The term hydranencephaly denotes major deficiency of the cerebral hemispheres. An early occlusion or developmental failure of both carotid arteries or of cerebral arteries may be the pathogenetic event: those parts of the brain receiving blood through the posterior cerebral circulation (brain stem, cerebellum, some of the occipital lobe, midbrain, and basal ganglia) are well developed, and one can demonstrate absence of the carotids by postmortem angiography. The cerebral hemispheres are reduced to a gliomatous membrane which lies pressed against the internal aspect of the cranium by the CSF, which fills the remaining space within the cranial cavity.

Hydranencephaly occurs as an isolated defect, not associated with malformations elsewhere, and virtually all cases are sporadic, involving about 1 per 5000 continuing pregnancies. Hydranencephaly usually is associated with polyhydramnios and is easily diagnosable on ultrasound; the differential diagnosis between hydrocephalus and holo-prosencephaly is illustrated in TABLE 3.

An ultrasonically normal telencephalon, in the first half of pregnancy, may de-velop later into hydranencephaly. In the most extreme cases of hydranencephaly, ter-mination of pregnancy or induction of premature labor might be requested, because of the progressive polyhydramnios and the hopeless prognosis. Although some hydra-nencephalic infants may survive for a few months, they do not develop neurologically after birth.

There are many more less severely affected children whose condition seems to rep-resent loss of tissue primarily from the anterior and middle cerebral artery territories (porencephaly). Some of these children live for years and may even acquire a few motor skills.

HOLOPROSENCEPHALY SEQUENCE

In the first weeks of embryonal development—the neural plate and neural groove stages—the brain consists of three recognizable parts: the prosencephalon, mesen-cephalon, and rhombencephalon. Between the time of neural tube closure and the fifth gestational week, the prosencephalon gives origin to telencephalon (cerebral hemi-spheres) and diencephalon (thalamus and hypothalamus); the mesencephalon forms the midbrain; and the rhombencephalon develops into metencephalon (pons and cerebel-lum) and myelencephalon (medulla oblongata). At the time of telencephalon/dien-cephalon differentiation, the prosencephalon also splits longitudinally—the longitudi-nal cerebral fissure—and the hemispheres develop on the lateral aspects of the fissure by progressive enlargement and hollowing of the cerebral vesicles. Remnants of the original septum lie in the fissure between the hemispheres.

Should the prechordal mesoderm fail to migrate normally the prosencephalon re-mains undivided. As a consequence, a common cerebral ventricle develops, cortex and thalamus form a single structure, and development of olfactory and optic bulbs is upset; there is abnormal differentiation and development of the nasofrontal process and the midline of the face (holoprosencephaly sequence).

Differing degrees of disorganization are reflected in the terms alobar, semilobar, and lobar holoprosencephaly.[1,2] The alobar (undivided) form is the most severe. The longi-

TABLE 3. Ultrasound—Differential Diagnosis of Dilated Cerebral Ventricles

Ultrasound Findings	Hydrocephalus	Hydranencephaly	Alobar Holoprosencephaly
Regular falx cerebri	+	−	−
Frontal cerebral tissue	+	−	+
Hypotelorism	−	−	+

tudinal cerebral fissure and the falx cerebri are completely absent, as is the septum pellucidum; the corpus callosum is absent or poorly developed; instead of two separate lateral ventricles there is a single midline prosencephalic cyst. In the semilobar (partially divided) form the posterior third of the prosencephalon has divided, and the frontoparietal region remains single. In the lobar (divided) form, the cerebral hemispheres are, for the greater part, separated. Only the most anterior aspect of the cerebrum remains as a single midline structure. In such cases there may also be fusion of the frontal or occipital horns of the lateral ventricles.

Arhinencephaly. The olfactory tracts and bulbs are lacking or, less frequently, rudimentary.

There are associated facial anomalies. Some facial malformation is consistently present: the more severe the holoprosencephaly defect the more severe the facial malformation.

Cyclotia. The ears are fused below the face (otocephaly); there is a midline orbit, a supraorbital proboscis, and a maxillary and mandibular defect. This is the most severe and rarest of the facial defects.

Cyclopia. The eyes and the bony orbits are fused, to a variable degree, and the normal nasal bones and soft tissues are absent. There is a supraorbital proboscis.

Ethmocephaly. Extreme hypotelorism, with a proboscis lying between the two orbits (TABLE 4).

Cebocephaly. Defect with close-set eyes and a flattened nose consisting of a single blindending nostril, with no sensory cells or fila olfactoria in the nasal mucosa.

Premaxillary agenesis. Hypotelorism, a hypoplastic nose and a very severe median cleft lip.

Cleft lip and palate. Either or both of these defects may be present (FIGS. 21 and 22).

Etiology is heterogeneous. Most cases are sporadic; in the few familial cases the inheritance pattern is usually unclear. Holoprosencephaly is associated with quite a few chromosome defects (chiefly, trisomy 13) and with maternal hyperglycemia (poorly controlled diabetes), and may constitute part of a multiple malformation syndrome (Váradi-Papp syndrome with autosomal recessive trait).[1,2]

Alobar holoprosencephaly is usually incompatible with postnatal life. Children with the semilobar or lobar forms are mentally and physically severely handicapped, and many will require long-term residential care, if they survive.

Prenatal Ultrasound Diagnosis

Ultrasound diagnosis is practicable. In the alobar form, no falx cerebri can be detected within the longitudinal fissure; in the other forms of holoprosencephaly it is present to a variable degree. The hypotelorism can be assessed by measurement of the interorbital distance, other midline facial defects can be detected, and the presence of cerebral tissue in the frontal areas and of normal subtentorial structures can be confirmed. Polyhydramnios is consistently present. The differential diagnosis of alobar holoprosencephaly, hydranencephaly, and hydrocephalus is given in TABLE 3.

INIENCEPHALY

The Greek word inion indicates occiput. Iniencephaly is a gross malformation of the occipital region, the spine, and central nervous system: the occipital bone itself and

TABLE 4. Normal Percentile Values for the Interorbital Distance (expressed in mm)[1]

Age (weeks)	5th Percentile	50th Percentile	95th Percentile
13	10	13	16
14	11	14	17
15	12	15	18
16	13	16	19
17	14	17	20
18	15	19	23
19	16	20	24
20	17	21	25
21	18	22	26
22	19	23	27
23	20	24	28
24	21	25	29
25	22	26	30
26	23	28	33
27	24	29	34
28	25	30	35
29	26	31	36
30	27	32	37
31	28	33	38
32	29	34	39
33	30	35	40
34	31	37	43
35	32	38	44
36	33	39	45
37	34	40	46
38	35	41	47
39	36	42	48
40	37	43	49

the cervical and thoracic vertebrae are partly or completely absent, remaining vertebrae are irregularly fused, with defective closure of the vertebral arches, and the neck is practically absent, with the facial skin continuing directly onto the chest. There is extreme lordosis in the cervicothoracic region, with a hyperextended "stargazing" head, and the trunk is shortened. The underlying nervous tissue (medulla, cervical, and thoracic spinal cord, etc.) is disorganized and there is usually an open spina bifida. Associated malformations may be present; polyhydramnios consistently occurs. The defect is more often seen in female fetuses. It is a condition incompatible with survival. Iniencephaly is usually sporadic, but occurs in some families with other neural tube defects; recurrence risks may be 1% or less. A definitive diagnosis requires ultrasound.[1,2]

It is important to differentiate iniencephaly from the Klippel-Feil anomaly. The latter is a viable condition in which there is fusion of most or all of the vertebral bodies in the cervical spine, extending sometimes to the thoracic region. The neck may be short and broad, with very reduced or no mobility. The underlying cord is often normal, but minor malformations frequently occur, with neurological sequelae (e.g., abnormal decussation of pyramidal tracts, with "mirror movements"). Open neural tube defects are not found. It is generally heterogeneous, most frequently with autosomal dominant inheritance, low penetrance, and variable expressivity.

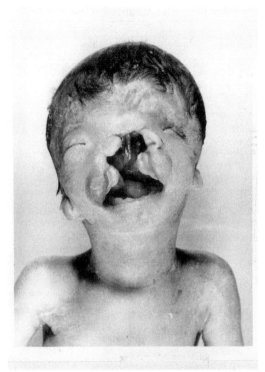

FIGURE 21. Cheilognathopalato-schisis in Váradi-Papp syndrome.

MICROCEPHALY

Microcephaly means small head, microencephaly small brain; when both are present the latter term is used, and this is always associated with developmental retardation.

Microcephaly may appear as an isolated defect or may result from insults during pregnancy or later (maternal PKU, irradiation, TORCH infections, perinatal asphyxia) or be associated with chromosomal abnormalities (trisomy 18) or malformation syndromes (Meckel's syndrome) or skeletal dysplasias. Isolated microencephaly may be inherited as an autosomal recessive trait. Autosomal dominant inheritance has also been reported.

The autosomal recessive forms can probably be seen on ultrasound before week 24 of gestation. Isolated biparietal diameter readings, even with certain dates, are less useful than serial measurements, at about fortnightly intervals, from the start of the second trimester; head/trunk ratios are also useful. Differentiation from craniosynostosis is important. In craniosynostosis the skull is small, but the brain is of normal size.

SUMMARY

Craniospinal (CSP) defects comprise the most frequent severe congenital anomalies; they pose major questions in prenatal diagnosis and genetic counseling. This entity includes three major types of defects: neural tube defects (NTD's), hydrocephalus

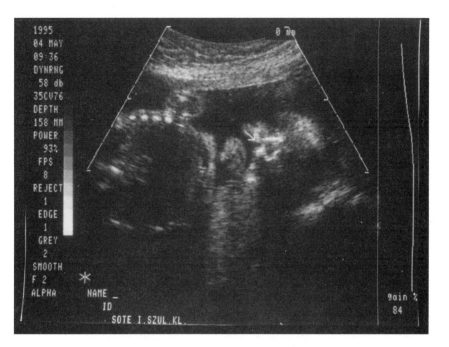

FIGURE 22. Cleft lip indicated by arrow.

(HC), and other craniospinal anomalies. Three major forms of the NTDs are anencephaly/ exencephaly, spina bifida, and encephalocele, where the first two account for 95% of all cases, and encephalocele for 5% of cases in Europe. The group of other CSP defects with clinical significance includes hydranencephaly, holoprosencephaly and associated disorders, microcephaly, and iniencephaly. The mechanism of abnormal neural development is still controversial: the most accepted theory is based on the multifactorial model of inheritance. NTDs in the majority of cases are isolated anomalies: only sequential concomitant anomalies are present. Isolated NTDs are inherited by the multifactorial trait of inheritance, whereas isolated HC cases have an etiology of monogenic inheritance in one-third of all cases; the rest follows the multifactorial trait. Risk of recurrence is primarily influenced by the degree and number of affected relatives, and the pathoanatomical severity of the disease. Prenatal recognition of these severe anomalies is one of the major challenges of proper pregnancy care. Screening includes the biochemical test—maternal serum AFP—and thorough ultrasound examination. By adequate administration of these screening tests the need for more invasive techniques such as amniocentesis obviously decreases. Appropriate timing and method of screening should result in a full range of possibilities of prenatal detection and, accordingly, allows for the termination of a pregnancy on the patient's wish. Screening of high-risk patients should always be done by highly trained staff of a prenatal diagnostic center.

REFERENCES

1. PAPP, Z. 1990. Obstetric Genetics. Hungarian Academic Press. Budapest.
2. PAPP, Z. 1992. Atlas of Fetal Diagnosis. Elsevier. Amsterdam.

3. SIEBERT, J. R., R. J. LEMIRE & M. M. COHEN. 1990. Aberrant morphogenesis of the central nervous system. Clin. Perinatol. **17:** 569–595.
4. PAPP, Z., K. CSÉCSEI, Z. TÓTH, K. POLGÁR & GY. SZEIFERT. 1986. Exencephaly in human fetuses. Clin. Genet. **30:** 440–444.
5. HENDRICKS, S. K., D. R. CYR, D. A. NYBERG, R. RAABE & L. A. MACK. 1988. Exencephaly. Clinical and ultrasonic correlation to anencephaly. Obstet. Gynecol. **72:** 898–901.
6. WILKINSH, L. & W. FREEDMAN. 1991. Progression of exencephaly to anenecephaly in the human fetus. An ultrasound perspective. Prenatal Diagn. **11:** 227–233.
7. VAN ALLEN, M.I., D.K. KALOUSEK, G.F. CHERNOFF, D. JURILOFF & M. HARRIS. 1993. Evidence for multi-site closure of the neural tube in humans. Am. J. Med. Genet. **47:** 723–743.
8. SELLER, M.J. 1995. Further evidence for an intermittent pattern of neural tube closure in humans. J. Med. Genet. **32:** 205–207.
9. CHERVENAK, F.A., C. DUNCAN, L.R. MENT, M. TORTONA, M. MCCLURE & J.C. HOBBINS. 1984. Perinatal management of meningomyelocele. Obstet. Gynecol. **63:** 376–380.
10. SIMPSON, J.L., J.L. MILLS, G.G. RHOADS, G.C. CUNNINGHAM, M.R. CONLEY & H.J. HOFFMAN. 1991. Genetic heterogeneity in neural tube defects. Ann. Genet. **34:** 279–286.
11. PAPP, CS., ZS. ÁDÁM, E. TÓTH-PÁL, O. TÖRÖK, V. VÁRADI & Z. PAPP. 1997. Risk of recurrence of craniospinal anomalies. J. Maternal-Fetal Med. **6:** 53–57.
12. PILU, G., N. RIZZO, L.F. ORSINI & L. BOVICELLI. 1986. Antenatal recognition of cerebral anomalies. Ultrasound Med. Biol. **12:** 319–326.
13. CAMPBELL, J. W.M. GILBERT, K.H. NICOLAIDES & S. CAMPBELL. 1987. Ultrasound screening for spina bifida: Cranial and cerebellar signs in a high-risk population. Obstet. Gynecol. **70:** 247–250.
14. BENACERRAF, B.R., J.M. STRYKER & F.D. FRIGOLETTO. 1989. Abnormal ultrasonography appearance of the cerebellum (banana sign). Indirect sign of spina bifida. Radiology **171:** 151–153.
15. PETRIKOVSKY, B.M. 1990. Fruit signs and neural tube defects. Prenatal Diagn. **10:** 134–134.
16. VAN DEN HOF, M.C., K.H. NICOLAIDES, J. CAMPBELL & S. CAMPBELL. 1990. Evaluation of the lemon and banana signs in 130 fetuses with open spina bifida. Am. J. Obstet. Gynecol. **162:** 322–327.
17. FLEMING, A.D., A.M. VINTZILEOS & W.E. SCORZA. 1991. Prenatal diagnosis of occipital encephalocele with transvaginal sonography. J. Ultrasound Med. **10:** 285–286.
18. HOBBINS, J.C. 1991. Diagnosis and management of neural tube defects today. N. Engl. J. Med. **324:** 690–691.
19. KOLLIAS, S.S., R.B. GOLDSTEIN, P.H. COGEN & R.A. FILLY. 1992. Prenatally detected myelomeningoceles. Sonographic accuracy in estimation of the spinal level. Radiology **185:** 109–112.
20. CASELLAS, M., M. FERRER, M. ROVIRA, F. PLA, M.A. MARTINEZ & L. CABERO. 1993. Prenatal diagnosis of exencephaly. Prenatal Diagn. **13:** 417–422.
21. LIMB, C.J. & L.B. HOLMES. 1994. Anenecephaly: Changes in prenatal detection and birth status, 1972 through 1990. Am. J. Obstet. Gynecol. **170:** 1333–1338.
22. PAPP, Z., Z. TÓTH, M. SZABÓ, K. CSÉCSEI & O. TÖRÖK. 1985. Prenatal screening for neural tube defects and other malformations by both serum AFP and ultrasound. *In* The Fetus as a Patient. A. Kurjak, Ed.: 167–180. Elsevier Science Publishers BV. Amsterdam.
23. NICOLAIDES, K.H., S.G. GABBE, S. CAMPBELL & R. GUIDETTI. 1986. Ultrasound screening for spina bifida: Cranial and cerebellar signs. Lancet **1:** 72–74.
24. TYRELL, S., D. HOWEL, M. BARK, E. ALLIBONE & R.J. LILFORD. 1988. Should maternal alpha-fetoprotein estimation be carried out in centres where ultrasound screening is routine? Am. J. Obstet. Gynecol. **158:** 1092–1099.
25. CAMPBELL, S. & P. SMITH. 1990. Routine screening for congenital abnormalities by ultrasound. Prenatal Diagn. **10:** 325–330.
26. CHITTY, L.S., G.H. HUNT, J. MOORE & M.O. LOBB. 1991. Effectiveness of routine ultrasonography in detecting fetal structural abnormalities in a low risk population. Br. Med. J. **303:** 1165–1169.
27. PLECHTER, B.A., C.D. AGNELLI, H.L. COHEN, L.P. LAWRENCE, G. SILVERBE & K.F. RAWLINSO. 1991. Sensitivity of ultrasound in detecting spina bifida. N. Engl. J. Med. **324:** 769–772.

28. WALD, N.J., H.S. CUCKLE, J.E. HADDOW, R.A. DOHERTY, G.J. KNIGHT & G.E. PALOMAKI. 1991. Sensitivity of ultrasound in detecting spina bifida. N. Engl. J. Med. **324:** 769–771.
29. MUECKLE, L.N. 1992. Prenatal screening for neural tube defects. A choice for all. Perspect. Biol. **36:** 87–96.
30. PLATT, L.D., L. FEUCHTBAUM, R. FILLY, L. LUSTIG, M. SIMON & G.C. CUNNINGHAM. 1992. The California Maternal Serum Alpha-Fetoprotein Screening Program: The role of ultrasonography in the detection of spina bifida. Am. J. Obstet. Gynecol. **166:** 1328–1329.
31. ROMERO, R. 1993. Routine obstetric ultrasound. Ultrasound Obstet. Gynecol. **3:** 303–307.
32. BERNASCHEK, G., I. STUEMPFLEN & J. DEUTINGER. 1994. The value of sonographic diagnosis of fetal malformations: Different results between indication-based and screening-based investigations. Prenatal Diagn. **14:** 807–812.
33. PAPP, Z., E. TÓTH-PÀL, Cs. PAPP, Z. TÓTH, M. SZABÓ, L. VERESS & O. TÖRÖK. 1995. Impact of prenatal mid-trimester screening on the prevalence of fetal structural anomalies: A prospective epidemiological study. Ultrasound Obstet. Gynecol. **6:** 320–326.
34. MILLS, J.L., G.G. RHOADS, J.L. SIMPSON, G.C. CUNNINGHAM, M.R. CONLEY, M.R. LASSMANN, M.E. WALDEN, O.R. DEPP & H.J. HOFFMANN. 1989. The absence of a relation between the periconceptional use of vitamins and neural tube defects. N. Engl. J. Med. **321:** 430–435.
35. SNYDER, R.D., A.F. FAKADEJ & J.E. RIGGS. 1991. Anencephaly in the United States, 1968–1987. The declining incidence among white infants. J. Child. Neurol. **6:** 304–305.
36. HOLMES, L. B. 1992. Prevention of neural tube defects. J. Pediatr. **120:** 918–919.
37. HOLMES-SIEDLE, M., R.H. LINDENBAUM & A. GALLIARD. 1992. Recurrence of neural tube defect in a group of at risk women. A 10-year study of Pregnavite forte-F. J. Med. Genet. **29:** 134–135.
38. FOX, A.M. 1993. Primary prevention of neural tube defects: Notice from HPB. Can. Med. Assoc. J. **149:** 1231–1232.
39. SCHORAH, C.J., N. HABIBZAD, J. WILD, R.W. SMITHELLS & M.J. SELLER. 1993. Possible abnormalities of folate and vitamin B(12) metabolism associated with neural tube defects. Ann. N.Y. Acad. Sci. **678:** 81–91.
40. WALD, N.J. 1993. Folic acid and the prevention of neural tube defects. Ann. N.Y. Acad. Sci. **678:** 112–129.
41. TÓTH-PÀL, E., Cs. PAPP & Z. PAPP. 1993. Computer follow-up system for obstetric genetic and neonatal care in Hungary. Int. J. Gynaecol. Obstet. **43:** 323–324.
42. WHITEVAN, M.C., J.M. CONNOR & M.A. FERGUSON-SMITH. 1990. Patient care before and after termination of pregnancy for neural tube defects. Prenatal Diagn. **10:** 497–505.
43. SILVER, R.K., M. MARZOCCHI, E.E. FARELL & D.G. McCLONE. 1989. The perinatal management of central nervous system anomalies. Clin. Perinatol. **16:** 939–953.

Influence of Prenatal Diagnosis on Congenital Heart Defects

GREGGORY R. DeVORE[a]

ALFIGEN The Genetics Institute, Pasadena, California, USA, and The Fetal Diagnostic Center, Salt Lake City, Utah, USA

ABSTRACT: The impact of prenatal detection of congenital heart defects (CHD) using the four-chamber screening examination cannot be accurately ascertained because of the wide range of detection rates that affect the cost associated with it. Assuming a screening ultrasound cost of $200 per examination, recent studies in which examiners not trained in fetal echocardiography obtained and interpreted the four-chamber view only identified 5.3% of CHD, for a cost of $476,190 per malformation. When the four-chamber screening examination was performed by an individual trained in fetal echocardiography, the detection rate increased to 55%, for a cost of $45,454 per malformation. This resulted in a savings of 90%, or $430,736. Because individuals trained in fetal echocardiography are not available to perform and interpret all of the heart screening examinations, another approach is for the fetal echocardiographer to review one to two minute video clips of the four-chamber and outflow tracts screening examination obtained by the individual performing the fetal screening examination. It is estimated that at a charge of $30 per video clip review, the cost to detect 50% of CHD would be $7,500 per defect. This would result in a reduction of 98% for the detection of CHD using current screening methods. This approach would increase the detection rate of CHD by 10-fold, remove the liability of missing CHD from the untrained individual performing the screening examination, and provide revenue to tertiary centers in which individuals skilled in fetal echocardiography could maximize their diagnostic skills.

INTRODUCTION

To ascertain the influence of prenatal diagnosis on congenital heart disease (CHD), large studies are required to compare the morbidity and mortality associated with CHD diagnosed prenatally and postnatally. To accomplish this the lesions must be similar in anatomy and functional impairment. In addition, the population of patients contributing to the study should be from a low-risk population undergoing screening ultrasound. Although two studies have suggested that prenatal diagnosis may decrease mortality as well as decrease the costs for health care, large population studies have not been conducted to ascertain the economic and medical benefits of prenatal diagnosis for CHD.[1,2]

In 1985 DeVore suggested that the four-chamber view of the fetal heart could be used to screen for major malformations of the cardiovascular system.[3] In the ensuing 12 years, investigators have reported their success in diagnosing correctly congenital heart defects *in utero.*[4–9] However, when the second trimester four-chamber view screening examination was implemented, the detection rates varied from 0 to 63%.[4–9] The main reason was the varied experience of the individuals performing and interpreting the four-chamber view screening examination.

[a] Address correspondence to Greggory R. DeVore, M.D., 4155 South Parkview, Salt Lake City, Utah 84124. E-mail: fetalecho@fetalecho.com

THE SCREENING EXAMINATION: DETECTION RATES AND COST

Prenatal Detection Rate of Congenital Heart Defects Less than 7%

In 1993 the RADIUS study demonstrated that routine screening examination of the four-chamber view performed at nontertiary centers identified 0% (0 of 17) of fetuses with CHD.[4] In 1995 Tegnander *et al.* reported the sensitivity of the four-chamber screening examination for detection of CHD in low-risk patients.[5] Heart defects were divided into two groups: noncritical and critical. Critical heart abnormalities were defined as those requiring surgery because they adversely affected cardiac function. The study was divided into two phases. In phase I the four-chamber view was not required to be imaged, whereas in phase II it was required as part of the screening examination. The incidence of heart defects in phase I (11 of 1000) was not significantly different from phase II (12 of 1000). In phase I 6.12% (3 of 49) of CHD were detected prenatally, of which all were critical (3 of 17; 18%). Of the 90 heart defects present in phase II, 6.6% (6 of 90) were detected during the second trimester, all of which were critical (6 of 23; 26%). In this study the incorporation of the four-chamber view did not significantly increase the detection rate between phase I and phase II of the study. In 1996 Buskens *et al.* reported findings from low-risk patients undergoing the four-chamber screening examination between 16 and 24 weeks of gestation.[6] Of the 44 cases of CHD, two were detected prenatally, for a detection rate of 4.5%. Combined data from these three studies demonstrated an overall detection rate for CHD of less than 7% for 17,401 screened low-risk patients (TABLE 1).

With the combined data from these three studies, the cost to detect CHD has been computed for a hypothetical population of 10,000 screened patients with an incidence of CHD of 8 per 1000 (TABLE 2). The cost per ultrasound ($200) is the same used by the authors of the RADIUS study.[4] With a detection rate of 5.3%, the cost to identify one fetus with CHD approaches one-half million dollars (TABLE 2).

TABLE 1. Prenatal Detection Rate of Congenital Heart Disease

Study	Fetuses Screened (n)	Identified Postnatally (n)	Incidence of CHD in the Population	CHD Detected Prenatally (n)	Prenatal Detection Rate (%)
LeFevre *et al.*[4]	4623	17	3.67/1000	0	0
Tegnander *et al.*[5]	7459	90	12/1000	6	6.7
Buskens *et al.*[6]	5319	44	7.5/1000	2	4.5
Total	17,401	151	8.7/1000	8	5.3

CHD, congenital heart disease.

TABLE 2. Cost to Identify One Fetus with Congenital Heart Disease

Screened patients (n)	10,000
Cost per ultrasound	$200
Total cost for screening	$2,000,000
Expected CHD (n)	80
Detected CHD (n)	4.2
Cost per detected CHD	$476,190

Prenatal Detection Rate of Congenital Heart Defects Greater than 45%

Since 1992 three studies have been reported in which investigators experienced in the recognition of CHD examined the four-chamber view and outflow tracts of the fetal heart during the second trimester.[7-9] Of the 143 fetuses with CHD, 55% were identified using only the four-chamber screening view, and 80% when the outflow tracts were included (TABLE 3). When the screening examination is performed by individuals with expertise in fetal echocardiography, the cost for detection of CHD is $45,454 for the four-chamber view, and $31,250 for the four-chamber and outflow tract views (TABLE 4). This represents a decrease of over 95% of cost when compared to studies in which the examiners had minimal experience interpreting the four-chamber view.[4-6]

From these data it appears that the examiner must have the necessary skill to not only acquire the ultrasound images of the fetal heart, but to interpret them as well. When the interpretation is done by a skilled examiner, the detection rate increases over 10-fold at a cost savings of over $430,000 per detected malformation.

IMPROVING THE DETECTION RATE FOR CONGENITAL HEART DEFECTS

To increase the detection rate for fetal CHD may be difficult to accomplish within health care systems as currently constituted. The reason for this is the wide variety of experience among ultrasound examiners. The following options, however, are potential solutions to the problem.

TABLE 3. Detecting Congenital Heart Disease Using the Four-Chamber View

Study	Study Patients with CHD (n)	Rate of Detection Using the Four-Chamber View (n)	(%)	Rate of Detection Using Four-Chamber and Outflow Tracts	Total Detected (%)
Achiron et al.[7]	23	11	48	18	78
Bromley et al.[8]	69	43	63	57	83
Kirk et al.[9]	51	24	47	40	78
Total	143	78	55	115	80

TABLE 4. Comparison of Costs Using Different Screening Examinations

Screening Examination	Cost per Ultrasound	Total Cost for Screening	Number of Expected CHD (n)	Detected CHD (n)	Cost per Detected CHD
Four-chamber view (n = 10,000)	$200	$2,000,000	80	44 (55%)	$45,454
Four-chamber and outflow tract views (n = 10,000)	$200	$2,000,000	80	64 (80%)	$31,250

Increase the Diagnostic Skills of the Screening Sonographer

This task requires an intensive program in which physicians/sonographers must become familiar with a myriad of congenital malformations of the cardiovascular system. When one considers the training required to become proficient in fetal echocardiography, it becomes impractical to expect a physician/sonographer to develop similar recognition and diagnostic skills without a great deal of effort. However, these individuals can be trained to acquire images of the fetal heart which could then be interpreted by those skilled in the recognition of CHD.

Review the Cardiovascular Screening Examination by Individuals Trained in Fetal Echocardiography

If the four-chamber and outflow tract views could be obtained by the physician/sonographer performing the initial screening examination of the fetus, recorded on videotape, and subsequently reviewed by an individual with expertise in fetal echocardiography, then it would be possible to screen a larger population of fetuses. This would be beneficial for all parties involved; the next section describes an approach which could be used to accomplish this task.

THE OFF-SITE FETAL ECHOCARDIOGRAPHIC SCREENING PROGRAM

Step 1: Imaging the Fetal Heart

Once the four-chamber view is imaged, the outflow tracts are identified by rotating the ultrasound transducer from the four-chamber view or by directing the ultrasound beam cephalad from the four-chamber view. The examiner can learn these skills by reviewing the literature, through hands-on training, or multimedia programs.[3,10-14]

Step 2: Recording the Cardiovascular Images Using a Standardized Protocol

Although the fetus may be in a number of fetal positions, it is imperative that the examiner orient the images of the four-chamber and outflow tract views in the same manner, irrespective of fetal position. This can be accomplished by flipping the image horizontally and/or vertically using software keys found on most ultrasound equipment.

Step 3: Recording the Screening Examination on Videotape

After the examiner identifies the four-chamber and outflow tract views, the videotape recorder is activated and the four-chamber-outflow tract sweep is begun.[10-14] This should take no longer than 60 seconds to accomplish. Once the sweep is completed, the videotape is stopped. Depending upon the number of examinations performed, the examiner may use a single videotape to accumulate all the examinations for one day, several days, or one week.

Step 4: Acquiring Patient Information for the Log Sheet

A log sheet is kept by the individual performing the screening examination of the fetal heart. The log sheet contains the patient's name, gestational age, and other pertinent information. In addition, the log sheet contains a column in which the fetal echocardiographer can place a check mark indicating whether the four-chamber and outflow tracts are normal, abnormal, or poorly imaged.

Step 5: Sending the Videotape and Log Sheet for Review by a Fetal Echocardiographer

At the completion of a series of examinations, the videotape and log sheet are sent to the fetal echocardiographer for review. Since the screening segments should be no longer than 60 seconds, the fetal echocardiographer can review the video segment and fill out the log sheet in less than five minutes. When the study is completed, a copy of the log sheet is kept by the fetal echocardiographer, and the videotape and original log sheet returned to the physician/sonographer performing the screening examination. If an abnormal screening examination is suspected, the patient is referred for a detailed fetal echocardiographic evaluation.

Cost for the Screening Program

The cost for review of the videotape of the screening examination of the fetal heart is $30 per examination. At this fee, the program is cost-effective for both the third-party payer as well as the fetal echocardiographer. Although the studies cited in this review identified 80% of CHD, for purposes of this analysis the cost will be based upon detection rates of 50, 60, 70, and 80% (TABLE 5). For a detection rate of 50%, the cost to detect one fetus with a heart defect is $7,500, which is 98% ($7,500/$476,190) lower than currently employed methods.

Cost-Effectiveness for the Fetal Echocardiographer

Because this program involves physicians with skills in fetal echocardiography, the question must be asked as to whether it would be cost-effective to undertake such a

TABLE 5. Cost-Effectiveness of Screening for Congenital Heart Defects

Number of Screened Patients	Cost per Ultrasound	Total Cost for Screening	Expected CHD (n)	CHD Detected (%)	Cost per Detected CHD
10,000	$30	$300,000	80	50 (40/80)	$7,500
10,000	$30	$300,000	80	60 (48/80)	$6,250
10,000	$30	$300,000	80	70 (56/80)	$5,357
10,000	$30	$300,000	80	80 (64/80)	$4,687

NOTE: Assuming a 50% detection rate, the cost to detect trisomy 21 using maternal triple marker screening modeled after the California Prenatal Screening Program in which one charge of $115 per patient provides all necessary services would be $191,666 per detected trisomy 21 $\{[(10,000_{\text{screened patients}})(\$115_{\text{per test}})]/6_{\text{trisomy 21 fetuses detected with screening}}\}$.

screening program. Physicians with skills in fetal echocardiography may be divided into four disciplines: pediatric cardiology, perinatology, obstetrics, and radiology. Assuming that the fetal echocardiographer reviews 10 cases per hour (6 min per case), the revenue generated would be $300 per hour. Because of the manner in which the program could be established, the overhead would be minimal. Translating this to one full-time equivalent, assuming a 40-h work week, the revenue generated for 50 weeks would be $600,000. This more than justifies the implementation of this type of service for a tertiary center in which individuals skilled in interpretation of fetal echocardiography could participate. The total number of examinations that could be reviewed would be 20,000 per year.

Cost-Effectiveness for the Third-Party Payer

There are two methods by which the third-party payer could implement the above program in a cost-effective manner. First, the third-party payer could incur the additional cost for the screening program with the hope of saving money as the result of decreased health care dollars spent postnatally.[1,2,15] A second choice would be to reduce the amount of money paid to the physician/sonographer performing the primary screening examination by $30 per patient. Although this would reduce the amount of revenue per ultrasound examination, it would also reduce the medical legal liability of the physician/sonographer responsible for the screening examination. Using the second approach would result in no additional expense incurred by third-party payers for the screening examination of the fetal heart.

DISCUSSION

Because of the low detection rate for CHD with screening ultrasound as currently practiced, a new approach must be considered to improve the prenatal detection rate before impact studies can be undertaken to ascertain the effect of prenatal diagnosis of CHD on neonatal morbidity, mortality, and health care finances. The concept outlined in this paper would enable a rapid deployment of improved prenatal echocardiographic diagnosis at no increased cost to third-party payers. Once the detection rate for CHD approaches 50%, which is similar to the detection rate of trisomy 21 with triple marker maternal serum screening, impact studies can be performed. Prenatal diagnosis of CHD could have an impact on those patients who would choose to terminate a pregnancy, as well as those who would choose to continue a pregnancy. For the latter patients, better care of the neonate could result in decreased morbidity, mortality, and health care dollars spent in the immediate neonatal period.[1,2] This becomes extremely important in rural areas where the diagnosis of CHD is often delayed and the cost for an emergency transport to a tertiary center could be avoided.

An additional benefit would be the monitoring of facilities performing the fetal screening examination. After 3,000 patients have been screened, the screening facility could be notified as to their primary detection rate for CHD. If it exceeded 50%, then the facility could be taken "off-line." If the detection rate dropped below 50%, then the facility would be placed back "on-line." This ensures quality assurance, which is required by laboratories performing biochemical screening or diagnostic tests. The same type of requirement should be applied to screening fetal ultrasound.

REFERENCES

1. CHANG, A.C., J.C. HUHTA, G.Y. YOON, D.C. WOOD, G. TULZER, A. COHEN, M. MENNUTI & W.I. NORWOOD. 1991. Diagnosis, transport, and outcome in fetuses with left ventricular outflow tract obstruction. J. Thorac. Cardiovasc. Surg. **102:** 841–848.

2. WU, J.L., M.P. LEUNG, J. KARLBERG, C. CHIU, J. LEE & C.K. MOK. 1995. Surgical repair of coarctation of the aorta in neonates: Factors affecting early mortality and re-coarctation. Cardiovasc. Surg. **3:** 573–578.

3. DEVORE, G.R. 1985. The prenatal diagnosis of congenital heart disease—A practical approach for the fetal sonographer. J. Clin. Ultrasound **13:** 229–245.

4. LEFEVRE, M.L., R.P. BAIN, B.G. EWIGMAN, F.D. FRIGOLETTO, J.P. CRANE & D. MCNELLIS. 1993. A randomized trial of prenatal ultrasonographic screening: Impact on maternal management and outcome. Am. J. Obstet. Gynecol. **169:** 483–489.

5. TEGNANDER, E., S.H. EIK-NES, O.J. JOHANSEN & D.T. LINKER. 1995. Prenatal detection of heart defects at the routine fetal examination at 18 weeks in a non-selected population. Ultrasound Obstet. Gynecol. **5:** 372–380.

6. BUSKENS, E., D.E. GROBBEE, I.M. FROHN-MULDER, P.A. STEWARD, R.E. JUTTMANN, J.W. WLADIMIROFF & J. HESS. 1996. Efficacy of routine fetal ultrasound screening of congenital heart disease in normal pregnancy. Circulation **94:** 67–72.

7. ACHIRON, R., J. GLASER, I. GELERNTER, J. HEGESH & S. YAGEL. 1992. Extended fetal echocardiographic examination for detecting cardiac malformations in low risk pregnancies. Br. Med. J. **304:** 671–674.

8. BROMLEY B., J.A. ESTROFF, S.P. SANDERS, R. PARAD, D. ROBERTS, F.D. FRIGOLETTO JR. & B.R. BENACERRAF. 1992. Fetal echocardiography: Accuracy and limitations in a population at high and low risk for heart defects. Am. J. Obstet. Gynecol. **166:** 1473–1481.

9. KIRK, J.S., T.W. RIGGS, C.H. COMSTOCK, W. LEE, S.S. YANG & E. WEINHOUSE. 1994. Prenatal screening for cardiac anomalies: The value of routine addition of the aortic root to the four-chamber view. Obstet. Gynecol. **84:** 427–431.

10. DEVORE, G.R. 1992. The aortic and pulmonary outflow tract screening examination in the human fetus. J. Ultrasound Med. **11:** 345–348.

11. DEVORE, G.R., R.L. DONNERSTEIN, C.S. KLEINMAN, L.D. PLATT & J.C. HOBBINS. 1982. Fetal echocardiography. I. Normal anatomy as determined by real-time–directed M-mode. Am. J. Obstet. Gynecol. **144:** 249–260.

12. HUHTA, J.C., D.J. HAGLER & L.M. HILL. 1984. Two-dimensional echoardigraphic assessment of normal fetal cardiac anatomy. J. Reprod. Med. **29:** 162–167.

13. SHIME, J., M. BERTRAND, S. HAGEN-ANSERT & H. RAKOWSKI. 1984. Two-dimensional and M-mode echocardiography in the human fetus. Am. J. Obstet. Gynecol. **148:** 679–685.

14. Internet Fetal Echocardiography. Internet address: http://www.fetalecho.com

15. WAITZMAN, N.J., P.S. ROMANO & R.M. SCHEFFLER. 1994. Estimate of the economic costs of birth defects. Inquiry **31:** 188–205.

Prenatal Diagnosis of Gastrointestinal Anomalies with Ultrasound

What Have We Learned?

DANIEL W. SKUPSKI[a]

The New York Hospital-Cornell Medical Center, Department of Obstetrics and Gynecology, 525 East 68th Street, Room J-130, New York, New York 10021, USA

ABSTRACT: The use of routine obstetric ultrasound has been shown to accurately diagnose fetal gastrointestinal anomalies, both during and after the midtrimester. These are among the most accurately diagnosed of all anomalies, comprising 5–7% of all fetal anomalies. From a review of the literature it is clear that the use of routine ultrasound allows: (1) the detection of multiple anomalies that are often present and affect outcome significantly, (2) preparation for delivery at a tertiary center where neonatal surgical experience will allow optimal outcome, and (3) decisions about mode and timing of delivery in cases where this is important, i.e., cases of omphalocele and gastroschisis.

INTRODUCTION

The last 20 years have seen major advances in the area of imaging with ultrasound, and in the diagnosis of fetal anomalies with ultrasound. With respect to the prenatal diagnosis of gastrointestinal anomalies, a number of questions remain unanswered despite many years of study. These include: (1) Can gastrointestinal tract defects be diagnosed by prenatal ultrasound? (2) Should prenatal care be altered based on the diagnosis? (3) Is there an optimal mode of delivery? and (4) Are there ultrasound findings that are predictive of poor outcome? Evidence-based medicine has led to the randomized controlled trial assuming an increased importance in decisions regarding both diagnostic tests and treatments in medicine. No randomized controlled trials are available to answer the above questions. The purpose of this article is to look at the combined experience in the literature in an effort to overcome the deficiency resulting from lack of controlled trials. In addition, we may be able to pinpoint the advances that are the most promising to allow us to focus the efforts of further research.

CAN GASTROINTESTINAL TRACT DEFECTS BE DIAGNOSED BY PRENATAL ULTRASOUND?

TABLE 1 shows the results of many published studies of the prenatal diagnosis of fetal anomalies, focusing on the sensitivity for the diagnosis of gastrointestinal tract defects. The five earlier studies,[1–5] published before 1993, show relatively small numbers of gastrointestinal defects in their series, with the one notable exception of the Belgian Multicentre Trial.[2] The sensitivity of prenatal ultrasound in the diagnosis of fetal gastrointestinal defects in these studies ranges from a low of 14% to a high of 86%. This wide range of sensitivities is due to a number of factors, including different types of

[a] E-mail: dwskupsk@mail.med.cornell.edu

TABLE 1. Sensitivity of Ultrasound in the Prenatal Diagnosis of Fetal Gastrointestinal Defects

Study and Year	Defects Detected (n)	Defects Present (n)	Sensitivity (%)
Helsinki (1990)	1	7	14
Levi (1991)	24	47	51
Chitty (1991)	4	7	57
RADIUS (1992)	2	5	40
Luck (1992)	7	8	86
Goncalves (1994)	10	21	48
Chambers (1995)	8	12	67
Papp (1995)	33	50	66
Carrera (1995)	60	74	81
IPIMC (1995)	170	690	25

gastrointestinal defects that were discovered in each of the studies, the differing experience of the investigators involved, and the timing of ultrasound during the pregnancy in each of the studies. The difference in sensitivity cannot be simply related to small numbers of patients, because the same wide range of sensitivities is seen in the latter five studies in TABLE 1.[6–10] In those studies published after 1993,[6–10] which include two very large prospective series, the sensitivity of prenatal ultrasound for the diagnosis of fetal gastrointestinal defects ranges from 25 to 81%.

The importance of the type of malformation in the ability to detect an anomaly is demonstrated in TABLE 2. This table shows the sensitivities of prenatal ultrasound in the diagnosis of specific types of gastrointestinal malformations for each of these studies where the data were provided in the text.[2,6–8,10] Omphalocele and gastroschisis are seen to be detectable in 47–61% of cases (universally detected in some studies), whereas esophageal atresia with or without tracheoesophageal fistula is detected in a very small percentage of cases (in all studies). In addition, an anomaly that has not been reported to be detected prior to 26 weeks' gestation is anal atresia or imperforate anus. Not surprisingly, anal atresia or imperforate anus is shown in TABLE 2 very unlikely to be detected in all studies. Important points that we have learned regarding studies of the sensitivity of prenatal ultrasound are that malformations should be listed by specific type

TABLE 2. Evaluation of Studies of the Prenatal Diagnosis of Fetal Gastrointestinal Defects by Specific Type of Malformation[a]

	Type of Malformation			
Study and Year	Omphalocele	Gastroschisis	Esophageal Atresia	Anal Atresia[b]
Levi (1991)	3/3 (100)	3/3 (100)	4/8 (50)	1/10 (10)
Goncalves (1994)	5/5 (100)	12/13 (92)	1/7 (14)	0/4 (0)
Chambers (1995)	3/3 (100)	4/4 (100)	2/4 (50)	0/0 (NA)
Papp (1995)	11/15 (73)	6/6 (100)	2/5 (40)	0/3 (0)
Baronciani (1995)	26/53 (49)	12/53 (52)	12/98 (12)	0/83 (0)
Total	48/79 (61)	37/79 (47)	21/122 (17)	1/100 (1)

[a]Numbers shown are the number of fetuses detected over the number of infants with the anomaly present after birth. Number in parentheses reflect percentages.
[b]Includes imperforate anus.

and by time of diagnosis during pregnancy. Some malformations are detectable; others are not. Some malformations are detectable early in pregnancy; others are detectable only late in pregnancy.

TABLE 3 reviews the current state of the art of prenatal ultrasound diagnosis of fetal gastrointestinal defects by type of malformation and time during pregnancy that they may be detected. A review of the literature reveals that of the malformations that are detectable and those that are not, many anomalies of the gastrointestinal tract fall in between; these are listed in the table as detectable in some cases.

All of the fetal gastrointestinal defects listed in TABLE 3 can be considered major anomalies, because they produce mortality or major morbidity (e.g., surgical treatment is necessary). It is important in any study of the prenatal diagnosis of fetal anomalies by ultrasound that the results are listed with several factors in mind: (1) Only major anomalies are included in calculations of sensitivity; (2) results are reported for each specific type of malformation; and (3) anomalies should be classified as detectable or not detectable. The focus of future study should be on major, detectable anomalies.[11] Most gastrointestinal anomalies fall into this category.

SHOULD PRENATAL CARE BE ALTERED BY THE DIAGNOSIS?

When a fetus is diagnosed with a gastrointestinal defect, the current literature supports the concept that prenatal care should be altered in at least as four ways: (1) Careful screening should occur to rule out multiple fetal anomalies; (2) preparation can be made for delivery to occur at a tertiary center where pediatric surgeons familiar with the neonate's condition are available; (3) close monitoring with ultrasound can occur prenatally in an effort to detect worsening condition of the fetus or ischemia or perforation of the bowel; and (4) elective delivery can be planned in the case of certain types of malformations (e.g., gastroschisis).

Fetuses with omphalocele will have multiple malformations in as many as 54% of cases, whereas those with gastroschisis will in 21%.[12] This knowledge requires that careful ultrasound screening by experienced sonologists is undertaken in order to make an accurate diagnosis. Accurate diagnoses are important so that parents may be accurately counseled regarding the prognosis and the likely course of disease for the infant

TABLE 3. Diagnosis of Fetal Gastrointestinal Anomalies by Ultrasound: Classification by Type of Anomaly and Time of Diagnosis

Disorder	Detectable < 24 weeks	Detectable > 24 weeks
Omphalocele	Yes	Yes
Gastroschisis	Yes	Yes
Bowel atresia	Yes[a]	Yes[a]
Anal atresia/Imperforate anus	No	Yes[a]
Esophaeal atresia	No[b]	No[b]
Pyloric stenosis	No[b]	No[b]
Volvulus/Intussusception	No	Yes[a]
Meconium ileus or peritonitis	Yes[a]	Yes[a]
Mesenteric cysts	Yes[a]	Yes[a]
Liver/Biliary anomalies	Yes[a]	Yes[a]
Hirschsprung's disease	No	No

[a]Detectable in some cases.
[b]A high index of suspicion can be present with indirect signs present on ultrasound.

after birth. In addition, if the diagnosis is able to be made in the early second trimester, the option of termination of pregnancy can be made available.

Although the literature is divided regarding the need for delivery at a tertiary center where pediatric surgery is available,[13,14] this option is important for two reasons. The first is that the neonatal medical and surgical problems encountered are more easily handled by the pediatric team when preparation is made in advance. The second is that prenatal referral avoids the panic that the parents may feel during an emergent neonatal transfer. It is difficult enough to handle the birth of an infant with an anomaly; panic is an unwelcome addition. Most physicians practicing at community hospitals cannot be expected to have the experience to adequately care for neonates with major anomalies. This is particularly true when, as in neonates with gastroschisis, the anomaly is physically difficult to control (loops of bowel may be difficult to contain).

Bowel ischemia or perforation may be evidenced by the rapid appearance of calcific masses, an increase in echogenicity, or an increase in bowel diameter. Intervention in the form of preterm iatrogenic delivery may be necessary. Thus, careful monitoring of the pregnancy with ultrasound every 2–4 weeks is an important adjunct in the prenatal management of gastrointestinal anomalies.

Elective delivery at 36 weeks is now being performed at several centers for fetuses with gastroschisis. This is because of data from one series that showed that 6 of 7 fetuses which progressed past 36 weeks were found to have hypoperistalsis after delivery (prolonged time of more than two weeks until oral feedings were tolerated).[15] Hypoperistalsis has the most serious and vexing morbidity requiring a prolonged period of total parental nutrition with its attendant complications.[15] It will not be avoided in every neonate, but a policy of elective delivery at 36 weeks will avoid iatrogenic complications of prematurity while providing the best chance for avoidance of hypoperistalsis.

IS THERE AN OPTIMAL MODE OF DELIVERY?

TABLE 4 shows the published trials of vaginal versus cesarean delivery for the specific malformation of gastroschisis.[16–21] It should be noted that five of the studies are retrospective case series, and one is a prospective case series. To date, no randomized controlled trials of mode of delivery for gastroschisis have been done. Three of these retrospective trials concluded that cesarean delivery was not beneficial compared to vaginal delivery, whereas three concluded that cesarean delivery was beneficial. Thus, the current data are not compelling that cesarean should be performed for the indication of fetal gastroschisis.

TABLE 4. Published Studies on Mode of Delivery in Fetuses with Gastroschisis[a]

Author	Cases (n)	Conclusion
Lenke (1983)	24	Cesarean beneficial
Sermer (1987)	8	Cesarean *not* beneficial
Fitzsimmons (1988)	16	Cesarean beneficial
Bethel (1989)	28	Cesarean *not* beneficial
Sakala (1993)	22	Cesarean beneficial
Novotny (1993)	69	Cesarean *not* beneficial

[a]All studies were retrospective case series except Fitzsimmons (1988), which was a prospective case series.

CAN OUTCOME BE PREDICTED BY SPECIFIC ULTRASOUND FINDINGS?

The prenatal ultrasound findings that have been suggested to be predictive of poor outcome or intestinal damage are echogenic bowel, maximum small bowel diameter, thickness of the bowel wall, rapid changes in echogenicity or small bowel diameter, and the appearance of a calcified mass in the abdomen.[15,22-26] In numerous case series to date, none of these findings has been sufficiently sensitive or specific to be useful. An example is the use of maximum small bowel diameter measurement, which has been studied in three large series (each using 24–30 patients).[15,22,23] The authors of these studies found diameters ranging from 10–18 mm as the cutoff for predicting poor outcome or intestinal damage. In addition, one of the studies found a very poor correlation between examiners (all experienced), who differed by as much as 5 mm when measuring the small bowel diameter in the same patient.[22]

It must be concluded that the use of prenatal ultrasound to predict poor outcome in fetuses with gastrointestinal anomalies is fraught with problems. Even very experienced sonographers and sonologists will have difficulty deciding when iatrogenic intervention is necessary. Despite this pessimistic conclusion after reviewing the literature, most experienced centers continue to attempt the prediction of bowel damage by the use of prenatal ultrasound. Isolated cases of the prediction of bowel damage continue to be diagnosed and timely intervention can benefit individual fetuses.

CONCLUSION

Routine ultrasound allows the (1) diagnosis of fetal gastrointestinal defects, (2) preparation for delivery to occur at a tertiary center where pediatric surgery is available, (3) timing of delivery at 36 weeks in cases of fetal gastroschisis, (4) detection of multiple anomalies, and (5) accurate differentiation between types of gastrointestinal defects. The last two will also allow accurate counseling of the parents regarding prognosis, and, if the diagnosis is made during the early second trimester, the option of termination of pregnancy. Much work remains to be done; specifically, randomized controlled trials or very large case series are needed to provide the vital information that is currently lacking in the case series already performed. In addition, the use of expert centers for routine ultrasound screening will decrease the chances of false positive diagnoses and avoid unnecessary parental emotional trauma.

REFERENCES

1. SAARI-KEMPPAINEN, A. *et al.* 1994. Fetal anomalies in a controlled one-stage ultrasound screening trial. A report from the Helsinki Ultrasound Trial. J. Perinat. Med. **22:** 279–289.
2. LEVI, S. *et al.* 1991. Sensitivity and specificity of routine antenatal screening for congenital anomalies by ultrasound: The Belgian Multicentric Study. Ultrasound Obstet. Gynecol. **1:** 102–110.
3. CHITTY, L.S. *et al.* 1991. Effectiveness of routine ultrasonography in detecting fetal structural abnormalities in a low risk population. Br. Med. J. **303:** 1165–1169.
4. CRANE, J.P. *et al.* 1992. A randomized trial of prenatal ultrasonographic screening: Impact on the detection, management, and outcome of anomalous fetuses. Am. J. Obstet. Gynecol. **171:** 392–399.
5. LUCK, C.A. 1992. Value of routine ultrasound scanning at 19 weeks: A four year study of 8849 deliveries. Br. Med. J. **304:** 1474–1477.
6. GONCALVES, L.F., P. JEANTY & J.M. PIPER. 1994. The accuracy of prenatal ultrasonography in detecting congenital anomalies. Am. J. Obstet. Gynecol. **171:** 1606–1612.
7. CHAMBERS, S.E. *et al.* 1995. Audit of a screening service for fetal abnormalities using early

ultrasound scanning and maternal serum alpha-fetoprotein estimation combined with selective detailed scanning. Ultrasound Obstet. Gynecol. **5:** 168–173.

8. PAPP, Z. *et al.* 1995. Impact of prenatal mid-trimester screening on the prevalence of fetal structural anomalies: A prospective epidemiological study. Ultrasound Obstet. Gynecol. **6:** 320–326.

9. CARRERA, J.M. *et al.* 1995. Routine prenatal ultrasound screening for fetal abnormalities: 22 years' experience. Ultrasound Obstet. Gynecol. **5:** 174–179.

10. BARONCIANI, D. *et al.* 1995. Ultrasonography in pregnancy and fetal abnormalities: Screening or diagnostic test? IPIMC 1986–1990 register data. Prenatal Diagn. **15:** 1101–1108.

11. SKUPSKI, D.W. *et al.* 1996. The impact of routine obstetric ultrasound screening in a low risk population. Am. J. Obstet. Gynecol. **175:** 1142–1145.

12. CALZOLARI, E. *et al.* 1995. Omphalocele and gastroschisis in Europe: A survey of 3 million births 1980–1990. Am. J. Med. Genet. **58:** 187–194.

13. ROBERTSON, F.M. *et al.* 1994. Prenatal diagnosis and management of gastrointestinal anomalies. Semin. Perinatol. **18:** 182–195.

14. NICHOLLS, G. *et al.* 1993. Is specialist centre delivery of gastroschisis beneficial? Arch. Dis. Child. **69:** 71–73.

15. LANGER, J.C. *et al.* 1993. Prenatal diagnosis of gastroschisis: Development of objective sonographic criteria for predicting outcome. Obstet. Gynecol. **81:** 53–56.

16. LENKE, R.R. & E. I. HATCH. 1986. Fetal gastroschisis: A preliminary report advocating the use of cesarean section. Obstet. Gynecol. **67:** 395–398.

17. SERMER, M. *et al.* 1987. Prenatal diagnosis and management of congenital defects of the anterior abdominal wall. Am. J. Obstet. Gynecol. **156:** 308–312.

18. FITZSIMMONS, J. *et al.* 1988. Perinatal management of gastroschisis. Obstet. Gynecol. **71:** 910–913.

19. BETHEL, C.A.I., J.H. SEASHORE & R.J. TOULOUKIAN. 1989. Cesarean section does not improve outcome in gastroschisis. J. Pediatr. Surg. **24:** 1–3.

20. SAKALA, E.P., L.N. ERHARD & J.J. WHITE. 1993. Elective cesarean section improves outcomes of neonates with gastroschisis. Am. J. Obstet. Gynecol. **169:** 1050–1053.

21. NOVOTNY, D.A., R.L. KLEIN & C.R. BOECKMAN. 1993. Gastroschisis: An 18-year review. J. Pediatr. Surg. **28:** 650–652.

22. BABCOOK, C.J. *et al.* 1994. Gastroschisis: Can sonography of the fetal bowel accurately predict postnatal outcome? J. Ultrasound Med. **13:** 701–706.

23. PRYDE, P.G. *et al.* 1994. Gastroschisis: Can antenatal ultrasound predict infant outcomes? Obstet. Gynecol. **84:** 505–510.

24. MULLER, F. *et al.* 1995. Hyperechogenic fetal bowel: An ultrasonographic marker for adverse fetal and neonatal outcome. Am. J. Obstet. Gynecol. **173:** 508–513.

25. LANGER, J.C. *et al.* 1989. Gastrointestinal obstruction in the fetus. Arch. Surg. **124:** 1183–1187.

26. BOND, S.J. *et al.* 1988. Severity of intestinal damage in gastroschisis: Correlation with prenatal sonographic findings. J. Pediatr. Surg. **23:** 520–525.

Does the Prenatal Diagnosis of Fetal Urinary Tract Anomalies Affect Perinatal Outcome?

LIL VALENTIN[a] AND KAREL MARŠÁL

Department of Obstetrics and Gynecology, University Hospital MAS, University of Lund, S-205 02 Malmö, Sweden

ABSTRACT: A review of the literature is presented. Congenital renal and urinary tract anomalies are described, and the possible consequences of detecting them *in utero* are discussed. Prenatal detection of lethal anomalies affords the parents the option of terminating the pregnancy. If termination of pregnancy is not an acceptable option for the parents, the antenatal knowledge of lethal fetal anomaly helps the clinician to avoid unnecessary obstetric intervention, e.g., cesarean delivery for fetal distress. In certain cases of nonlethal renal and urinary tract anomalies, antenatal detection may influence both obstetric and postnatal management. It seems reasonable to anticipate that this might improve the prognosis of some children in terms of better preservation of kidney function. However, no scientific evidence is available to support such a statement. There are no randomized trials evaluating the outcome of congenital renal and urinary tract anomalies using different prenatal and postnatal diagnostic and therapeutic approaches. It is hoped that further research will lead to more rational antenatal and postnatal management protocols.

INTRODUCTION

Anomalies of the fetal urinary tract are relatively easily accessible for antenatal diagnosis by ultrasonography. Using modern high-resolution ultrasound scanners, it is possible to visualize the fetal kidneys as early as in the first trimester of gestation both transabdominally[1] and transvaginally.[2] Collection of fluid in the urinary tract, e.g., in cases of renal pelvis dilatation (pyelectasis), is especially recognizable in the ultrasound image. Anomalies of the fetal urinary tract correspond to 20–25% of all anomalies diagnosed antenatally using ultrasonography.[3–5] A high detection rate is reported, even at routine ultrasound examination in pregnancy. Levi *et al.*[3] found the sensitivity for malformations of the urogenital tract to be 67%, Stoll *et al.*[6] 59%, and Carrera *et al.*[4] 91%. The latter study demonstrated between 1970 and 1991 an improvement with time in the detection rate due to the improved technical quality of ultrasound equipment and the increased skills and experience of the examiners.

The fetal urinary tract should always be scrutinized at ultrasound examinations in the second and third trimester. Both fetal kidneys, fetal bladder, and the amount of amniotic fluid should be systematically evaluated. The following ultrasound features give a strong suspicion of congenital urinary tract anomaly: presence of oligohydramnios, urinary tract dilatation, renal cysts, abnormal echogenicity or size and shape of the kidneys, and possible associated abnormalities indicating a syndrome.[7]

It might be anticipated that the antenatal diagnosis of an anomaly in the fetal urinary tract would be an advantage, because it allows for planned delivery and early postnatal treatment. However, the antenatal evaluation of possible renal function impairment is often difficult, and management depends on the gestational age at which the anomaly is detected. Early diagnosis of severe renal anomalies, e.g., bilateral renal

---

[a] Corresponding author. E-mail: Lil.Valentin@obst.mas.lu.se

agenesis, gives the option of terminating the pregnancy. Most minor anomalies, e.g., isolated pyelectasis, are not detectable until late in pregnancy, and usually they do not necessitate any intervention before birth. Nevertheless, the antenatal knowledge of such anomalies makes it possible to follow up the infants with regard to urinary tract morphology and function. This enables identification of clinically important pathological changes in the infants, which otherwise might have remained unrecognized for months after birth. In certain cases, early postnatal surgical intervention may be important for the preservation of renal function.

In this paper, we present a short review on the antenatal diagnosis of congenital renal and urinary tract anomalies and then focus on the most common intrauterine diagnosis of urinary tract disease, hydronephrosis. We will try to answer the question of whether it is of benefit to the patient to have fetal pyelectasis diagnosed *in utero*. Unfortunately, it will be necessary to consider only indirect evidence of possible beneficence, because a strict scientific evidence based on randomized controlled trials is practically impossible to obtain, due to the low incidence of congenital urinary tract disease in neonates.

FETAL RENAL ANOMALIES

Renal Agenesis

Bilateral renal agenesis is a rare (0.3 per 1000 births)[8] but lethal condition, characterized at fetal ultrasound examination by severe oligohydramnios, nonvisualization of the fetal bladder and kidneys, and often also a small thorax.[9] There are possible pitfalls in the prenatal diagnosis—enlarged fetal adrenals being mistaken for kidneys, not revealed ectopic kidneys, and oligohydramnios due to other causes. Unilateral renal agenesis is found in about 1‰ of autopsies.[10] At prenatal diagnosis of absent kidney, the possibility of ectopic kidney must always be considered. Most individuals with a single kidney are asymptomatic; however, associated genital anomalies may occur. There is a male predominance for both bilateral and unilateral renal agenesis.

Renal Cystic Disease

Infantile polycystic kidney disease (Potter type I) is a very rare anomaly, which may become clinically manifest at various ages, but uniformly leads to death from renal failure. The ultrasonographic feature of infantile polycystic kidneys is bilaterally enlarged hyperechogenic kidneys of normal shape.[11] In severe cases, the urinary bladder cannot be visualized and there is severe oligohydramnios. The kidney enlargement is progressive and may be found before 20 weeks of gestation. Nevertheless, the finding of normal kidneys at that time of gestation does not exclude later manifestation of the disease. *Multicystic kidney disease* (Potter type II) may be bilateral, unilateral or segmental, i.e., limited to a localized portion of the kidney. If both kidneys are affected, then the condition is lethal and characterized at antenatal ultrasound examination by bilaterally enlarged multicystic kidneys, oligohydramnios, and nonvisible fetal bladder.[12] Unilateral multicystic kidney disease (round cysts of variable size, normal amount of amniotic fluid) can be clinically silent, but in many cases it causes a palpable neonatal abdominal mass, and in 20–45% it is associated with contralateral urinary tract anomaly, e.g., hydronephrosis or renal hypoplasia. *Adult polycystic kidney disease* (Potter type III) is a common cause of renal failure late in life, usually in the fourth or fifth decade. However, the gross anatomical lesions, i.e., the renal cysts, may be present and detectable by ultrasound already in fetuses and newborns.[13] The sonographic features are similar to those of infantile polycystic kidney disease—enlarged echogenic kidneys, or sometimes multiple cysts. Amniotic fluid volume is usually normal, and the fetal bladder is visible because the kidneys are still functioning *in utero.* A unilateral finding of renal cysts does not exclude the diagnosis of adult polycystic kidney disease in the fetus.

In the sonographic differential diagnosis of an enlarged fetal kidney, the possibility should be considered of congenital renal tumor, e.g., mesoblastic nephroma.[14]

Is Detecting Congenital Renal Disease in Utero *Worth It?*

At present, there is no way of improving the prognosis for fetuses with impending or established renal failure when this is due to a lethal kidney malformation, e.g., bilateral renal agenesis, infantile polycystic kidney disease, or bilateral multicystic kidney disease. Whether parents prefer to know about the fatal condition of their child before or after birth probably varies between parents. Some will certainly consider the option of terminating the pregnancy in such cases. Even when termination of pregnancy is not an option for the parents, it might be psychologically advantageous to know about the anomaly before birth. It has been shown that the identification of fetal malformation before birth may help the parents to adjust emotionally.[15] In addition, in some cases, the antenatal knowledge of lethal fetal anomaly helps the clinician to avoid unnecessary obstetric intervention, e.g., cesarean delivery for fetal distress.

In cases of antenatal diagnosis of a nonlethal kidney anomaly, the prognosis is usually difficult to make. Unilateral multicystic kidney disease may be completely asymptomatic, but it may lead to complications, such as hypertension, infection, or malignant transformation. Whether to manage the infants with unilateral multicystic kidney disease conservatively or to perform nephrectomy prophylactically is still a matter of controversy.

Counseling parents of a fetus with adult polycystic kidney disease is a delicate matter, because there is little to be done to improve the outcome. Possibly, timely treatment of hypertension can be initiated in some cases. Otherwise, it must be suspected that the knowledge of having a disease probably leading to premature death and suboptimal quality of life may be a psychological burden for the individual.

FETAL HYDRONEPHROSIS

Dilatation of a part or of all of the fetal urinary tract is the most common anomaly of the fetal urogenital system, accounting for 87% of fetal renal anomalies.[16] Actually, it is the most common fetal abnormality revealed by antenatal ultrasound.[4] Congenitally dilated renal pelvis (hydronephrosis or pyelectasis) is usually unilateral with preponderance in male fetuses. The incidence of fetal pyelectasis reported in the literature varies between 2[17] and 15[18] per 1000 fetuses, these figures being very much dependent on the definition of pyelectasis used. Unfortunately, no consensus exists as to what should be considered significant fetal pyelectasis. The diameter of the renal pelvis can be measured as the largest anteroposterior diameter in a transverse section,[19] or as the average of the anteroposterior and transverse diameters (L. Chitty, personal communication). In addition, the anteroposterior pelvic diameter can be related to the anteroposterior dimension of the kidney. Normally, the ratio between the diameters should not exceed 0.35.[20] Ratios between 0.35 and 0.50 are considered "mild hydronephrosis"; ratios of more than 0.50 usually indicate progressive disease.[21] Some authors use different definitions of fetal pyelectasis at different gestational ages, e.g., anteroposterior diameter ≥ 4 mm before 20 weeks, ≥ 5 mm between 20 and 30 weeks, and ≥ 7 mm between 30 and 40 weeks.[22] However, there seems to be agreement in the literature that the finding of an anteroposterior diameter of the fetal kidney pelvis exceeding 10 mm should be considered important.[19] The risk of finding significant urinary tract pathology after birth is much greater if the pelvis dilatation increases during pregnancy than if the dilatation remains unchanged.[23] If the dilatation resolves, the risk is very small. The possible presence of calyceal dilatation, hyperechogenic kidney parenchyma, and cystic changes in the kidney increase the risk of finding significant pathology after birth.[19]

The cause of congenital hydronephrosis may be ureteropelvic junction obstruction, ureterocele, ureteral stricture, ureterovesical junction obstruction, vesicoureteral reflux, urethral obstruction (usually due to posterior urethral valve) or, very rarely, megacystis-microcolon-intestinal hypoperistalsis syndrome. The detailed description of various pathological processes and their antenatal ultrasonographic features can be found in specialized textbooks.[24,25] The examiner should always try to identify the cause of fetal pyelectasis to be able to provide the parents with adequate information about the prognosis. Unfortunately, the antenatal examination does not always give the answer as to the underlying disease. Besides, in many cases no pathological process explaining the antenatal pyelectasis is found postnatally, and the dilatation of the urinary tract may disappear after birth.

If fetal pyelectasis is unilateral, the amniotic fluid volume is usually normal. If the process is bilateral and the renal function is impaired, there will be oligohydramnios and no urine in the fetal bladder. In some cases, the dilated urinary tract may rupture leading to paranephric urinoma or urinary ascites.[26]

Fetal pyelectasis is frequently found at routine ultrasound examination (TABLE 1). As mentioned above, the incidence reported is dependent on the definitions of fetal pyelectasis used. Moreover, they depend on the number of routine scans per pregnancy and on the gestational age at which the examinations are performed. In the multicenter Eurofetus study,[5] the average gestational age at diagnosis of 738 minor urinary tract anomalies (of which 62% were hydronephrosis) was 28.7 weeks (FIG. 1). The corresponding gestational age for 129 major anomalies (bilateral renal agenesis, polycystic kidneys, extrophy of urinary bladder, etc.) was 23.3 weeks.

The incidence of significant pathology of the urinary tract after birth given in TABLE 1 includes ureteropelvic junction obstruction, ureterocele, ureterovesical junction obstruction, vesicoureteral reflux, posterior urethral valve, congenital megaureter, multicystic, polycystic or dysplastic kidney, renal agenesis, and duplex or ectopic kidney. The incidence depends on how the diagnosis was defined by the pediatricians and on the length of follow-up in infancy. This is illustrated in FIGURE 2, which describes the postnatal follow-up of 37 infants who had pyelectasis detected in 1994 at routine fetal ultrasound examination at the Department of Obstetrics and Gynecology, University Hospital Lund, Sweden (I. Helin, personal communication). After one year, six children had been operated upon (diagnoses: two multicystic dysplastic kidney, one duplex kidney with ectopic ureter, and three significant congenital hydronephrosis); in one infant a rudimentary kidney had disappeared; 28 infants had been declared healthy, and two children were still being followed (one with pyelectasis > 10 mm, one with unconfirmed suspicion of cystic kidneys).

The positive predictive value of fetal pyelectasis with regard to significant urinary tract pathology varies in the literature between 12 and 77% (TABLE 1). In 1.5–9% of the cases, the prenatal diagnosis of pyelectasis was wrong: the sonographic finding corresponded to cystic or dysplastic kidneys, or even to dilated intestines. Livera and coworkers[18] followed 6,292 infants for 18 months and found the sensitivity and specificity of routine fetal ultrasound examination at 28 weeks to be 88 and 99%, respectively.

TABLE 1. Incidence of Fetal Pyelectasis and Significant Urinary Tract Anomalies in Infants Who Underwent Routine Antenatal Ultrasound Examination

Study	Pregnant Population (n)	Gestational Age at Examination (weeks)	Definition of Pyelectasis	Incidence of Fetal Pyelectasis (per 1000)	Significant Postnatal Urinary Tract Pathology[a] (per 1000)	Positive Predictive Value (%)
Arger et al.[47]	3,530	19–42	Diameter ≥ 5 mm	9	2	32
Helin & Persson[17]	11,986	16 and 33	Not stated	2	1	60
Livera et al.[18]	6,292	28	Diameter ≥ 10 mm	15	6.6	47
Rosendahl[27]	4,586	18 and 34	Anteroposterior diameter ≥ 10 mm	4	3	77
Paduano et al.[48]	9,707	Not stated	Not stated	5	2.7	54
Scott & Renwick[49]	242,628	Majority: 16	Not stated	2	0.8	45
Engström et al.[50]	4,902	16	Not stated	6	2.9	52
Morin et al.[23]	5,900	<24	Anteroposterior diameter 4–10 mm	5	0.8	12
Walsh & Dubbins[51]	15,927	18	Anteroposterior diameter ≥ 5 mm	5	0.8	19
Chitty, L. (personal communication)	108,373	<26	Mean diameter[b] 5–15 mm	8	—	—
Valentin, L. (unpublished data)	27,904	17 and 33	Anteroposterior diameter ≥ 10 mm	6	0.9–3.6	23–74

[a] Significant postnatal urinary tract pathology: Ureteropelvic junction obstruction, vesicoureteral reflux, posterior urethral valve, congenital megaureter, multicystic kidney, polycystic kidney, dysplastic kidney, renal agenesis, duplex kidney, ectopic kidney.
[b] Mean diameter: (anteroposterior + transverse diameter)/2.

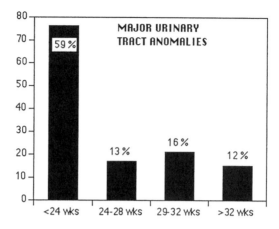

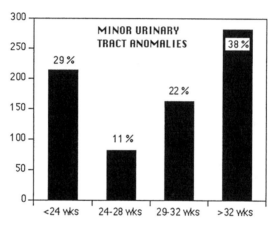

FIGURE 1. Gestational age at ultrasound diagnosis of 129 major *(upper graph)* and 738 minor *(lower graph)* fetal urinary tract anomalies. (Data from Eurofetus Study Report.[5])

Rosendahl[27] found in the unselected population of 4,586 fetuses the sensitivity of 85% and specificity 99.9%; in the multicenter Eurofetus study comprising 190,000 pregnancies, the corresponding figures were 88 and 99.9%. The positive predictive values of prenatal ultrasound were similar in a preselected population when ultrasound examination was performed on indication (TABLE 2).

Fetal Pyelectasis and Chromosomal Abnormalities

The reported incidence of chromosomal abnormalities associated with antenatally diagnosed fetal hydronephrosis varies greatly between the studies—from 0 in 161 fetuses (Valentin, unpublished data) to 5 in 43 fetuses[28] (TABLE 3). In a large European study, Ferguson-Smith & Yates[29] found that the risk of fetal chromosomal aberrations increased three times when an isolated renal abnormality was present, and 30 times when

FETAL PYELECTASIS

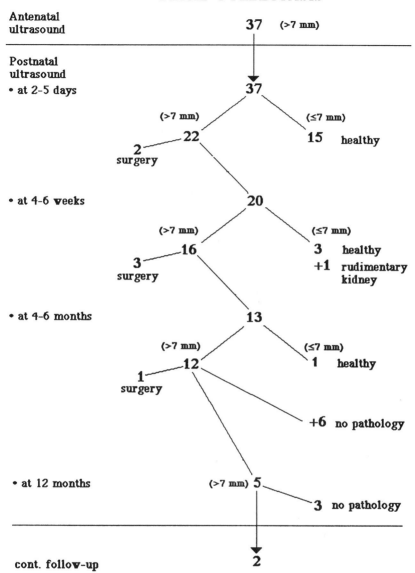

FIGURE 2. Postnatal follow-up of 37 fetuses with unilateral renal pyelectasis diagnosed antenatally in 1994 at the Departments of Obstetrics and Gynecology, and Pediatrics, University of Lund, Sweden (based on I. Helin, personal communication). Figures in brackets denote the anteroposterior diameter of renal pelvis. Indications for surgery: Multicystic dysplastic kidney ($n=2$), duplex kidney ($n=1$), congenital hydronephrosis ($n=3$).

TABLE 2. Incidence of Fetal Pyelectasis and Significant Urinary Tract Anomalies in Infants Who Underwent Antenatal Ultrasound Examination on Indication

Study	Pregnant Population (n)	Gestational Age at Examination (weeks)	Definition of Pyelectasis	Incidence of Fetal Pyelectasis (per 1000)	Significant Postnatal Urinary tract Pathology[a] (per 1000)	Positive Predictive Value (%)
Johnson et al.[52]	7,530	>20	Length ≥ 9 mm	6	1.6	26
Gunn et al.[53]	3,856	>28	Length ≥ 15 mm	81	14.3	13

[a] Significant postnatal urinary tract pathology: Ureteropelvic junction obstruction, vesicoureteric junction obstruction, distending vesicoureteral reflux, posterior urethral valve, congenital megaureter, multicystic dysplastic kidney, renal hypoplasia, renal agenesis.

TABLE 3. Chromosomal Abnormalities in Fetuses with Pyelectasis Detected at Ultrasound Examination

Study	Chromosomal Abnormalities	
	(n)	(%)
Reuss et al.[28]	5/43	11.6
Benacerraf et al.[22]	7/210	3.3
Scott & Renwick[49]	4/421	0.9
Gunn et al.[53]	2/301	0.7
Morin et al.[23]	5/127	3.9
Chitty, L. (personal communication)		
No risk factors:	3/1000	0.3
Risk factors:	10/100	1.0
Valentin, L. (unpublished data)	0/161	0

there were additional abnormalities. Similarly, Chitty (personal communication) did not find any increased risk of chromosomal abnormalities in fetuses with isolated mild pyelectasis. However, in cases with additional risk factors, e.g., maternal age above 37 years or additional fetal malformations, the risk of chromosomal abnormality was as high as 10%. In mild pyelectasis, the most commonly associated chromosomal abnormality is trisomy 21.[22,29] In cases of severe hydronephrosis, multicystic kidney or renal agenesis, the most frequent chromosomal aberrations are trisomies 13 and 18.[29]

Antenatal Management of Fetal Pyelectasis Diagnosed by Ultrasound

A finding of fetal pyelectasis should initiate a detailed sonographic evaluation of the degree of dilatation, level of possible obstruction, amount of amniotic fluid, appearance of the contralateral kidney, and possible other associated anomalies. In cases of severe hydronephrosis or presence of other risk factors, fetal karyotype should be assessed. All the above factors, together with the gestational age at diagnosis and subsequent course as pregnancy continues, are of importance in judging the prognosis, clinical management, and counseling the parents. As precise an antenatal diagnosis as possible should be attempted, even if, admittedly, it is often impossible to determine before birth the cause of urinary tract dilatation.

Unilateral fetal pyelectasis of mild degree without any other associated anomalies or risk factors and with normal contralateral kidney does not seem to necessitate karyotyping or other extensive antenatal evaluation. One antenatal follow-up ultrasound examination at about 30 to 35 weeks is suitable to determine the possible progression of the hydronephrosis. The obstetric management should not be influenced in these cases. However, postnatal workup is indicated.

Fetuses with *bilateral hydronephrosis* should be followed up with repeated scans in order to assess the amount of amniotic fluid and possible progress of hydronephrosis. Information on fetal sex is sometimes useful; among fetuses with urethral obstruction, there is a preponderance of males when the obstruction is caused by the posterior urethral valve[30] and of females in cases of megacystis-microcolon-intestinal hypoperistalsis syndrome.[31] Karyotyping should be offered in all cases of urethral obstruction, and in cases with associated anomalies or other risk factors. Fetuses with distal obstruction of the urinary tract have chromosomal abnormalities in up to 44% of cases.[32] Evaluation of fetal renal function should be attempted, because evidence of functional impairement might call for preterm delivery and early surgery after birth, or for fetal therapy. Merrill and Weiner[33] consider as a candidate for antenatal intervention the fetus whose obstruction is severe enough to compromise pulmonary and renal development, but not so severe that the damage is irreversible after antenatal relief of the obstruction. Fetal renal function can be evaluated by analyzing fetal urine obtained via ultrasound-guided puncture of the fetal bladder, by following the amniotic fluid volume and the ultrasound appearance of fetal kidneys. Normal ranges have been established for fetal urinary electrolytes and osmolality,[34] and for urine microproteins.[35] Increased urinary sodium and calcium[36] and beta 2-microglobulin[37] were the best predictors of fetal renal failure. Recently, nuclear magnetic resonance spectroscopy of fetal urine was used to differentiate between different degrees of fetal renal function impairment.[38]

Several research groups performed urinary diversion *in utero* in an attempt to prevent renal damage and lung hypoplasia in cases associated with oligohydramnios. Vesicoamniotic shunts,[39] open fetal surgery,[40] and fetoscopic surgery[41] have been used in fetal intervention. All intrauterine procedures are associated with technical difficulties and risks, and thus far the clinical results have not been convincing. The main problem of fetal therapy for obstructive uropathy seems to be the selection of suitable cases. Repeated ultrasound-guided punctures of the fetal bladder with longitudinal evaluation of urinary osmolality and concentrations of sodium, calcium, and beta 2-microglobulin, as well as ultrasound evaluation of bladder filling, may facilitate identification of fetuses who might benefit from *in utero* therapy.[42] At present, it is recommended that only cases of urethral-level obstruction diagnosed before lung maturity, associated with oligohydramnios and otherwise normal fetuses with preserved renal function, should be considered for vesicoamniotic shunting.[33,43]

Postnatal Management of Infants with Pyelectasis Diagnosed in Utero

The first neonatal ultrasound examination should be performed within one week after birth, but not in the first 48 hours, because at that time the hydronephrosis might be transiently absent. This is probably due to a relative dehydration and low glomerular filtration rate following birth.[44] If the primary ultrasound examination is normal, usually a second one is done after one month to confirm that there is no pyelectasis or other abnormality. Thereafter, no further follow-up is necessary. If a significant renal pyelectasis is confirmed after birth, a full radiologic workup is done, including voiding cystourethrogram, intravenous pyelogram, and renal scintigram. FIGURE 3 gives an example of a follow-up program used for fetuses with pyelectasis diagnosed at routine third trimester obstetric ultrasound examination at the Departments of Obstetrics and Gynecology, and Pediatrics in Malmö, Sweden.

There is no agreement regarding how long infants with antenatally diagnosed pyelectasis should be followed. Sometimes, repeated examinations are necessary to arrive at a diagnosis and, in some cases, to indicate surgery. No consensus exists among pediatricians as to what constitutes significant congenital urinary tract obstruction. Consequently, indications for surgical correction vary widely. It has been suggested that congenital urinary obstruction in children should be defined as "impaired urinary drainage which, if uncorrected, will limit the ultimate functional potential of a developing kidney."[45] However, a standardized way of assessing the functional potential of kidneys has not yet been defined.

Infection secondary to dilatation of the urinary tract can damage the kidney. Therefore, most pediatricians initiate prophylactic treatment with antibiotics in infants with congenital hydronephrosis. The prophylaxis can be given directly after birth to all newborns who had significant pyelectasis *in utero*, or at the first ultrasound examination in the neonatal period to those who have persistent hydronephrosis (FIG. 3).

MANAGEMENT OF FETAL PYELECTASIS

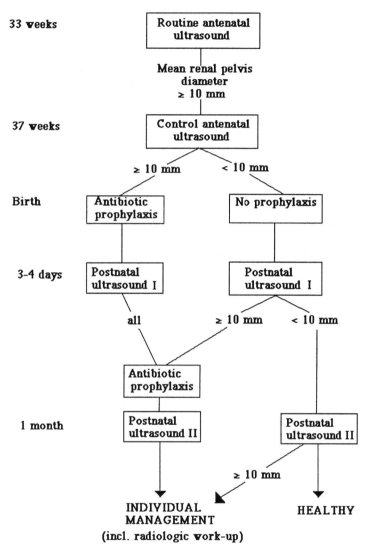

FIGURE 3. Management program for the fetuses with renal pyelectasis diagnosed at third trimester routine ultrasound examination. Departments of Obstetrics and Gynecology, and Pediatrics, University Hospital, Malmö, Sweden.

Is Detection of Fetal Pyelectasis Worth It?

The finding of pyelectasis *in utero* is a signal for other fetal anomalies and chromosomal aberrations. An early finding of multiple malformations or chromosomal abnormalities gives the parents the option of termination of the pregnancy. In cases of continuing the pregnancy, the knowledge of the presence of malformation in the fetus offers psychological advantages, provided that the parents receive proper counseling and support.[15] In cases of severe hydronephrosis, the antenatal follow-up might influence the obstetric management and the timing of delivery. Only in very few fetuses with urethral obstruction will intervention *in utero* improve the prognosis.

In the majority of cases, various degrees of unilateral pyelectasis are found *in utero*, which do not necessitate extensive antenatal workup. However, the knowledge of fetal urinary tract dilatation allows early postnatal investigation, diagnosis, and treatment. The therapy can be surgical or observational, with or without antibiotic prophylaxis.[45] It seems reasonable to anticipate that early treatment would lead to better preservation of kidney function and fewer complications such as urinary tract infections and stones. However, no scientific evidence is available to support such a statement. To our knowledge, no randomized trials have been made that evaluate the outcome of perinatal obstructive uropathies using different diagnostic and therapeutic approaches. Still, some indirect evidence exists of potential benefits of diagnosing urinary tract anomalies *in utero*. Before the ultrasound era, many cases of hydronephrosis in infants due to obstruction or reflux were not diagnosed until there was manifest urosepsis.[46] Nowadays, in centers with ongoing programs for routine antenatal ultrasound examination, this is very rarely observed. Helin (personal communication) analyzed the numbers of infants hospitalized in the first months of life because of acute pyelonephritis at the Department of Pediatrics in Lund, Sweden. He compared two periods of time, with and without third trimester routine obstetric ultrasound examinations and found that the number of infants hospitalized per year was twice as high when fewer antenatal diagnoses of fetal pyelectasis were made.

When estimating the benefits of antenatal detection of fetal pyelectasis, possible negative effects of false positive diagnoses must be considered. Many of the antenatal dilations of the urinary tract are not confirmed after birth, or they are not associated with any significant postnatal pathology (TABLE 1). In the Eurofetus study,[5] the percentage of false positive findings regarding urinary tract anomalies (defined as the cases with fetal pyelectasis not having significant urinary tract anomaly after birth) was as high as 17%. After an antenatal false positive diagnosis of urinary tract disease, the pregnant woman and her child are subjected to a number of investigations, which retrospectively might be considered unnecessary. Probably the insignificant antenatal ultrasound finding poses a psychological burden on the parents. Luckily, in most cases of isolated unilateral pyelectasis detected *in utero*, follow-up consists only of one antenatal and two postnatal ultrasound examinations. McNeil and Torstensson[15] demonstrated that the potential negative effects of false positive diagnoses can be limited by proper counseling. In their study, at follow-up interview 3–6 years after delivery, only one of 11 women with a false positive finding of fetal pyelectasis expressed some bitterness, and all 11 women valued positively ultrasound examinations in pregnancy. The current mental health of the women was fully comparable with that of control women with correct negative ultrasound findings.

CONCLUSIONS

Early prenatal ultrasound diagnosis of fetal lethal renal anomalies affords the parents the option of terminating the pregnancy. In most other cases of fetal renal anomalies, the prognosis and postnatal course are usually not influenced by the antenatal diagnosis. Bilateral fetal obstructive uropathy diagnosed *in utero* calls for detailed antenatal evaluation and repeated examinations for assessment of fetal renal function. The obstetric management might be directed by the antenatal findings. At present, the importance of fetal therapy in cases of bilateral hydronephrosis is not known, the main problem being the difficulty in selecting cases suitable for intervention. The antenatal finding of isolated unilateral fetal pyelectasis does not influence the obstetric management; however, it enables postnatal follow-up, early diagnosis, and initiation of conservative or surgical therapy. Postnatal antibiotic prophylaxis probably improves the prognosis for infants with congenital renal pyelectasis. False positive antenatal findings do not seem to be a major clinical problem, provided proper counseling of the parents is offered. There is a need for further investigation of congenital urinary tract anomalies in order to improve the understanding of underlying pathological processes and the prognostic value of antenatal ultrasound features. It is hoped that further research will lead to improved accuracy of postnatal diagnosis, better means of assessing postnatal renal function, and, consequently, to more rational antenatal and postnatal management protocols.

ACKNOWLEDGMENT

We thank Dr. Ingemar Helin for supplying us with information on his results of pediatric follow-up of fetuses with pyelectasis.

REFERENCES

1. GREEN, J. J. & J. C. HOBBINS. 1988. Abdominal ultrasound examination of the first trimester fetus. Am. J. Obstet. Gynecol. **159:** 165–175.
2. ROSATI, P. & L. GUARIGLIA. 1996. Transvaginal sonographic assessment of the fetal urinary tract in early pregnancy. Ultrasound Obstet. Gynecol. **7:** 95–100.
3. LEVI, S., Y. HYJAZI, J.-P. SCHAAPS, *et al.* 1991. Sensitivity and specificity of routine antenatal screening for congenital anomalies by ultrasound: The Belgian multicentric study. Ultrasound Obstet. Gynecol. **1:** 102–110.
4. CARRERA, J. M., M. TORRENTS, C. MORTERA, *et al.* 1995. Routine prenatal ultrasound screening for fetal abnormalities: 22 years' experience. Ultrasound Obstet. Gynecol. **5:** 174–179.
5. EUROFETUS STUDY REPORT. 1995. Cost-effectiveness of antenatal screening for fetal malformation by ultrasound. S. Levi, H. Grandjean & T. Lebrun, Eds. Vol. 1. European Union, Direction Generale XII. Brussels.
6. STOLL, C., B. DOTT, Y. ALEMBIK, *et al.* 1995. Evaluation of routine prenatal diagnosis by a registry of congenital anomalies. Prenatal Diagn. **15:** 791–800.
7. GRANNUM, P. 1990. The Genitourinary tract. *In* Diagnostic Ultrasound of Fetal Anomalies: Text and Atlas. D. A. Nyberg, B. S. Mahony & D. H. Pretorius, Eds.: 433–491. Mosby Year Book. St. Louis, MO.
8. POTTER, E. L. 1965. Bilateral absence of ureters and kidneys: Report of 50 cases. Obstet. Gynecol. **25:** 3–12.
9. DUBBINS, P. A., A. B. KURTZ, R. J. WAGNER, *et al.* 1981. Renal agenesis: Spectrum of in utero findings. J. Clin. Ultrasound **9:** 189–193.
10. LONGO, V. J. & G. J. THOMPSON. 1952. Congenital solitary kidney. J. Urol. **68:** 63–68.
11. ROMERO, R., M. CULLEN, P. JEARNTY, *et al.* 1984. The diagnosis of congenital renal anomalies with ultrasound. II. Infantile polycystic kidney disease. Am. J. Obstet. Gynecol. **150:** 259–262.
12. STUCK, K. J., S. A. KOFF & T. M. SILVER. 1982. Ultrasonic features of multicystic dysplastic kidney: Expanded diagnostic criteria. Radiology **143:** 217–221.
13. PRETORIUS, D. H., M. E. LEE, M. L. MANCO-JOHNSON, *et al.* 1987. Diagnosis of autosomal

dominant polycystic kidney disease in utero and in the young infant. J. Ultrasound Med. **6:** 249–255.

14. GIULIAN, B. B. 1984. Prenatal ultrasonographic diagnosis of fetal renal tumors. Radiology **152:** 69–70.

15. MCNEIL, T. F. & G. TORSTENSSON NIMBY. 1997. Psychological aspects of screening. *In* Textbook of Perinatal Medicine. A. Kurjak, Ed. The Parthenon Publishing Group. London. In press.

16. MANDELL, J., B. R. BLYTH, C A. PETERS, *et al.* 1991. Structural genitourinary defects detected in utero. Radiology **178:** 193–196.

17. HELIN, I. & P.-H. PERSSON. 1986. Prenatal diagnosis of urinary tract abnormalities by ultrasound. Pediatrics **78:** 879–883.

18. LIVERA, L. N., D. S. K. BROOKFIELD, J. A. EGGINTON, *et al.* 1989. Antenatal ultrasonography to detect fetal renal abnormalities: a prospective screening programme. Br. Med. J. **298:** 1421–1423.

19. GRIGNON, A., R. FILION, D. FILIATRAULT, *et al.* 1986. Urinary tract dilation in utero: Classification and clinical applications. Radiology **160:** 645–647.

20. JEANTY, P. & R. ROMERO. 1984. Obstetrical Ultrasound. McGraw-Hill. New York. p. 143.

21. KLEINER, B., P. W. CALLEN & R. A. FILLY. 1987. Sonographic analysis of the fetus with ureteropelvic junction obstruction. Am. J. Radiol. **148:** 359–363.

22. BENACERRAF, B. R., J. MANDELL, J. A. ESTROFF, *et al.* 1990. Fetal pyelectasis: A possible association with Down Syndrome. Obstet. Gynecol. **76:** 58–60.

23. MORIN, L., M. CENDRON, T. M. CROMBLEHOLME, *et al.* 1996. Minimal hydronephrosis in the fetus: Clinical significance and implications for management. J. Urol. **155:** 2047–2049.

24. ROMERO, R., G. PILU, P. JEANTY, A. GHIDINI & J. C. HOBBINS. 1988. Prenatal Diagnosis of Congenital Anomalies. Appleton & Lange. Norwalk, CT.

25. NYBERG, D. A., B. S. MAHONY & D. H. PRETORIUS. 1990. Diagnostic Ultrasound of Fetal Anomalies: Text and Atlas. Mosby Year Book. St. Louis, MO.

26. CALLEN, P. W., D. BOLDING, R. A. FILLY, *et al.* 1983. Ultrasonographic evaluation of fetal paranephric pseudocysts. J. Ultrasound Med. **2:** 309–312.

27. ROSENDAHL, H. 1990. Ultrasound screening for fetal urinary tract malformations. A prospective study in general population. Eur. J. Obstet. Gynecol. Reprod. Biol. **36:** 27–33.

28. REUSS, A., P. A. STEWART, J. W. WLADIMIROFF, *et al.* 1988. Non-invasive management of fetal obstructive uropathy. Lancet **2:** 949–951.

29. FERGUSON-SMITH, M. A. & J. R. W. YATES. 1984. Maternal age specific rates for chromosome aberrations and factors influencing them: Report of a collaborative European study on 52,965 amniocenteses. Prenatal Diagn. **4:** 5.

30. STEINHARDT, G., W. HOGAN, E. WOOD, *et al.* 1990. Long-term survival in an infant with urethral atresia. J. Urol. **143:** 336–337.

31. MANCO, L. H. & P. OSTERDAHL. 1984. The antenatal sonographic features of megacystis-microcolon-intestinal hypoperistalsis syndrome. J. Clin. Ultrasound **12:** 595–598.

32. HOLZGREVE, W. & M. EVANS. 1993. Nonvascular needle and shunt placements for fetal therapy. West. J. Med. **159:** 333–340.

33. MERRILL, D. C. & C. P. WEINER. 1997. Urinary tract obstruction. *In* Fetal Therapy. Invasive and Transplacental. N. M. Fisk & K. J. Moise, Jr., Eds.: 273–286. Cambridge University Press. Cambridge, UK.

34. NICOLINI, U., N. M. FISK, C. H. RODECK, *et al.* 1992. Fetal urine biochemistry: An index of renal maturation and dysfunction. Br. J. Obstet. Gynaecol. **99:** 46–50.

35. LIPITZ, S., G. RYAN, C. SAMUELL, *et al.* 1993. Fetal urine analysis for the assessment of renal function in obstructive uropathy. Am. J. Obstet. Gynecol. **168:** 174–179.

36. NICOLAIDES, K. H., H. H. CHENG, R. J. M. SNIJDERS, *et al.* 1992. Fetal urine biochemistry in the assessment of obstructive uropathy. Am. J. Obstet. Gynecol. **166:** 932–937.

37. MANDELBROT, L., Y. DUMEZ, F. MULLER, *et al.* 1991. Prenatal prediction of renal function in fetal obstructive uropathies. J. Perinat. Med. **19:** 283–297.

38. EUGÈNE, M., F. MULLER, M. DOMMERGUES, *et al.* 1994. Evaluation of postnatal renal function in fetuses with bilateral obstructive uropathies by proton nuclear magnetic resonance spectroscopy. Am. J. Obstet. Gynecol. **170:** 595–602.

39. MANNING, F. A., M. R. HARRISON & C. RODECK. 1986. Catheter shunts for fetal hydronephrosis and hydrocephalus. Report of the International Fetal Surgery Registry. N. Engl. J. Med. **315:** 336–340.
40. HARRISON, M. R., M. S. GOLBUS, R. A. FILLY, *et al.* 1982. Fetal surgery for congenital hydronephrosis. N. Engl. J. Med. **306:** 591–593.
41. QUINTERO, R. A., M. P. JOHNSON, R. ROMERO, *et al.* 1995. In utero percutaneous cystoscopy in the management of fetal lower obstructive uropathy. Lancet **346:** 537–540.
42. JOHNSON, M. P., T. P. BUKOWSKI, C. REITLEMAN, *et al.* 1994. In utero surgical treatment of fetal obstructive uropathy: A new comprehensive approach to identify appropriate candidates for vesicoamniotic shunt therapy. Am. J. Obstet. Gynecol. **170:** 1770–1779.
43. ESTES, J. M. & M. R. HARRISON. 1993. Fetal obstructive uropathy. Semin. Pediatr. Surg. **2:** 129–135.
44. LAING, F. C., V. D. BURKE, V. W. WING, *et al.* 1984. Postpartum evaluation of fetal hydronephrosis: Optimal timing for follow-up sonography. Radiology **152:** 423–424.
45. PETERS, C. A. 1995. Urinary tract obstruction in children. J. Urol. **154:** 1874–1884.
46. GINSBURG, C. M. & G. H. MCCRACKEN. 1982. Urinary tract infections in young infants. Pediatrics **69:** 409–412.
47. ARGER, P. H., B. G. COLEMAN, M. C. MINTZ, *et al.* 1985. Routine fetal genitourinary tract screening. Radiology **156:** 485–489.
48. PADUANO, L., L. GIGLIO, B. BEMBI, *et al.* 1991. Clinical outcome of fetal uropathy. I. Predictive value of prenatal echography positive for obstructive uropathy. J. Urol. **146:** 1094–1096.
49. SCOTT, J. E. S. & M. RENWICK. 1993. Urological anomalies in the northern region fetal abnormality survey. Arch. Dis. Child. **68:** 22–26.
50. ENGSTRÖM, E., S. BERG, H. LILJA, *et al.* 1995. Behöver barn med antenatalt vidgade urinvägar särskild uppföljning? Hygiea, Svenska Läkaresällskapets Handlingar **104:** 327.
51. WALSH, G. & P. A. DUBBINS. 1996. Antenatal renal pelvis dilatation: A predictor of vesicoureteral reflux? Am. J. Radiol. **167:** 897–900.
52. JOHNSON, C. E., J. S. ELDER, N. E. JUDGE, *et al.* 1992. The accuracy of antenatal ultrasonography in identifying renal abnormalities. Am. J. Dis. Child. **146:** 1181–1184.
53. GUNN, T. R., D. MORA & P. PEASE. 1995. Antenatal diagnosis of urinary tract abnormalities by ultrasonography after 28 weeks' gestation: Incidence and outcome. Am. J. Obstet. Gynecol. **172:** 479–486.

Surgical Treatment for Fetal Disease

The State of the Art

CRAIG T. ALBANESE[a] AND MICHAEL R. HARRISON

Fetal Treatment Center, Department of Surgery, University of California, San Francisco, 513 Parnassus Avenue, HSW-1601, San Francisco, California 94143-0570, USA

ABSTRACT: Sophisticated imaging and fetal sampling techniques have defined the natural history and pathophysiologic characteristics of many previously mysterious conditions of newborn. Although most prenatally diagnosed malformations are best managed by appropriate medical and surgical therapy after delivery, an increasing number of simple anatomic abnormalities with predictably devastating developmental consequences have been successfully corrected before birth. Many of the technical intricacies of open fetal surgery have been solved, but preterm labor remains an omnipresent risk to the mother and fetus. The recent development of minimally invasive techniques to treat the fetus prenatally has significantly lessened preterm labor. Minimally invasive surgical techniques, in combination with new tocolytic strategies, promise to extend the indications for fetal surgical intervention.

Over the past two decades, sophisticated ultrasonographic imaging and fetal sampling techniques have had a tremendous impact on the study of abnormal fetal development. Although most prenatally diagnosed malformations are best managed by appropriate medical and surgical therapy after planned delivery near term, an increasing number of simple anatomic abnormalities with predictably devastating developmental consequences have been successfully corrected before birth. In the 1980s, the pathophysiology of several potentially correctable fetal lesions was elucidated using a variety of animal models. Concomitantly, the natural history of these abnormalities was determined by serial observation of human fetuses, selection criteria for prenatal intervention were developed, and anesthetic, tocolytic, and surgical techniques for hysterotomy and fetal surgery were refined.[1-3] In the 1990s, this investment in basic and clinical research has benefited an increasing number of fetal patients.

FETAL SURGERY TECHNIQUES

There are numerous technical aspects of open and minimally invasive fetal surgery (FETENDO) that have evolved over 15 years of experimental and clinical work.[1-14] In the operating room, the mother is positioned to avoid inferior vena caval compression by the gravid uterus, and she and her baby are anesthetized with a halogenated agent. Maternal monitoring is accomplished with routine noninvasive monitors plus central venous and arterial catheters.

[a] Corresponding author. E-mail: craig@itsa.ucsf.edu

74

Open Fetal Procedures

The uterus is exposed through a low, transverse abdominal incision. Ultrasonography is used to localize the placenta and inject the fetus with a narcotic and a paralytic agent. Depending on the position of the placenta, the uterus is opened either anteriorly or posteriorly using absorbable staples that provide hemostasis and seal the membranes. Specially designed backbiting clamps, along with the staples, provide uterine hemostasis and aid in exposure of the pertinent fetal part. A miniaturized pulse oximeter records fetal pulse rate and oxygen saturation intraoperatively. Warm lactated Ringer's solution is continuously infused around the fetus. After fetal repair, a radiotelemeter is implanted in a submuscular pocket before closing the fetal incision. This provides postoperative monitoring of fetal heart rate, temperature, and amniotic pressure. The uterine incision is closed with two layers of absorbable sutures and fibrin glue. Amniotic fluid is restored with warm lactated Ringer's solution.

Minimally Invasive Fetal Procedures (Fetal Endoscopy or FETENDO)

Maternal positioning and monitoring, anesthesia, and maternal abdominal incision to expose the uterus are as described above. Intraoperative sonography maps the placental position and guides trocar placement. Up to five trocars have been used to perform FETENDO procedures. Continuous irrigation to optimize visibility is performed using a pump irrigation system via the sheath of the telescope. The fetus is monitored by transuterine ultrasonography. A miniaturized telemeter that can be placed into the amniotic cavity via a trocar site has been developed and is presently being tested. Each uterine puncture site is closed with one or two absorbable sutures and fibrin glue.

POSTOPERATIVE MANAGEMENT OF MOTHER AND FETUS

Postoperative management takes place in the Fetal Intensive Care Unit. Maternal arterial pressure, central venous pressure, urine output, and oxygen saturation are continuously monitored. Fetal well-being and uterine activity are recorded externally by a tocodynamometer and by a radiotelemeter implanted at surgery which continuously records the fetal ECG, temperature, and intra-amniotic pressure.[9] Patient-controlled analgesia and/or continuous epidural analgesics ease maternal stress and aid tocolysis. When labor is controlled and the fetus stable (usually several days), the patient is transferred to the obstetric ward where radiotelemetric monitoring continues until discharge (usually one week). Outpatient monitoring and tocolysis continue and fetal sonograms are performed at least weekly. Cesarean delivery is performed when membranes rupture or labor cannot be controlled, usually before 36 weeks' gestation.

PRETERM LABOR

Breeching the uterus, whether by puncture or incision, incites uterine contractions. In spite of technical advances, preterm labor is in the Achilles' heel of fetal therapy. The regimen of preoperative indomethacin, intraoperative deep halogenated inhalation anesthesia, and postoperative indomethacin, magnesium sulfate, and betamimetics, which was first perfected in sheep and monkeys,[4,5] has proven inadequate for extensive procedures in humans. Although halogenated inhalation agents provide satisfactory anesthesia for mother and fetus, the depth of anesthesia necessary to achieve intraoperative uterine relaxation can produce fetal and maternal myocardial depression and effect placental perfusion.[6] Indomethacin can constrict the fetal ductus arteriosus, and the combination of magnesium sulfate and betamimetics can produce maternal pulmonary edema. Fluid restriction to avoid this complication can compromise maternal-placental-fetal circulation and contribute to recalcitrant preterm labor. The search for a more effective and less toxic tocolytic regimen led to the demonstration in monkeys that exogenous nitric oxide ablates preterm labor induced by hysterotomy.[7] For the last two years, we have used intravenous nitroglycerin (a nitric oxide donor) intraoperatively and postoperatively. It is a potent tocolytic, but requires careful control to avoid serious complications.[8,9]

THE RISKS AND BENEFITS

For the fetus, the risk of the procedure is weighed against the benefit of correction of a lethal or debilitating defect. The risks and benefits for the mother are more difficult to assess. Maternal safety is paramount because most fetal malformations do not directly threaten the mother's health. However, she must bear significant risk and discomfort from the procedure and the tocolytic therapy. She may choose to accept the risk to aid her unborn fetus and to alleviate her own burden in raising a child with a severe malformation.

Since open fetal surgery has rarely been attempted elsewhere, the 75 cases performed at the University of California, San Francisco (UCSF) Fetal Treatment Center through June 1997 provide the best data on maternal outcome (TABLE 1). No maternal deaths and few postoperative maternal complications have occurred, but there has been considerable morbidity, primarily related to preterm labor and its treatment.[3,15] There were no infections. Eleven patients required blood transfusions. In our early experience, two patients developed amniotic fluid leaks through the hysterotomy site requiring repair, and five patients developed amniotic fluid leaks from the vagina. All patients experienced labor after hysterotomy, and treatment of preterm labor accounted for most of the morbidity. Eleven patients developed pulmonary edema while receiving high doses of tocolytic drugs. Although reversible, this complication emphasized the need for close monitoring in an intensive care setting.[8,9] Because the mid-gestation hysterotomy is not in the lower uterine segment, delivery after fetal surgery and all future deliveries should be by cesarean section. Early in our series, five uterine scar dehiscences occurred in subsequent pregnancies allowed to labor; uterine closure and neonatal outcome were excellent in all cases. Finally, the ability to carry and deliver subsequent pregnancies does not appear to be jeopardized by fetal surgery. Twenty-seven mothers have attempted pregnancy after fetal surgery; 25 conceived and delivered normal children. Two, both of whom had a strong preoperative history of infertility, failed to conceive.

FETAL PROBLEMS AMENABLE TO SURGICAL CORRECTION BEFORE BIRTH

The only anatomic malformations that warrant consideration are those that lethally interfere with fetal organ development and that, if alleviated, would allow normal development to proceed (TABLE 2). At present, only a small number of life-threatening malformations have been successfully corrected. A few others should be considered for treatment as their prenatal pathophysiology (natural history) is unraveled. As minimally invasive interventional techniques continue to be developed and proven safe, along

TABLE 1. Maternal Outcome with Open and Endoscopic Fetal Surgery[a]

Variable	Median	Range
Maternal age (year)	27	18–43
Gestational age of fetus (week)	26.0	17–28
Operative time, total (min)	135.4	69–365
Operative time, fetal repair (min)	32	5–92
Blood loss (mL)	455	150–2500
Interval to delivery (week)	4.5	1–15
Subsequent pregnancy history (n)		
Term cesarean delivery, healthy	27[b]	
Currently pregnant	2	
Not attempted, not desired, too early, etc.	30	

[a]Data from the University of California, San Francisco, Fetal Treatment Center, 75 cases through June 1994.
[b]Three women each had two subsequent pregnancies.
(Adapted from Harrison.[56])

with improvements in the treatment and/or prevention of preterm labor, prenatal treatment of select nonlethal anomalies may be considered.

Urinary Tract Obstruction

Fetal urethral obstruction produces pulmonary hypoplasia and renal dysplasia, and these often fatal consequences can be ameliorated by urinary tract decompression before birth.[16] The natural history of untreated fetal urinary tract obstruction is well documented, and selection criteria based on fetal urine electrolyte and B_2 microglobulin levels and the sonographic appearance of the fetal kidneys have proven reliable.[17,18] Of all fetuses with urinary tract dilation, as many as 90% do not require intervention. However, fetuses with bilateral hydronephrosis due to urethral obstruction who develop oligohydramnios require treatment. If the lungs are mature, the fetus can be delivered early for postnatal decompression. If the lungs are immature, the bladder can be decompressed *in utero* by a catheter shunt placed percutaneously under sonographic guidance,[19] by open fetal vesicostomy,[20] by fetoscopic vesicostomy,[21] or by placement of a wire mesh stent that may solve the technical problems historically encountered with shunts (malfunction, dislodgment, abdominal wall disruption).[22] Experience treating several hundred fetuses in many institutions suggests that selection is good enough to avoid inappropriate intervention, and that restoration of amniotic fluid can prevent the development of fatal pulmonary hypoplasia. It is not clear whether decompression can reverse renal functional damage.

Cystic Adenomatoid Malformation

Although congenital cystic adenomatoid malformation (CCAM) often presents as a benign pulmonary mass in infancy or childhood, some fetuses with large lesions die *in utero* or at birth from hydrops and pulmonary hypoplasia.[23] The pathophysiology of hydrops and the feasibility of resecting the fetal lung have been studied in animals.[24,25] Experience managing 111 cases suggests that most lesions can be successfully treated after birth, and that some lesions resolve or significantly regress before birth.[26] Al-

TABLE 2. Malformations Which May Benefit from Treatment before Birth

Defects	Effect on Development (Rationale for Treatment)	Result without Treatment	Recommended Treatment
Life-threatening			
Urinary obstruction (urethral valves)	Hydronephrosis Lung hypoplasia	Renal failure Pulmonary failure	Percutaneous catheter Fetoscopic vesicostomy Open vesicostomy Fetoscopic valve ablation
Cystic adenomatoid malformation	Lung hypoplasia/ hydrops	Fetal hydrops/demise	Open pulmonary lobectomy
Diaphragmatic hernia	Lung hypoplasia	Pulmonary failure	Open complete repair Bowel exteriorization Temporary tracheal occlusion
Sacrococcygeal teratoma	High output failure	Fetal hydrops/demise	Resect tumor Fetoscopic vascular occlusion[a]
Twin–twin transfusion syndrome	Vascular steal through placenta	Fetal hydrops/demise	Open fetectomy Fetoscopic laser division of placental vessels Fetoscopic umbilical cord ligation
Aqueductal stenosis	Hydrocephalus	Brain damage	Ventriculoamniotic shunt Open ventriculoperitoneal shunt[a]
Complete heart block	Low output failure	Fetal hydrops/demise	Percutaneous pacemaker Open pacemaker
Pulmonary/aortic obstruction	Ventricular hypertrophy	Heart failure	Percutaneous valvuloplasty Open valvuloplasty[a]
Tracheal atresia/ stenosis/obstruction by tumor	Overdistension by lung fluid	Hydrops/demise	Fetoscopic tracheostomy[a] Open tracheostomy[a] *Ex utero* intrapartum treatment
Nonlethal			
Myelomeningocele	Spinal cord damage	Paralysis, neurogenic bladder	Fetoscopic coverage[a] Open repair[a]
Clefting/lip and palate	Facial defect	Persistent deformity	Fetoscopic repair[a] Open repair[a]

[a]Not yet attempted in human fetuses.
(From Harrison.[56])

though only a few fetuses with very large lesions will develop hydrops before 26 weeks, almost all of these progress rapidly and die *in utero*. Careful sonographic surveillance of large lesions is necessary to detect the first signs of hydrops because fetuses that develop hydrops (less than 10% of all fetuses with CCAMs) can be successfully treated by emergency resection of the cystic lobe *in utero*. When hydrops is accompanied by placentomegaly and signs of maternal preeclampsia, it is too late for fetal intervention. Early in our experience, this clinical scenario was responsible for two postoperative fetal deaths. Fetal pulmonary lobectomy has proven to be surprisingly simple and quite successful. Twelve fetuses have undergone open surgical resection of the massively enlarged pulmonary lobe. Six of these had rapid resolution of hydrops, impressive *in utero* lung growth bilaterally, and normal postnatal growth and development with a follow-up of 52–84 months.[27,28] For lesions with single, large cysts, thoracoamniotic shunting has also been successful.[29]

Diaphragmatic Hernia

Congenital diaphragmatic hernia (CDH) is an anatomically simple defect that is correctable after birth by removing the herniated viscera from the chest and closing the diaphragm. Although less severely affected babies survive with modern postnatal surgical care including extracorporeal membrane oxygenation support (ECMO), the majority of babies die despite all intervention because their lungs are underdeveloped (hypoplastic) and associated pulmonary hypertension is present. Because retrospective estimates of mortality for congenital diaphragmatic hernia vary widely and are flawed by a "hidden mortality" of unknown magnitude, we prospectively studied 52 fetuses with potentially correctable, isolated diaphragmatic hernias diagnosed before 24 weeks. The mortality was 58% despite the best postnatal care including ECMO.[30] Babies who die *in utero* and soon after birth contribute to a substantial hidden mortality. Salvage of these severely affected babies remains an unsolved problem.

The pulmonary hypoplasia of diaphragmatic hernia is reversible after repair, but weeks or months are required. After birth, pulmonary support with ECMO is limited to one or two weeks and cannot save severely affected babies. We have shown experimentally that repair before birth, when the lungs can grow while the fetus remains on placental support, is physiologically sound and technically feasible.[31] Repair *in utero* has proven to be a formidable challenge, particularly when the left lobe of the liver is incarcerated in the chest, because reduction of the liver compromises umbilical blood flow.[32,33] Many technical problems associated with this difficult repair led to the development of the "congenital diaphragmatic hernia two-step," a carefully orchestrated approach that allows the reduction of viscera, reconstruction of the diaphragm, and enlargement of the abdomen to accept the returned viscera.[34] The efficacy, safety, and cost-effectiveness of *in utero* repair have been prospectively evaluated in a National Institutes of Health–sponsored trial. The results indicate that children in whom the liver is not incarcerated in the left hemithorax can be successfully treated by *in utero* repair.[35] However, *in utero* repair in this group has not led to an increased survival compared to matched controls who received standard postnatal therapy.

When an isolated fetal CDH is diagnosed prior to 24 weeks' gestation, the family has three choices: (1) terminate the pregnancy; (2) carry to term and deliver in a tertiary neonatal center for intensive care with an expected mortality of 58%, considerable morbidity, and an average cost of $161,000; or (3) attempt prenatal intervention. The family's dilemma in choosing management is particularly difficult because the natural history of fetal CDH is quite variable, because no direct biochemical or imaging parameters exist that reliably predict postnatal lung function. We have recently established a new sonographic prognostic measure of severity, the lung-to-head ratio (LHR).[36] It is determined by measuring right lung volume, corrected for gestational age by dividing by the head circumference; the greater the mediastinal shift, the greater the ipsilateral and contralateral lung compression, and the lower the LHR. An LHR < 1.0 is highly predictive of a poor postnatal outcome. It is known that fetuses who herniate late in gestation (> 25 weeks) will do well with modern postnatal surgical and neonatal care after delivery at a tertiary center. Conversely, fetuses with early herniation, severe mediastinal shift, low LHR, dilated intrathoracic stomach (gastric outlet obstruction produces polyhydramnios and gastric dilation), and herniated liver have a poor outlook. Fetuses with herniated liver have never been successfully repaired using the two-step technique *in utero* despite extensive efforts using a variety of techniques. Indeed, it took many years to recognize the significance of liver herniation and to be able to reliably predict it sonographically. For fetuses deemed unfixable by virtue of liver herniation, we have developed experimentally and now tested clinically a new approach to improving fetal lung development. We have shown in lamb fetuses that impeding the normal egress of fetal lung fluid by controlled tracheal obstruction enlarges the hypoplastic lungs and pushes the viscera back into the abdomen.[37-39] Initial experience with this new procedure, which we call PLUG (Plug the Lung Until It Grows) suggests that temporary occlusion of the fetal trachea accelerates fetal lung growth and ameliorates the often fatal pulmonary hypoplasia associated with severe CDH. We initially achieved clinical prenatal tracheal occlusion using open fetal surgical techniques. Presently, we have developed a fetoscopic approach, used in the last six patients, that has proven safe and efficacious and has resulted in less preterm labor and lower maternal morbidity.[13,14]

Sacrococcygeal Teratoma

Most neonates with sacrococcygeal teratoma (SCT) survive and malignant invasion is unusual. However, the outcome for SCT diagnosed prenatally (by sonogram or elevated alpha-fetoprotein) is less favorable. A subset of fetuses (less than 20%) with large tumors develop hydrops from high output failure secondary to high blood flow through the extremely vascular tumor. Because hydrops progresses very rapidly to fetal demise, frequent sonographic follow-up is mandatory. Excision of the tumor reverses this pathophysiology[40] and has been successful in two patients.[41,42] Attempts to interrupt the vascular steal by sonographically guided or fetoscopic techniques are being investigated.

Twin–Twin Transfusion Syndrome

In some twin pregnancies, abnormal chorionic blood vessels in the placenta connect the circulation of the two fetuses. These placental abnormalities are associated with perinatal mortality as high as 75% for twin–twin transfusion syndrome (anatomically normal twins) and for acardiac–acephalus twin syndrome. Serial amniocenteses of the polyhydramniotic sac have proven effective in stabilizing the pathophysiologic imbalance in many cases. Interrupting the abnormal placental vascular connections may improve outcome in severe cases. This has been accomplished by occluding the umbilical circulation percutaneously, by dividing the abnormal placental vessels endoscopically using a laser probe, and by removing the abnormal fetus by hysterotomy.[43,44] All of these techniques have proven successful in small series, and the optimal approach has not yet been determined.

Heart Block

Most fetuses with structurally normal hearts who develop complete heart block associated with maternal collagen-vascular disease will survive without intervention. A few with very slow rates (< 50 per minute) may develop hydrops and die *in utero*. If low output failure cannot be reversed by increasing the heart rate with beta agonists or by treatment with steroids, a pacemaker can be placed by open or percutaneous techniques. This has proven effective experimentally, but has only been attempted a few times.[45]

Aqueductal Stenosis

Obstruction to the flow of cerebrospinal fluid dilates the ventricles, compresses the developing brain, and eventually compromises neurologic function. For severe cases with progression *in utero,* decompressing the ventricles may ameliorate the adverse effects on the developing brain. However, percutaneously placed ventriculo-amniotic shunts have not improved outcome,[19] and a moratorium is being observed until the natural history is clarified, selection criteria developed, and better fetal shunting techniques developed.[46]

Pulmonary/Aortic Obstruction

A few simple structural cardiac defects which interfere with development may benefit from prenatal correction. For example, if obstruction to blood flow across the pulmonary or aortic valve interferes with development of the ventricles or the pulmonary or systemic vasculature, relief of the anatomic obstruction may allow normal development with improved outcome. Although this pathophysiology remains to be proven experimentally, stenotic fetal heart valves have been dilated by a balloon catheter placed percutaneously,[47] and several centers are developing experimental techniques to correct fetal heart defects.[48]

Tracheal Atresia/Stenosis

Fetuses with congenital high airway obstruction syndrome (CHAOS) have large echogenic lungs due to overdistention by lung fluid. Fetal tracheostomy may prevent development of fetal hydrops.[49]

At delivery, fetuses with an intrinsic or extrinsic obstruction can have the airway repaired and secured while the fetus remains on placental support before dividing the cord. We developed this *ex utero* intrapartum treatment (EXIT procedure) to deliver fetuses with CDH who had their trachea occluded, and have applied it successfully to fetuses with large neck tumors.[50]

Myelomeninogocele

The incidence of myelomeningocele is decreasing because it can be detected early in gestation by alpha-fetoprotein screening or sonography, and may be prevented by folate supplementation. Although it has been assumed that the spinal cord is intrinsically defective, recent studies suggest that neurologic impairment after birth may be due to exposure of the spinal cord *in utero.* We have shown in fetal lambs that exposure of the spinal cord causes neurologic damage that can be prevented or ameliorated by repairing the anatomic defect *in utero.*[51,52] Although we are developing techniques for repair experimentally, clinical application for this nonfatal defect is not yet justified. The natural history of myelomeningocele in human fetuses must first be elucidated, particularly the time in gestation when the lower-extremity neurologic damage occurs.

Cleft Lip and Palate

The observation that fetal wounds heal without scar formation has stimulated interest in the possibility of correcting cleft lip and palate *in utero* in order to avoid scarring, mid-facial growth restriction, and secondary nasal deformity. However, the theoretical benefits of repair are unproven and do not yet justify the risks of intervention for this nonlethal anomaly.[53]

THE PAST AND FUTURE OF FETAL INTERVENTION

Although only a few fetal defects are amenable to surgical treatment at present, the enterprise of fetal surgery has produced some unexpected "spin-offs" that have interest beyond this narrow therapeutic field. For pediatricians, neonatologists, sonologists, and dysmorphologists, the natural history and pathophysiology of many previously mysterious conditions in the newborn have been clarified by following the development of the disease *in utero*. For obstetricians, perinatologists, and fetologists, techniques developed in experimental work in lambs and monkeys will prove useful in caring for other high-risk pregnancies, for example, an absorbable stapling device developed for fetal surgery has been applied to cesarean sections;[11] radiotelemetric monitoring has applications outside fetal surgery;[12] and videoendoscopic techniques (FETENDO), which allow fetal manipulation without hysterotomy, will greatly extend the indications for fetal intervention.[13,14,43,54] Finally, the intensive effort to solve the vexing problem of preterm labor after hysterotomy for fetal surgery[6] has yielded new insight into the role of nitric oxide in myometrial contractions, and has spawned interest in treating spontaneous preterm labor with nitric oxide donors.[55] Fetal surgery research has yielded advances in fetal biology with implications beyond fetal therapy. The serendipitous observation that the fetus heals incisions without scar has provided new insights into the biology of wound healing and stimulated efforts to mimic the fetal process postnatally.

The great promise of fetal therapy is that for some diseases the earliest possible intervention (i.e., before birth) will produce the best possible outcome, that is, the best quality of life for the resources expended. However, the promise of cost-effective, preventive fetal therapy can be subverted by misguided clinical applications, for example, a complex *in utero* procedure that "half saves" an otherwise doomed fetus for a life of intensive (and expensive) care. Enthusiasm for fetal intervention must be tempered by reverence for the interests of the mother and her family, by careful study of the disease in experimental fetal animals and untreated human fetuses, and by a willingness to abandon therapy that does not prove effective and cost-effective in properly controlled trials.

ACKNOWLEDGMENTS

This therapeutic venture was made possible by the many heroic families who have gone beyond their own harrowing ordeal to support this enterprise, by our wonderful colleagues at the UCSF Fetal Treatment Center, Russell Jennings, Scott Adzick, Alan Flake, Lori Howell, Jody Farrell, Vilma Zarate, and a host of talented and enthusiastic research fellows, by the financial support of the National Institutes of Health, the March of Dimes, the G. Harold and Leila Y. Mathers Charitable Foundation, by the enlightened third-party payors who recognized their responsibility to pay for fetal treatment, by the UCSF Medical Center and the Fetal Treatment Center who donated their services to cover those patients whose insurance denied payment, and by American Airlines, United Airlines, and the March of Dimes/UCSF Kids 'n Moms House for covering travel and lodging expenses of these families in time of need.

REFERENCES

1. HARRISON, M.R., M.S. GOLBUS & R.A. FILLY, Eds. 1990. The Unborn Patient: Prenatal Diagnosis and Treatment, 2nd edit. W.B. Saunders Co. Philadelphia, PA.
2. HARRISON, M.R. & N.S. ADZICK. 1990. The fetus as a patient: Surgical considerations. Ann. Surg. **213:** 279–291.
3. HARRISON, M.R. 1993. Fetal surgery. West. J. Med. **159:** 341–349.
4. ADZICK, N.S. & M.R. HARRISON. 1994. Fetal surgical therapy. Lancet **343:** 897–902.
5. HARRISON, M.R., J. ANDERSON, M.A. ROSEN, N.A. ROSS & A.F. HENDRICKX. 1982. Fetal surgery in the primate. I. Anesthetic, surgical, and tocolytic management to maximize fetal-neonatal survival. J. Pediatr. Surg. **17:** 115–122.
6. SABIK, J.F., R.S. ASSAD & F.L. HANLEY. 1993. Halothane as an anesthetic for fetal surgery. J. Pediatr. Surg. **28:** 542–546.
7. JENNINGS, R.W., T.E. MACGILLIVRAY & M.R. HARRISON. 1993. Nitric oxide inhibits preterm labor in the rhesus monkey. J. Maternal-Fetal Med. **2:** 170–175.
8. BEALER, J.F., H.E. RICE, N.S. ADZICK & M.R. HARRISON. Acute non-cardiac pulmonary edema complicating nitroglycerin tocolysis following open fetal surgery. Obstet. Gynecol. Submitted.
9. HARRISON, M.R., K.J. VANDERWALL, J.F. BEALER, A.P. METKUS, N.S. ADZICK, M.A. ROSEN, I.K. AUER & M.A. HEYMANN. Nitroglycerin suppresses preterm labor after hysterotomy and fetal surgery. Am. J. Obstet. Gynecol. Submitted.
10. HARRISON, M.R. & N.S. ADZICK. 1993. Fetal surgical techniques. Semin. Pediatr. Surg. **2:** 136–142.
11. BOND, S.J., M.R. HARRISON, R.N. SLOTNICK, J. ANDERSON, A.W. FLAKE & N.S. ADZICK. 1989. Cesarean delivery and hysterotomy using an absorbable stapling device. Obstet. Gynecol. **74:** 25–28.
12. JENNINGS, R.W., N.S. ADZICK, M.T. LONGAKER & M.R. HARRISON. 1993. Radiotelemetric fetal monitoring during and after open fetal surgery. Surg. Obstet. Gynecol. **176:** 59–64.
13. VANDERWALL, K.J., S.W. BRUCH, M. MEULI, T. KOHL, Z. SZABO, N.S. ADZICK & M.R. HARRISON. 1996. Fetal endoscopic ('FETENDO') tracheal clip. J. Pediatr. Surg. **31:** 1101–1104.
14. HARRISON, M. R., G. B. MYCHALISKA, C. T. ALBANESE, et al. 1998. Correction of congenital diaphragmatic hernia in utero. IX: Fetuses with poor prognosis (liver herniation and low lung-to-head ratio) can be saved by fetoscopic temporary tracheal occlusion. J. Pediatr. Surg. In press.
15. LONGAKER, M.T., M.S. GOLBUS, R.A. FILLY, M.A. ROSEN, S.W. CHANG & M.R. HARRISON. 1991. Maternal outcome after open fetal surgery. JAMA **265:** 737–741.
16. ADZICK, N.S., M.R. HARRISON, A.W. FLAKE & P.L. GLICK. 1985. Fetal urinary tract obstruction: Experimental pathophysiology. Semin. Perinatol. **9:** 79–80.
17. NICOLAIDES, K.H., H.H. CHENG, R.J.M. SNIJDERS & C.F. MONIZ. 1992. Fetal urine biochemistry in the assessment of obstructive uropathy. Am. J. Obstet. Gynecol. **166:** 932–937.
18. JOHNSON, M.P., T.P. BUKOWSKI, C. REITLEMAN, N.B. ISADA, P.G. PRYDE & M.I. ERAUS. 1994. In utero surgical treatment of fetal obstructive uropathy: A new comprehensive approach to identify appropriate candidates for vesicoamniotic shunt therapy. Am. J. Obstet. Gynecol. **170:** 1770–1779.
19. MANNING, F.A., M.R. HARRISON, C.H. RODECK, et al. 1986. Special report. Catheter shunts for fetal hydronephrosis and hydrocephalus. N. Engl. J. Med. **315:** 336–340.
20. CROMBLEHOLME, T.M., M.R. HARRISON, J.C. LANGER, et al. 1988. Early experience with open fetal surgery for congenital hydronephrosis. J. Pediatr. Surg. **23:** 1114–1121.
21. MACMAHAN, R.A., P.M. RENOU, P.A. SHEKELTON & R.J. PATERSON. 1992. In utero cystotomy. Lancet **340:** 1234.
22. ESTES, J.M. & M.R. HARRISON. 1993. Fetal obstructive uropathy. Semin. Pediatr. Surg. **2:** 129–135.

23. ADZICK, N.S., M.R. HARRISON, P.L. GLICK, et al. 1985. Fetal cystic adenomatoid malformation: Prenatal diagnosis and natural history. J. Pediatr. Surg. **20:** 483–488.
24. RICE, H.E., J.M. ESTES, M.H. HEDRICK, J.F. BEALER, M.R. HARRISON &I N.S. ADZICK. 1994. Congenital cystic adenomatoid malformation: A sheep model of fetal hydrops. J. Pediatr. Surg. **29:** 692–696.
25. ADZICK, N.S., L.M. HU, P. DAVIES, A.W. FLAKE, L.M. REID & M.R. HARRISON. 1986. Compensatory lung growth after pneumonectomy in the fetus. Surg. Forum **37:** 648.
26. MACGILLIVRAY, T.E., M.R. HARRISON, R.B. GOLDSTEIN & N.S. ADZICK. 1993. Disappearing fetal lung lesions. J. Pediatr. Surg. **28:** 1321–1325.
27. HARRISON, M.R., N.S. ADZICK, R.W. JENNINGS, et al. 1990. Antenatal intervention for congenital cystic adenomatoid malformation. Lancet **336:** 965–967.
28. ADZICK, N.S., M.R. HARRISON, A.W. FLAKE, et al. 1993. Fetal surgery for cystic adenomatoid malformation of the lung. J. Pediatr. Surg. **28:** 806–812.
29. BLOTT, M., K.H. NICOLAIDES & A. GREENOUGH. 1988. Posntnatal respiratory function after chronic drainage of fetal pulmonary cyst. Am. J. Obstet. Gynecol. **159:** 858–859.
30. HARRISON, M.R., N.S. ADZICK, J.M. ESTES & L.J. HOWELL. 1994. A prospective study of the outcome of fetuses with congenital diaphragmatic hernia. JAMA **271:** 382–384.
31. HARRISON, M.R., N.A. ROSS & A.A. DELORIMIER. 1981. Correction of congenital diaphragmatic hernia in utero. III. Development of a successful surgical technique using abdominoplasty to avoid compromise of umbilical blood flow. J. Pediatr. Surg. **16:** 934–942.
32. HARRISON, M.R., J.C. LANGER, N.S. ADZICK. et al. 1990. Correction of congenital diaphragmatic hernia in utero. V. Initial clinical experience. J. Pediatr. Surg. **25:** 47–57.
33. HARRISON, M.R., N.S. ADZICK, A.W. FLAKE, et al. 1993. Correction of congenital diaphragmatic hernia in utero: VI. Hard-earned lessons. J. Pediatr. Surg. **28:** 1411–1418.
34. HARRISON, M.R., N.S. ADZICK, A.W. FLAKE & R.W. JENNINGS. 1993. The CDH two-step: A dance of necessity. J. Pediatr. Surg. **28:** 813–816.
35. HARRISON, M.R., N.S. ADZICK, K.M. BULLARD, J.A. FARRELL, L.J. HOWELL, M.A. ROSEN, A. SOLA, J.D. GOLDBERG & R.A. FILLY. 1997. Correction of congenital diaphragmatic hernia in utero. VII: A prospective trial. J. Pediatr. Surg. **32:** 1637–1642.
36. LIPSHUTZ, G.S., C.T. ALBANESE, V.A. FELDSTEIN, R.W. JENNINGS, H.T. HOUSELEY, R. BEECH, J.A. FARRELL & M.R. HARRISON. 1997. Lung-to head ratio predicts survival in prenatally diagnosed congenital diaphragmatic hernia. J. Pediatr. Surg. **32:** 1643–1646.
37. DIFIORE, J.W., D.O. FAUZA, D. SLAVIN, C.A. PETERS, J.C. FACKLER & J.M. WILSON. 1994. Experimental fetal tracheal ligation reverses the structural and physiologic effects of pulmonary hypoplasia in congenital diaphragmatic hernia. J. Pediatr. Surg. **29:** 248–257.
38. HEDRICK, M.H., J.M. ESTES, K.M. SULLIVAN, J.F. BEALER, J.A. KITTERMAN, A.W. FLAKE, N.S. ADZICK & M.R. HARRISON. 1994. Plug the lung until it grows (PLUG): A new method to treat congenital diaphragmatic hernia *in utero*. J. Pediatr. Surg. **29:** 612–617.
39. HARRISON, M.R., N.S. ADZICK, A.W. FLAKE, et al. 1996. Correction of congenital diaphragmatic hernia in utero. VIII: Response of the hypoplastic lung to tracheal. J. Pediatr. Surg. **31:** 1339–1348.
40. LANGER, J.C., M.R. HARRISON, K.G. SCHMIDT, et al. 1989. Fetal hydrops and death from sacrococcygeal teratoma: Rationale for fetal surgery. Am. J. Obstet. Gynecol. **160:** 1145–1150.
41. GRAF, J.L., R. BEECH, R.W. JENNINGS, C.T. ALBANESE & M.R. HARRISON. 1997. Successful fetal sacrococcygeal teratoma resection in a hydropic fetus. J. Pediatr. Surg. In press.
42. GRAF, J.L., H.T. HOUSELY, C.T. ALBANESE, N.S. ADZICK & M.R. HARRISON. 1997. A surprising histologic evolution of preterm sacrococcygeal teratomas. J. Pediatr. Surg. In press.
43. DE LIA, J.E., D.P. CRUIKSHANK & W.R. KEYE. 1990. Fetoscopic neodymium: YAG laser occlusion of placental vessels in severe twin-twin fusion syndrome. Obstet. Gynecol. **75:** 1046–1053.
44. FRIES, M.H., J.D. GOLDBERG & M.S. GOLBUS. 1992. Treatment of acardiac-acephalic twin gestations by hysterotomy and selective delivery. Obstet. Gynecol. **79:** 601–604.
45. ESTES, J.M., N.H. SILVERMAN, G.S. VAN HARE, et al. *In utero* placement of an epicardial pacemaker for the treatment of congenital heart block. Submitted.
46. HUDGINS, R.J., M.S.B. EDWARDS, R.B. GOLDSTEIN, et al. 1988. Natural history of fetal ventriculomegaly. Pediatrics **82:** 692.

47. ALLAN, L.D., D. MAXWELL & M. TYNAN. 1991. Progressive obstructive lesions of the heart—An opportunity for fetal therapy. Fetal Ther. **6:** 173–177.
48. HANLEY, F.L. 1994. Fetal cardiac surgery. Adv. Cardiac Surg. **5:** 47–74.
49. MARTINEZ-FERRO, M., M.H. HEDRICK, A.W. FLAKE, M.R. HARRISON & N.S. ADZICK. 1994. Prenatal diagnosis of congenital high airway obstruction (CHAOS): Potential for perinatal intervention. J. Pediatr. Surg. **29:** 271–274.
50. MYCHALISKA, G.B., J.F. BEALER, J.L. GRAF, M.A. ROSEN, N.S. ADZICK & M.R. HARRISON. 1997. Operating on placental support: The ex utero intrapartum treatment procedure J. Pediatr. Surg. **32:** 227–231.
51. MEULI, M., C. MEULI-SIMMEN, C.D. YINGLING, K.B. HOFFMAN, M.R. HARRISON & N.S. ADZICK. 1995. A new model of myelomeningocele: Studies in the fetal lamb. J. Pediatr. Surg. **30:** 1034–1037.
52. MEULI, M., C. MEULI-SIMMEN, G.M. HUTCHINS, C.D. YINGLING, K.M. HOFFMAN, M.R. HARRISON & N.S. ADZICK. 1995. *In utero* surgery rescues neurologic function at birth in sheep with spina bifida. Nature Med. **1:** 342–347.
53. LONGAKER, M.T., D.J. WHITBY, N.S. ADZICK, L.B. KABAN & M.R. HARRISON. 1991. Fetal surgery for cleft lip: A plea for caution. Plast. Reconstr. Surg. **88:** 1087–1092.
54. ESTES, J.M., T.F. MACGILLIVRAY, M.H. HEDRICK, N.S. ADZICK & M.R. HARRISON. 1992. Fetoscopic surgery for the treatment of congenital anomalies. J. Pediatr. Surg. **27:** 950–954.
55. LEES, C., S. CAMPBELL, E. JAUNIAUX, *et al.* 1994. Arrest of preterm labor and prolongation of gestation with glyceryl trinitrate, a nitric oxide donor. Lancet **343:** 1325–1326.
56. HARRISON, M.R. 1996. Fetal surgery. Am. J. Obstet. Gynecol. **174:** 1255–1264.

Routine Ultrasound Screening of Congenital Anomalies

An Overview of the European Experience

SALVATOR LEVI

Ultrasound Laboratory, Department of Obstetrics and Gynecology, Centre Hospitalier Universitaire Brugmann, and Université Libre de Bruxelles, Place A. Van Gehuchten 4, B1020 Brussels, Belgium

ABSTRACT: Results from ultrasound in low-risk pregnant women are significant when routine screening is performed on a large population because the anomalies are rare. Professionals expect from routine ultrasound objective information that cannot usually be obtained by clinical procedures. Parents seek reassurance about the absence of fetal congenital anomalies and overall fetal health. Therefore, Europeans view routine ultrasound as a part of obstetrical care, capable of filling important gaps by delivering much key information for improving obstetrical practice. Fetal anomalies screening (FAS) requires higher education and qualifications than obstetrical ultrasound. The health insurance systems support ultrasound screening and allow its spread in most European countries; approximately 98% of pregnant women are examined by ultrasound and, frequently, two to three times (usually once per trimester). Detection rate of congenital anomalies is about 28% in geographical areas (private practice and hospitals), 60 to 80% in Ob/Gyn's ultrasound labs. Routine ultrasound screening policy has not proved to result in an immoderate use of ultrasound; on the contrary, chaotic use of routine ultrasound can lead to an unproductive and excessive number of scans. New trends in FAS, such as the early detection of fetal defects and chromosomal anomalies, bring more arguments for routine screening. Effectiveness should increase by enhancing education and training and the systematic referral for FAS to accredited laboratories.

BRIEF HISTORICAL COMMENT: FROM PRIMARY SCANS TO FETAL SCREENING

The diagnostic capability of ultrasound was first reported by Dussik, in Vienna in 1942,[1] and was brought into its present application in 1953 by Wild, a British surgeon operating in Minneapolis, Minnesota. Ultrasound for use in obstetrics and gynecology was developed in Glasgow by Donald and Brown and introduced in 1958 in a historical paper published in The Lancet.[2]

The first fetal anomaly displayed by ultrasound was reported shortly thereafter in 1961 by Donald—who reported on the majority of ob/gyn ultrasound cases— describing a case of fetal hydrocephaly;[3] acrania was subsequently shown by Sunden in Sweden in 1964,[4] and Campbell, in the United Kingdom, published reports on anencephaly in 1972[5] and spina bifida in 1975.[6] The first kidney anomaly was described by Garrett in Australia in 1970.[7]

The screening of low-risk pregnancies for common obstetrical conditions, e.g., fetal age, number, growth and so forth, together with placental localization and amniotic fluid, was initiated in several laboratories, including ours in Brussels, from 1972 onward. The widely accepted use of ultrasound in obstetrics occurred in the late 1970s.

We acknowledge Grennert *et al.* for the publication of their screening experience of a general population in Sweden in 1978;[8] the authors pointed out the benefits of ultrasound screening for the management of pregnancy and fetal outcome, as well as accurate pregnancy dating and early twin detection. Several reports on obstetrical ultrasound screening in low-risk populations were published afterward; randomized series—mainly issued from Scandinavia—usually showed benefits, although not consistently significant because of the low frequency of the anomalies and the small size of the samples.[9-13]

The accuracy of ultrasound for screening fetal malformations in high-risk populations was evaluated during the early 1980s in Europe by Kurjak *et al.,*[14] Campbell and Pearce,[15] Gembruch and Hansmann,[16] and, in the United States, by Sabbagha *et al.* in 1985.[17] Screening for congenital anomalies in a large series was realized from the late 1970s by Campbell and Pearce[15] and then in Sweden and the United States.[18-20] Systematic routine ultrasound for identification of congenital anomalies were performed in strictly low-risk pregnancies during 1984 to 1985,[21] and then in larger populations.[22-35]

WHAT DO PROFESSIONALS AND PARENTS EXPECT FROM ROUTINE ULTRASOUND?

Professionals

Professionals primarily expect routine ultrasound to complement the clinical examination of the pregnant woman with objective information that cannot usually be obtained by clinical means or by inoffensive techniques. Ultrasound screening is a quick, harmless, painless procedure, which can be completed in a doctor's office or in maternity care units, and offers varied information as well as precise numerical values; among them are the determination of gestational age, fetal and placental position, the estimation of fetal size and growth, and of amniotic fluid volume; the detection of fetal congenital defects and of maternal uterine anomalies. The sum of these items completes the patient history, physical examination and assessment of blood analyses, all necessary for pregnancy management. Ultrasound can be repeated for monitoring these essential conditions. Furthermore, the parents like the examination. Ultrasound screening not only reassures the parents, but also the professionals in charge of the pregnant woman because clinical examination can only recognize a small proportion among the possible anomalies, and even a smaller fraction in due time: for example, from fetal growth restriction to congenital defects, from oligohydramnios to placenta previa. For appropriate care of their patients, professionals anticipate possible delayed clinical signs. Early signs of pregnancy disturbances lead to counseling, managing therapy, or termination of the pregnancy.

Parents

The parents, and particularly the mother, usually have an ambiguous feeling about the desired pregnancy: an amalgam of happiness and fear. They are happy to anticipate the arrival of their baby, yet fear any kind of anomaly that can alter their happiness. Fear is usually induced either by their personal experience of disturbed pregnancies, or by any information dispatched by the media or family and friends, i.e., by any person anxious to share their particular and subjective know-how about pregnancy. Therefore, they thirst for reassurance about the absence of fetal congenital anomalies, of any physical and mental fetal health disturbance. The parents expect to be informed about their baby's health and about possible anomalies; when anomalies are present, they want to know the prognosis, possible treatment, and recovery. They require the right to decide from among the possible options when the time for decision arrives.

Ultrasound screening is a means to start answering many of the questions arising from fears or due to an established disturbed pregnancy.

EUROPEANS CLAIM ROUTINE ULTRASOUND IS A PART OF OBSTETRICAL CARE

The use of obstetrical ultrasound in Europe and in the United States is somewhat different. Whereas the Europeans have chosen promptly to scan pregnant women on a routine basis, very quickly reaching high compliance rates, in the USA there is still debate about routine versus indicated ultrasound. We should lessen this apparent difference by emphasizing that the positive indications apply to a large majority of pregnant women, who have the ultrasound later than those scanned as soon they are known to be pregnant if routine screening policies are in use.

Up until now, the difficulty showing significant differences and settling the methodology quarrel can be explained by the lack of clear statistics; this gives rise to a dose of subjectivity about the benefits of routine ultrasound during pregnancy. The paucity of definite figures is not due to a conjectural weak detection power of ultrasound when screening pregnancies; it is because of the difficulty comparing pregnant women having and those not having had competent ultrasound performed at the fundamental stages of pregnancy. Indeed, the use of ultrasound started so abruptly, lacking a sufficient time period before a correct evaluation could be done. Had this evaluation been done in the early 1970s, before ultrasound's take-off, the result might have been inconclusive. Indeed, imaging capabilities are still improving dramatically, year after year, being significantly at higher levels since the introduction of gray-scaling and real-time; we also should take into account the expanding experience of a growing number of ob/gyn sonologists, the disciples of Donald and of their own disciples.

The insufficiency of positive figures is also due to difficulties linked to statistical rules, involving the individual low prevalence of many factors that occasionally disturb the course of a pregnancy. A large number of pregnant women has to be studied to harvest statistically significant figures about outcome, in screened and unscreened groups. Furthermore, outcome depends on how procedures involved in reacting to positive ultrasound screening and diagnosis are used to modify subsequently the outcome.

Obstetricians/gynecologists were among the first in the medical profession to recognize ultrasound as an unique tool. Health insurance systems have accepted its routine use in obstetrics—and indeed energized it—so that routine obstetrical ultrasound is offered to and paid for all pregnant patients. Several consensus conferences took place in Europe,[36] all emphasizing the likely favorable role of ultrasound screening: for example, in Germany,[37] Great Britain,[38] and France.[39]

In contrast, the National Institutes of Health in the United States acknowledged the prominent role of ultrasound, but only when indicated, and refused the principle of screening.[40]

OBSTETRICAL ULTRASOUND SCREENING

Obstetrical ultrasound was promptly considered as *the* technique formerly lacking in the routine practice that was capable of filling important gaps by delivering key information and completely updating obstetrical practices. Several studies in Europe, including randomized series, were intended to proceed from case reports—hence somewhat restricted demonstrations—to figures issued from series, constituting an objective presentation of evidence of the advantage of ultrasound for the management of pregnancies.

FETAL ANOMALIES SCREENING

Although obstetrical ultrasound is easy to perform with minimal training and average good-quality equipment, ultrasound for fetal anomalies screening (FAS) requires education and expertise. Steps following the screening and detection are the diagnosis and prognosis which require more education and expertise in congenital anomalies, supported by high-quality equipment and links with experts in other related fields such as genetics and surgery.

The specialty of obstetrics/gynecology has become increasingly complex, including the practice of ultrasound. No one can be an expert in everything; therefore specialization is necessary, within an adequately organized health system. Each participant should perform the tasks he/she is qualified for; each individual should be qualified in areas where he/she has commitments. Ultrasound practice and education in Europe are described in the last section of this paper. Screening pregnancies by ultrasound includes examinations at the first level, which should include an overview on fetal anatomy, in addition to the standard examination. Doctors who avoid the difficult and time-consuming screening for fetal malformations, scanning only for the basic information usually collected, should systematically refer their patients for anatomical examination aimed at detecting congenital anomalies. At the second level—more typical of hospital ultrasound expertise—the basic screening is completed with one or more FAS sessions.

ROLE OF HEALTH INSURANCE SYSTEMS IN THE USE OF ULTRASOUND SCREENING

Screening is supported by health insurance systems in most European countries; almost all pregnant women (approximately 98%) have ultrasound, and thus one of the conditions for effective screening is met. The number of allotted sessions is commonly two or three for each uncomplicated pregnancy (e.g., usually one per trimester). When ultrasound is indicated for a specific reason that was not routine, such as evaluation of gestational age and detection of multiple pregnancies, one or more extra ultrasound sessions can be approved. Ultrasound indicated for any condition carrying a high-risk of congenital anomaly can replace or be added to the routine scans. Other conditions, such as fetal growth restriction, can be monitored by ultrasound and require several additional ultrasound sessions.

PATIENTS' DEMAND AND WILLINGNESS TO PAY

Despite financial coverage of obstetrical ultrasound by health insurance systems, some patients ask for more ultrasound, with such requests usually based on a particular anxiety. These costs are normally charged to the patient. Charges for obstetrical ultrasound are, as a rule, lower in Europe than in the United States. The patients may find ultrasound screening of special value and are ready to pay for it.[41]

EFFICIENCY OF FETAL ANOMALIES SCREENING IN EUROPEAN PRACTICE

The routine application of FAS in the 15 countries of the European Union, as well as others including those of the former Soviet Union, is not uniform. Obstetrical ultrasound and FAS are done almost everywhere in the European Union, in private offices and in hospital ultrasound laboratories, unless particular regulations assign FAS to accredited laboratories. Results of FAS can thus vary considerably, depending on the place where it is performed. Professionals in private offices are generally less experienced in ultrasound than those in hospital labs. Hospital labs usually include experienced ob/gyn sonologists who oversee trainees, residents, consultants, and sonographers (usually trained midwives). Their average experience in ultrasound and fetal anomalies is good, although significant variations are found because of different levels of experience.

Experienced consultants and senior personnel have particular tasks: ascertaining the detected anomalies and formulating the final diagnosis, both for hospital patients and for referred patients, who were previously screened elsewhere. Although dissimilarities exist among the states in the European Union, the differences do not exceed an acceptable level and should not alter the overall impression about the efficiency of FAS as it is generally practiced. In addition to papers published in journals, two main databases can be used for evaluation of FAS in Europe: the Eurocat and the Eurofetus databases.

- Eurocat is a register that records congenital anomalies in 30 geographical areas from 15 countries, most from the European Union, for the epidemiological surveillance of births with defects. The program, started in 1979, gathers data from approximately 300,000 births and 5,000 congenital anomalies per year.[42]
- Eurofetus is a database obtained from information collected prospectively from ultrasound laboratories practicing routine obstetrical ultrasound and FAS; the ultrasound units involved are located in ob/gyn departments from 60 hospitals in 14 countries. About 4,600 congenital anomalies were recorded.[30] Because large numbers are necessary for statistical analysis and because the prevalence is only 2–3% of births, this kind of study may yield significant information. The study includes 30 kinds of congenital anomalies, or classes of anomalies, which correspond to the most frequently recorded defects.

Published papers have dealt with screening in hospitals and, as far as we know, figures about ultrasound in private offices as a single entity have never been reported. However, there are papers where the results from private and hospital practice are mixed, with the population selection based on a relatively large geographical area, a province for instance. By examining papers about screening in ultrasound labs, one can deduce some information about screening in private practice. Let us take the example of a regional ultrasound screening—ultrasound labs and private office ultrasound practice—that pertains to a single region covered by the Eurocat database. Private practice includes almost all obstetrical ultrasound, thus not necessarily FAS as a systematic procedure. Outcome was checked during a 5-year period, from 1991 to 1995; it included all pregnant women who were a part of a population of 743,742 (versus 9,890,000 for the entire corresponding country), and who delivered in the area ($n = 41,074$ within the five years). The study was retrospective and no particular program for screening was followed; it can thus be considered as a view of ultrasound practice in the region concerned.[43] The number of malformed fetuses during the entire period was 1,172, that is, a prevalence[a] of 2.8%, representing severe, major, and minor[b] malformations, with the exception of chromosomal anomalies.

The ultrasound detection rate was 23.3% of all congenital anomalies, including patients who did not have ultrasound (presumably less than 10%). The overall sensitivity seems low, but was especially concerned with the detection of fatal congenital anomalies,[b] since 46% of detected cases had termination of pregnancy (TOP); the relative high number of TOP represents only 11% of the total of congenital anomalies. During this period, 12 fetuses that had anencephaly were detected and the pregnancies terminated (100%); of 26 fetuses with spina bifida, only 13 were detected, 7 pregnancies terminated, and 16 born alive; 12 of 19 congenital diaphragmatic anomalies were detected and 7 pregnancies terminated. Among the congenital heart defects (CHD), 10% only were detected, yet we should emphasize that the CHD account for 34% of the total number of reported anomalies, including a great proportion of benign defects. The total number of chromosomal anomalies in this group was 122, and 72 were Down syndrome. Thirty-two chromosomal anomalies were detected by ultrasound. Taking into account the proportion of low-risk pregnancies scanned, primarily by hospital ultrasound labs, and the sensitivity reached, the detection rate from ultrasound in private offices should not exceed 10%.

Ultrasound screening in hospitals has been evaluated in several papers; however, only a selection of them is reported here. The selection was made with respect to the strict low-risk characteristics of the screened population (i.e., patients not submitted to any selection, and with no specific indication for ultrasound, showing a standard prevalence and distribution of congenital anomalies, which correspond to similar findings in geographical-area populations).[42,43,30] Together, they accumulated 53,869 pregnant women at low-risk with 1,196 congenital anomalies (2.0%); 552 were detected (46.1%).[25-28,31]

EUROFETUS

Eurofetus results might appear less impressive than those of some European ultrasound units, but not when the same basic figures—linked to methodology—are encountered. The average sensitivity is 61.4% for major and minor anomalies; sensitivity is 73.7% for a large group of "major" congenital anomalies only, corresponding to

---

[a] The above-mentioned prevalence is supposed to be the closest figure of the average congenital anomalies in a common population of pregnant women in Europe. That prevalence found in a large and not-selected population sample from a geographical area cannot be suspected to include exceedingly high proportions of congenital anomalies or of high-risk patients. However, they could be underestimated, because of some anomalies systematically discarded for the registration and because of inadequate inspection of newborn infants.

The variety of published prevalence rates in studies on ultrasound screening and their influence in altering figures have been discussed elsewhere (Levi[67]).

[b] Major and minor anomalies are terms habitually used yet lacking any explicit definition. More precise terminology should be "lethal anomalies"; "noncurable anomalies"; "serious" meaning curable severe anomalies frequently necessitating repeated operations; "mild" and "minor" anomalies, corresponding to less severe and to minor operations. The suggested terminology should better define the broad scope of the gravity of encountered congenital anomalies. It could possibly be simplified by using "fatal" anomalies for the two first categories, "serious," "mild," and "minor" for those necessitating heavy to light surgical procedures, and "not significant" for those not requiring significant therapeutic measures. If the standard denomination remains, "major" should apply to all classes except the "not significant" one.

37.5% of the 4,615 recorded congenital anomalies.[31] Galvanized by the figures obtained by highly successful teams participating in the collaborative study, the weaker performing units should rapidly approach the average sensitivity and should then increase and reach approximately 75%.

In fact, it has been shown that significant improvements occur with time. Therefore, expectations in ultrasound screening can be great. Indeed, sensitivity of routine ultrasound screening, operated by the same groups, significantly increases at successive intervals, as shown by these examples: sensitivity has augmented between the years:

- 1986 and 1990, from 25 to 71% (single lab result)[44]
- 1980–1984 and 1990–1991, from 85 to 96% (about 14,000 cases of mixed high- and low-risk pregnancies)[45]
- 1984–1989 and 1990–1992, from 40 to 51% (about 25,500 patients at low-risk pregnancies); the most spectacular improvement was a twofold increase before 23 weeks of the detection rate of CHD, central nervous system, and urinary tract[31]
- 1991 and 1995, from 20 to 29%[43]
- 1980 and 1992, a 31% average increase, in the same geographical areas; sensitivity was recorded for six specific anomalies from 8,800 abnormal fetuses. The sensitivity range increased from 37–57% to 65–82% depending upon the anomaly.[42]

The policy in the United States[40] that recommends an ultrasound scan only when indicated has created a problem in terms of routine screening. However, serious concerns have been raised about the ability of the indication-based obstetrical ultrasound to detect fetal anomaly early enough for therapeutic options;[46] yet only one prospective study (RADIUS) was made in an attempt to answer the question as to the adequacy of routine versus indicated obstetrical ultrasound for FAS.[47] The study is special in having included a control group, a situation that is now almost impossible in Europe, because ultrasound is so popular that pregnant women would not accept, for the most part, being in a control group. The American study was comparable in some ways to the quoted European studies, for example, by its large population of low-risk pregnancies certified by strict selection and a congenital anomaly prevalence of 2.3%. In addition, the method was similar to the European multicentric and hospital-based studies in that it entrusted the scans to ultrasound laboratories and ultrasound professionals. The American study was different from the European geographical area-based studies where a great proportion of examinations was done by non-ultrasound professionals.

The RADIUS study clearly demonstrates that screening, although not of high performance (35% before birth, 17% before 24 weeks) detects many more congenital anomalies than indicated ultrasound, and that the clinical judgment of the physician is not effective in detecting congenital anomalies because, in the control group, only 11% were detected prenatally and 5% before 24 weeks. The RADIUS study also has brought arguments for having FAS done where experienced sonologists and sonographers do the scanning, since sensitivity is tripled in more experienced labs compared to the others.

A retrospective study of FAS, also done in the United States, similarly reinforced, in our view, arguments in favor of routine FAS.[48] The study included 6,616 fetuses; among the fetuses with congenital anomalies, 287 had prenatal ultrasound examination and 96 had not. The high prevalence of CA (5.8%) is in accordance with the high number of abnormal pregnancies delivered in this tertiary perinatal facility. FAS was not done in low-risk pregnancies. Among the patients at high-risk and examined by ultrasound, the sensitivity for congenital anomalies was similar (53%) to that by routine FAS in low-risk pregnancies elsewhere.[30,31] The tertiary ultrasonography done on patients with a fetus with CA was done because of definite evidence of possible congenital anomalies: 31% had a prior abnormal ultrasound and 15% had a history of high risk for CA, including elevated maternal serum alpha fetoprotein. Finally, in this population of scanned and unscanned pregnant women, the overall sensitivity was 40%, to be compared to nearly 96% when doing systematic FAS in similar conditions, i.e., mixed low-risk and high-risk pregnancies.[45]

An additional example concerning routine versus indicated ultrasound can be found in Eurocat registers[42] in which prenatal diagnosis is mentioned for some congenital anomalies. Ultrasound screening—but not necessarily including FAS—is performed in the great majority of, but not all, participating areas. Among 673 fetuses with bilateral renal agenesis, nearly 60% were detected when routine ultrasound was done (FAS+), and 4% when FAS was not completed (FAS–). Among 2,116 fetuses with spina bifida, nearly 50% were detected in FAS+ areas, versus 2% (FAS–). Among 1,268 fetuses with hydrocephaly, nearly 60% were detected in FAS+ areas versus 2% (FAS–). Among 966 fetuses with cystic kidney disease, nearly 70% were detected in FAS+ areas versus 3% (FAS–). Among 727 fetuses with omphalocele, nearly 60% were detected in FAS+ areas versus 2% (FAS–); this latter example, related to its significant association with chromosomal abnormality, emphasizes the importance of the detected congenital anomaly as an indication for karyotyping, allowing diagnoses of unsuspected chromosomal anomaly.

Routine ultrasound screening policy does not lead to an immoderate use of ultrasound; indeed, the average number of scans was 2.1 in the screened group versus 1.8 in the control group.[12] On the contrary, more random use of routine ultrasound can lead to an excess, which is not necessarily beneficial to the patient's health and is probably of low cost-efficiency. An illustration of nonroutine use of screening that can lead to an excessive numbers of scans per patient was found in two different geographical area populations: one included nearly 50% of the pregnant women having had four to nine ultrasounds[49] with a poor detection result; the other had 40% of pregnant women with four to six and more ultrasounds during their pregnancy.[50]

NEW TRENDS IN FETAL ANOMALIES SCREENING

Early Detection of Fetal Defects

Until recently, the first trimester screening was aimed at checking the validity of menstrual gestation age, the fetal localization, and possible gemellity. The new trend in fetal anomaly screening includes the first trimester scan (11–14 weeks) for a full fetal anatomy check. This first scan, using vaginal and abdominal routes, allows an especially good and quick anatomical visualization. It leads to an earlier detection of many severe anomalies, early diagnoses, and therapeutic options. Unless positive for anomaly, it has anyway to be completed about eight weeks later because the first trimester screening does not completely replace the standard midtrimester scan for structural anomalies; the later scan is required in order to catch anomalies missed at prior examination.

Chromosomal Anomalies

The first trimester ultrasound, in addition to the above-mentioned considerations, allows the search of morphological details that enlarge the FAS area to chromosomal anomalies.[51] The finding of chromosomal abnormality shows the usefulness and efficiency of ultrasound screening. Identification of cases at risk of chromosomal anomalies, and particularly trisomy 21, seems more accurate with ultrasound screening than with hormones presently used for screening. Two aspects of the policies, already accepted in Europe, that include two and three routine scans for each pregnancy, address the issues of the efficiency of screening:

- The systematization of ultrasound screening authorizes the examination of a broad range of maternal ages, corresponding to diversified risks of having a chromosomal anomaly—which is not the original primary goal of ultrasound screening—yet this is becoming one of the most important goals.
- The distribution of the ultrasound sessions allows the detection of the signs corresponding to chromosomal anomaly at the time they are visible, because they frequently disappear during the period established for screening for structural anomalies.[52]

Systematic Referral for Low-Risk Screening

An ultrasound finding of fetal congenital anomalies in low-risk pregnancies cannot be considered as an easy task because it requires skill, training, and experience in screening for a catalogue of anomalies as discussed above.

The consequences of detection of a congenital anomaly are important. Major *and* minor anomalies are to be searched for; both carry significant issues, such as catching chromosomal abnormalities and associated multiple anomalies to form an aggravated prognosis. This evidence should be used to apply the best possible method for screening. Experience and published figures show clearly that in Europe—taking into account cost and availability for systematic examination of patients—the hospital ultrasound labs can and should fulfill this mission reliably and with efficiency (compared to overall sensitivity and costs in geographical area-based population screening).[53] Such a policy should also allow for scan performances at the most favorable periods for FAS, e.g., end of first trimester and mid-second trimester of pregnancy. Considering the findings of the King's College group[51,54-56] and taking into account abnormal nuchal lucency, fetal heart rate and maternal age, first trimester screening—operated by well-trained personnel—should significantly improve the detection of Down syndrome to a 80% detection rate. Eurocat data[42] have recorded 1,827 fetuses with trisomy 21 during the 1980–1992 period, among 2,080,000 pregnant women aged less than 35 years; using the above-mentioned detection rate, 1,462 of 1,827 chromosomal anomalies should thus be detected, with less than 5% false positives, i.e., less than 104,000 irrelevant punctures in the population concerned. On the other hand, the systematic karyotyping in the 232,000 pregnant women, aged 35 and more, will diagnose 1,472 cases of Down syndrome (100%), at the cost of 232,000 punctures for the population concerned, i.e., irrelevant for 230,528 of them. Although the results of Nicolaides' team have to be confirmed, cost-benefit of first trimester ultrasound should be significantly affected by these figures.

WHO IS PERFORMING ULTRASOUND SCREENING IN EUROPE?

Ultrasound screening is mainly performed by obstetrician/gynecologists, and much less frequently by trained midwives in hospitals, and sporadically by radiologists; the respective frequency is according to the country. Pregnant women, referred for suspicious anomalies by their ob/gyn practitioner, are sent to ob/gyns experienced in ultrasound. As a matter of course, particular certification is not yet required everywhere. Notwithstanding, programs for qualification in obstetrical ultrasound, and more often basic and postgraduate courses, are organized everywhere in Europe;[57-59] we regret that they are not compulsory, although they are firmly considered as a requisite by the professionals. Programs for FAS qualification—a matter where competency is a basic requirement—are rare. Therefore, education is first the responsibility of the person concerned and of the teachers during a residency, for example. Because education is assumed to be a continuous process, competency in screening will persist and improve.

It is important to remember the results of several comparisons, previously cited, that show significant positive screening results in places where ultrasound professionals are in charge of FAS.[60–66]

Training in FAS requires much time, many occurrences, close supervision or management, and extreme motivation; all of these requisites, fulfilled or not, depend on the place of training. An effort is made in Europe to promote formal education in ultrasound screening training.[58] European certified courses leading to the European certificate of expertise in obstetrical ultrasound and prenatal diagnosis—as decided by the European Association of Perinatal Medicine—should be in the forefront of organizing and improving ultrasound screening. Organized on a broad international basis, it can meet the requirement of the European regulations authorizing European citizens to have their professional practice anywhere in the European Union.

In summary, outstanding training in ultrasound is imperative for making prenatal diagnoses, because ultrasound is one of the major tools in prenatal diagnosis.

REFERENCES

1. Dussik, K.T. 1942. Über die Möglichkeit hochfrequente mechanische Schwingungen als diagnostiches Hilfsmittel zu verwenden. Z. Neurol. Psychiat. **174:** 153–168.
2. Donald, I., J. McVicar & T.G. Brown. 1958. Investigation of abdominal masses by pulsed ultrasound. Lancet **1:** 1188–1194.
3. Donald, I. & T.G. Brown. 1961. Demonstration of tissue interfaces within the body by ultrasonic echo sounding. Br. J. Radiol. **34:** 539–546.
4. Sunden, B. 1964. On the diagnostic value of ultrasound in obstetrics and gynaecology. Acta Obstet. Gynecol. Scand. **43(Suppl. 6).**
5. Campbell, S., E.M. Holt, F.D. Johnstone & P. May. 1972. Anencephaly: Early ultrasonic diagnosis and active management. Lancet **2:** 1226–1227.
6. Campbell, S., J. Pryse-Davies, J.T.M. Coltart, M.J. Seller & J.D. Singer. 1975. Ultrasound in the diagnosis of spina bifida. Lancet **1:** 1065–1068.
7. Garrett, W.J., G. Grunwald & D.E. Robinson. 1970. Prenatal diagnosis of fetal polycystic kidney by ultrasound. Aust. N. Z. J. Obstet. Gynaecol. **10:** 7–9.
8. Grennert, L., P.H. Persson & G. Gennser. 1978. Benefits of ultrasonic screening of a pregnant population. Acta Obstet. Gynecol. Scand. Suppl. **78:** 5–14.
9. Bakketeig, L.S., G. Jacobsen, C.J. Brodtkorb, S.H. Eik-Nes, M.K. Ulstein, P. Balstad & N.P. Jorgensen. 1984. Randomised controlled trial of ultrasonographic screening in pregnancy. Lancet **2:** 207–210.
10. Bucher, H.C. & J.G. Schmidt. 1993. Does routine ultrasound scanning improve outcome in pregnancy? Meta-analysis of various outcome measures. Br. Med. J. **307:** 13–17.
11. Persson, P.H. & S. Kullander. 1983. Long-term experience of general ultrasound screening in pregnancy. Am. J. Obstet. Gynecol. **146:** 942–947.
12. Saari-Kemppainen, A., O. Karjalainen, P. Ylostalo & O.P. Heinonen. 1990. Ultrasound screening and perinatal mortality: Controlled trial of systematic one-stage screening in pregnancy. Lancet **336:** 387–391.
13. Waldenstrom, U., S. Nilsson, O. Fall, O. Axelsson, G. Eklund & S. Lindeberg. 1988. Effects of routine one-stage ultrasound screening in pregnancy: A randomised controlled trial. Lancet **2:** 585–588.
14. Kurjak, A., P. Kirkinen, V. Latin & B. Rajhvajn. 1980. Diagnosis and assessment of fetal malformations and abnormalities by ultrasound. J. Perinat. Med. **8:** 219–235.
15. Campbell, S. & J.M. Pearce. 1983. Ultrasound visualization of congenital malformations. Br. Med. J. **39:** 322–331.

16. GEMBRUCH, U. & M. HANSMANN. 1984. Gezielte sonographische Ausschlussdiagnostik fetaler fehlbildungen in risikogruppen. Gynäkologe **17**: 19–32.

17. SABBAGHA, R.E., Z. SHEIKH, R.K. TAMURA, S. DALCOMPO, J.L. SIMPSON, R. DEPP & A.B. GERBIE. 1985. Predictive value, sensitivity, and specificity of ultrasonic targeted imaging for fetal anomalies in gravid women at high-risk for birth-defects. Am. J. Obstet. Gynecol. **152**: 822–827.

18. HILL, L. M., R. BRECKLE & W. C. GEHRKING. 1985. Prenatal detection of congenital malformations by ultrasonography. Am. J. Obstet. Gynecol. **151**: 44–50.

19. KULLENDORFF, C.M., L.T. LARSSON & C. JORGENSEN. 1984. Advantage of antenatal diagnosis of intestinal and urinary tract malformations. Br. J. Obstet. Gynaecol. **91**: 144–147.

20. LI, T.C.M., R.A. GREENES, M. WEISBERG, D. MILLAN, M. FLATLEY & L. GOLDMAN. 1988. Data assessing the usefulness of screening obstetrical ultrasonography for detecting fetal and placental abnormalities in uncomplicated pregnancy: Effects of screening a low-risk population. Med. Decision Making **8**: 48–54.

21. LEVI, S. & P. CROUZET. 1986. An ultrasound mass screening for structural fetal anomalies detection. J. Ultrasound Med. **5**: 102.

22. BROCKS, V. & J. BANG. 1991. Routine examination by ultrasound for the detection of fetal malformations in a low risk population. Fetal Diagn. Ther. **6**: 37–45.

23. CHAMBERS, S.E., R.T. GEIRSSON, R.J. STEWART, C. WANNAPIRAK & B.B. MUIR. 1995. Audit of a screening service for fetal abnormalities using early ultrasound scanning and maternal serum alpha fetoprotein estimation combined with selective detailed scanning. Ultrasound Obstet. Gynecol. **5**: 168–173.

24. CHITTY, L.S., G.H. HUNT, J. MOORE & M.O. LOBB. 1991. Effectiveness of routine ultrasonography in detecting fetal structural abnormalities in a low-risk population. Br. Med. J. **303**: 1165–1169.

25. CONSTANTINE, G. & J. MCCORMACK. 1991. Comparative audit of booking and mid-trimester ultrasound scans in the prenatal diagnosis of congenital anomalies. Prenatal Diagn. **11**: 905–914.

26. D'OTTAVIO, G., Y.J. MEIR, M.A. RUSTICO, G. CONOSCENTI, A. MAIERON, L. FISCHER-TAMARO & G.P. MANDRUZZATO. 1995. Pilot screening for fetal malformations: Possibilities and limits of transvaginal sonography. J. Ultrasound Med. **14**: 575–580.

27. D'OTTAVIO, G., M.A. RUSTICO, Y.J. MEIR, L. FISCHER-TAMARO, N.R. MAIERON & G. CONOSCENTI. 1996. Lo screening delle malformazioni fetali mediante ecografia transvaginale. *In* Congreso Nazionale SIEOG, Eco '96. M. Campogrande, Ed.: 40–45.

28. EIK-NES, S.H., H.G. BLAAS, T. KISERUD, E. TEGNANDER, O.J. JOHANSEN & C. ISAKSEN. 1992. Detection of fetal developmental disorders in a nonselected population. Presented at the Second World Congress of Ultrasound in Obstetrics and Gynecology, Bonn, 1992.

29. LEVI, S., P. CROUZET, J.P. SCHAAPS, P. DEFOORT, R. COULON & M. DEBRIER. 1989. Ultrasound screening for fetal malformations. Lancet **1**: 678.

30. LEVI, S., H. GRANDJEAN & B. DERVAUX. 1995. Cost effectiveness of antenatal screening for fetal malformation by ultrasound. An evaluation of antenatal mass screening by ultrasound for the diagnosis of birth defects (1990–1993). Supported by the European Union, contract MR4*-0225-B, Brussels.

31. LEVI, S., J.P. SCHAAPS, P. DE HAVAY, R. COULON & P. DEFOORT. 1995. End-result of routine ultrasound screening for congenital anomalies: The Belgian multicentric study 1984–92. Ultrasound Obstet. Gynecol. **5**: 366–371.

32. LUCK, C.A. 1992. Value of routine ultrasound scanning at 19 weeks—A 4-year study of 8849 deliveries. Br. Med. J. **304**: 1474–1478.

33. ROSENDAHL, H. & S. KIVINEN. 1989. Antenatal detection of congenital malformations by routine ultrasonography. Obstet. Gynecol. **73**: 947–955.

34. SAARI-KEMPPAINEN, A., O. KARJALAINEN, P. YLOSTALO & O.P. HEINONEN. 1994. Fetal anomalies in a controlled one-stage ultrasound screening trial: A report from the Helsinki Ultrasound Trial. J. Perinat. Med. **22**: 279–289.

35. SHIRLEY, I.M., F. BOTTOMLEY & V.P. ROBINSON. 1992. Routine radiographer screening for fetal abnormalities by ultrasound in an unselected low-risk population. Br. J. Radiol. **65**: 564–569.

36. CARRERA, J.M. & G.C. DI RENZO. 1993. Recommendations and protocols for prenatal di-

agnosis. Report of the European Study Group on Prenatal Diagnosis, European Association of Perinatal Medicine, Barcelona.

37. Prenatal Care Guidelines of the Federal Republic of Germany issued on October 31, 1979. 1986. *In* Ultrasound Diagnosis in Obstetrics and Gynecology. M. Hansmann, B.J. Hackeloer, A. Staudach & B. Wittmann, Eds.: 349 Springer Verlag. Berlin.

38. ROYAL COLLEGE OF OBSTETRICIANS AND GYNAECOLOGISTS. 1984. Report of the RCOG Working party on routine ultrasound examination in pregnancy. RCOG. London.

39. TOURNAIRE, M., G. BREART, E. PAPIERNIK & M. DELECOUR. 1987. Apport de l'échographie en obstétrique (annexe au rapport). Collège National des Gynécologues et Obstétriciens français. Paris.

40. NATIONAL INSTITUTES OF HEALTH, DEPARTMENT OF HEALTH AND HUMAN SERVICES, Public Health Service. 1984. Diagnostic ultrasound; imaging in pregnancy. Report of a consensus development conference, National Institutes of Health. NIH publication 84-667. Bethesda, MD.

41. BERWICK, D.M. & M.C. WEINSTEIN. 1985. What do patients value—Willingness to pay for ultrasound in normal pregnancy? Med. Care **23**: 881–893.

42. EUROCAT WORKING GROUP. 1995. Surveillance of congenital anomalies in Europe 1980–1992 (report 6). European Union Project, Institute of Hygiene and Epidemiology, Brussels.

43. GILLEROT, Y. 1995. European Registers of congenital abnormalities and twins (EUROCAT): Registre Hainaut-Namur 1991–95. Loverval, Belgium.

44. LEVI, S. & Y. HYJAZI. 1992. Sensitivity of routine ultrasonographic screening for congenital anomalies during the last 5 years. J. Ultrasound Med. **11**: 188.

45. CARRERA, J.M., M. TORRENTS, C. MORTERA, V. CUSI & A. MUNOZ. 1995. Routine prenatal ultrasound screening for fetal abnormalities: 22 years' experience. Ultrasound Obstet. Gynecol. **5**: 174–179.

46. HEGGE, F.N., R.W. FRANKLIN, P.T. WATSON & B.C. CALHOUN. 1989. An evaluation of the time of discovery of fetal malformations by an indication based system for ordering obstetric ultrasound. Obstet. Gynecol. **74**: 21–24.

47. CRANE, J.P., M.L. LEFEVRE, R.C. WINBORN, J.K. EVANS, B.G. EWIGMAN, R.P. BRAIN, F.D. FRIGOLETTO, D. MCNELLIS & THE RADIUS STUDY GROUP. 1994. A randomized trial of prenatal ultrasonographic screening: Impact on the detection, management, and outcome of anomalous fetuses. Am. J. Obstet. Gynecol. **171**: 392–399.

48. GONCALVES, L.F., P. JEANTY & J.M. PIPER. 1994. The accuracy of prenatal ultrasonography in detecting congenital anomalies. Am. J. Obstet. Gynecol. **171**: 1606–1612.

49. LYS, F., P. DE WALS, I. BORLEE-GRIMEE, A. BILLIET, M. VINCOTTE-MOLS & S. LEVI. 1989. Evaluation of routine ultrasound examination for the prenatal diagnosis of malformation. Eur. J. Obstet. Gynecol. Reprod. Biol. **30**: 101–109.

50. BLONDEL, B., C. DU MAZAUBRUN & G. BREART. 1996. Enquête Nationale Périnatale. Rapport de fin d'études. INSERM U 149. Paris.

51. SNIJDERS, R.J.M. & K.H. NICOLAIDES. 1996. Ultrasound markers for fetal chromosomal defects. Parthenon Publishing Group. New York.

52. BROMLEY, B. & B.R. BENACERRAF. 1995. The resolving nuchal fold in second trimester fetuses: Not necessarily reassuring. J. Ultrasound Med. **14**: 253–255.

53. LEVI, S. 1997. Impact économique du dépistage échographique prénatal de quelques anomalies congénitales. Presented at L'Echographie ultrasonore: l'année de l'évaluation, Société francophone pour l'application des ultrasons à la médecine et à la biologie. Paris.

54. HYETT, J.A., P.L. NOBLE, R.J.M. SNIJDERS, N. MONTENEGRO & K.H. NICOLAIDES. 1996. Fetal heart rate in trisomy 21 and other chromosomal abnormalities at 10–14 weeks of gestation. Ultrasound Obstet. Gynecol. **7**: 239–244.

55. NICOLAIDES, K.H., M.L. BRIZOT & R.J.M. SNIJDERS. 1994. Fetal nuchal translucency: Ultrasound screening for fetal trisomy in the first trimester of pregnancy. Br. J. Obstet. Gynaecol. **101**: 782–786.

56. NOBLE, P.L., H.D. ABRAHA, R.J.M. SNIJDERS, R. SHERWOOD & K.H. NICOLAIDES. 1995. Screening for fetal trisomy 21 in the first trimester of pregnancy: Maternal serum free B-hCG and fetal nuchal translucency thickness. Ultrasound Obstet. Gynecol. **6**: 390–395.

57. ARDUINI, D. 1994. Teaching ultrasonography in the field of obstetrics and gynecology. Ultrasound Obstet. Gynecol. **4:** 1–2.
58. ISUOG EDUCATION COMMITTEE. 1996. Update on proposed minimum standards for ultrasound training for residents in Ob/Gyn. Ultrasound Obstet. Gynecol. **8:** 363–365.
59. WLADIMIROFF, J.W. 1992. ISUOG in a united Europe and beyond. Ultrasound Obstet. Gynecol. **2:** 383.
60. DE LA FUENTE, P. 1997. Personal communication.
61. DI RENZO, G.C. 1997. Personal communication.
62. HOLZGREVE, W. 1997. Personal communication.
63. MANDRUZZATO, G. P. 1997. Personal communication.
64. MONTENEGRO, N. 1997. Personal communication.
65. PAPP, Z. 1997. Personal communication.
66. ROSENDAHL, H. 1997. Personal communication.
67. LEVI, S. Screening procedures in perinatology. *In* A Textbook of Perinatal Medicine. A. Kurjak, Ed. Parthenon Publishing Group. London. In press.

Quality Assurance in Obstetric and Gynecologic Ultrasound

The Hungarian Model

ISTVÁN SZABÓ,[a,c] LÁSZLÓ CSABAY, ZOLTÁN TÓTH,[b] OLGA TÖRÖK,[b]
AND ZOLTÁN PAPP

[a]I. Department of Obstetrics and Gynecology, Semmelweis University Medical School,
Budapest, Hungary
[b]Department of Obstetrics and Gynecology, University Medical School, Debrecen,
Hungary

ABSTRACT: The majority of physicians performing obstetric scans are radiologists
and obstetricians. The radiologist is well trained in imaging but lacks the obstetric background required to interpret information obtained from the scan. The obstetrician is
qualified in obstetric knowledge but often lacks the formal imaging training necessary
to optimize the pictures. In Hungary, nearly 100% of the physicians who perform obstetric and gynecologic scans are obstetricians. In order to create a standard and to hold
together the practitioners in obstetrics and gynecology, as well as to eliminate the serious consequences of clinical malpractice, we organized the Hungarian Society of Ultrasound in Obstetrics and Gynecology in 1992. The Society was established according
to the standards of the most skilled obstetricians and gynecologists. In addition to working out the conditions and the standards, the Society provides for its members continuous education, postgraduate training, and monitors the knowledge and level of practitioners.
We have established three levels of qualification. Each level requires a medical un-
dergraduate degree. The levels range from basic (A), intermediate (B), to specialist (C).
To receive the certificate every user and ultrasound laboratory have to fulfill requirements
based on skill as well as equipment and circumstances. The certificates are valid for one
year. Every year the practitioner must pass a special examination at the appropriate level.
By doing so, the Society provides its members with not only professional support, but ethical and legal security as well.

INTRODUCTION

Ultrasound has revolutionized the practice of obstetrics and gynecology. The widespread availability of ultrasound equipment has enabled physicians and sonographers
to apply this technology widely in many patients. Because of this widespread availability, assurance of quality in ultrasound use is sometimes erratic.[1–5] Some recent trials have clearly demonstrated that, if ultrasound examination is to be performed, it
must be of high quality. The following paper describes attempts in Hungary to maintain a high standard of quality in ultrasound use.

[c] Address correspondence to István Szabó, M.D., I. Department of Obstetrics and Gynecology,
Semmelweis University Medical School, Baross utca 27, Budapest, Hungary, H-1088.

THE HUNGARIAN MODEL

In Hungary, obstetrician-gynecologists have traditionally performed ultrasound examinations. Although obstetrician-gynecologists are very knowledgeable in fetal anatomy, physiology, and the clinical application of the ultrasound information, they often lack formal imaging training, which is necessary to optimize the images obtained. Before the advent of quality assurance in the use of ultrasound, a medical degree, enthusiasm, and enough money to buy an ultrasound machine were all that was required.

In order to assure the quality of ultrasound examinations, the Hungarian Society of Ultrasound in Obstetrics and Gynecology was organized in 1992 by one of the authors (Z.P.).[6] The Society has grown from 249 members in 1992 to 587 members in 1996. Membership in the Society is intended to include all practitioners of obstetric and gynecologic ultrasound (currently 522 obstetricians, 49 midwives, 6 radiologists, 6 neonatologists, and 4 others). The Society is directed by a supervisory board. This board comprises a president, a secretary general, an accountant, and 11 members (nine obstetricians and two sonographers).

Three levels of ultrasound examinations were established for laboratories and examiners. Level 1 ultrasound examinations are performed in private clinics, outpatient clinics, and prenatal care units; level 2 ultrasound examinations in district or regional hospitals; and level 3 ultrasound examinations in university departments.

Level 1 ultrasound examinations are performed by all practitioners, including physicians, residents, midwives, and sonographers; level 2 examinations by obstetricians, radiologists and neonatologists; and level 3 ultrasound examinations by obstetricians with specialized training in genetics, developmental dysmorphology, and physiology.

A certification process was introduced so that the level of the ultrasound examination and the license number would be clearly stated on the ultrasound report. The three types of licenses corresponded to the three levels of ultrasound examination. For level 1 ultrasound examinations, it is required that the patient be referred for consultation if there are suspicious or abnormal ultrasound findings (License A). For level 2 ultrasound examinations, second opinions in management are provided (License B). For level 3 ultrasound examinations, second or third opinions are provided, with the management of cases requiring special laboratory back-up (License C).

TABLE 1 presents the guidelines for the performance of obstetric and gynecologic ultrasound examinations. First-trimester, third-trimester, and intrapartum ultrasound examinations can be performed by examiners with Licenses A, B, or C. Second-trimester examinations, however, are limited to those practitioners with Licenses B or C. Suspicious or abnormal findings must be evaluated by those who hold Licenses B or C. Specialized prenatal invasive procedures are limited to those with License C. Gynecologic ultrasound examinations, which complement the gynecologic examination, can be performed by examiners with Licenses A, B, or C. Specialized gynecologic invasive procedures are limited to those with Licenses B or C.

The Society has developed the minimal training requirements for the three licenses. For License A, three months of training (400 obstetric and 200 gynecologic scans) under strict supervision are required. There is a written examination after a postgraduate course, together with oral and practical examinations. In addition, there is a postgraduate education requirement of at least one ultrasound course per year. In 1995, the College of Hungarian Obstetricians and Gynecologists accepted the training requirements for License A for all residents starting their training in obstetrics and gynecology.

License B requires five years of training (5,000 obstetric and 2000 gynecologic ultrasound examinations), two written examinations after two postgraduate courses, together with oral and practical examinations. There is a postgraduate education requirement of at least one advanced ultrasound course or congress per year.

TABLE 1. Guidelines for Performance of Obstetric and Gynecologic Ultrasound Scanning

Procedure	License
Routine screening	
I First trimester (8–12 weeks)	A, B, or C
Number and size of embryos, viability	
Pregnancy dating	
Uterus, adnexae	
Ectopic pregnancy	
II Second trimester (18–20 weeks)	Only B or C
amniotic fluid, placenta	
fetal anatomy and measurements	
III Third trimester (28–32 weeks)	A, B, or C
Amniotic fluid, placenta	
Fetal anatomy and measurements	
Checking IUGR	
IV Before term (38 weeks) or intrapartum	A, B, or C
Amniotic fluid, placenta	
Fetal position, well-being	
Diagnostic scanning	
I Pelvic (gynecologic) scanning, complementary to the gynecologic examination	A, B, or C
II Gynecologic invasive procedures	B or C
III Suspicious and abnormal findings on routine screening	B or C
IV Prenatal invasive procedures	C

License C is granted only after requirements for Licenses A and B have been fulfilled, together with specialized training in a tertiary center. Academic productivity must be evident, including at least one presentation per year at advanced courses or congresses.

Members of the Society must apply every year for renewal of certification. In 1993, 287 of 478 or 60% (117 License A, 136 License B, 34 License C); in 1994, 350 of 519 or 67.4% (146 License A, 166 License B, 38 License C); in 1995, 324 of 585 or 55.4% (143 License A, 142 License B, 39 License C); and in 1996, 368 of 587 or 62.3% (150 License A, 179 License B, 39 License C) of the members of the Society received license certification.

The Hungarian Society of Ultrasound in Obstetrics and Gynecology performs an important educational role that helps assure quality. National congresses are held every two years and four special theoretical courses are held annually. The Society encourages the teaching of the clinical use of ultrasound within university curricula, including biophysics, radiology, obstetrics and gynecology, and clinical genetics. The Society directly assures quality by making regular evaluations of the quality and condition of equipment and evaluates false-positive and false-negative cases of its members.

Certificates are issued when requirements for licensure are fulfilled. These certificates must be renewed yearly, with evidence of further postgraduate education. The Society aids doctors who wish to advance the level of ultrasound examinations that they perform and provides professional, legal, and ethical support for its members.

In conclusion, assuring the quality of ultrasound examinations is a worldwide concern for all physicians who perform ultrasound examinations, and for all patients who receive them. It is hoped that our Hungarian experience will be helpful to physicians in other countries in their efforts to establish and maintain quality ultrasound use. It is our strong belief that quality assurance in ultrasound examinations is an essential dimension of modern obstetrics and gynecology.

REFERENCES

1. PLATT, L.D. 1991. Leveling out. Ultrasound Obstet. Gynecol. **1:** 83–84.
2. BENACERRAF, B.R. 1993. Who should be performing fetal ultrasound? Ultrasound Obstet. Gynecol. **3:** 1–2.
3. CHERVENAK, F.A. & L.B. McCULLOUGH. 1993. The importance of ethics to the practice of obstetric ultrasound. Ann. Med. **23:** 271–273.
4. ARDUINI, D. 1994. Teaching ultrasonography in the field of obstetrics and gynecology. Ultrasound Obstet. Gynecol. **4:** 1–3.
5. SKUPSKI, D.W., F.A. CHERVENAK & L.B. McCULLOUGH. 1995. Routine obstetric ultrasound. Int. J. Gynaecol. Obstet. **50:** 233–242.
6. PAPP, Z. 1996. Quality assurance in obstetric and gynecological ultrasound in Hungary. Ultrasound Obstet. Gynecol. **7:** 305–306.

Eurofetus: An Evaluation of Routine Ultrasound Screening for the Detection of Fetal Defects[a]

Aims and Method

SALVATOR LEVI[b,c] AND NUNO AIRES MONTENEGRO[d]

[b]*Obstetrics-Gynecology Diagnostic Ultrasound Unit, Centre Hospitalier Universitaire Brugmann and Université Libre de Bruxelles, Place A. Van Gehuchten 4, B-1020 Brussels, Belgium*

[d]*Department of Obstetrics/Gynecology and Ultrasound Laboratory, Hospital Sãn João, P-4200 Porto, Portugal*

ABSTRACT: The aims of this study are (1) to evaluate the efficiency of ultrasound in detecting CA in low-risk populations of pregnant women by routine screening performed in hospital ultrasound labs (level II); (2) to highlight the areas where improvement could be obtained; (3) to determine efficient timing and number of examinations; (4) to evaluate the psychological returns of detection and nondetection of CA; and (5) to evaluate the cost-effectiveness ratio of antenatal screening of CA. A European collaboration was supposed to help in meeting these objectives because results concerning the analysis of individual CAs or groups of CAs can only be statistically significant when their number is sufficiently large. It was estimated that it was necessary to collect nearly 5,000 CA; this corresponds to about 200,000 pregnant women, the prevalence of malformations at birth being estimated at 2.5%. These conditions yield worthy conclusions, given the following circumstances: a large variety of CA, the extremely low incidence of each CA, the multiple approaches for diagnosis and management, the manifold classes of defects, the differences in gestational age when anomalies are detectable and detected. We study prospectively (1) the reliability of ultrasound in detecting antenatal malformations by recording all CA, ultrasonically suspected and not; (2) the gestational age of anomaly recognition; (3) the response to antenatal diagnosis of CA; (4) the individual outcome of pregnancies; (5) the financial cost of the screening program; and (6) the psychological consequences for the parents.

BACKGROUND OF THE COLLABORATIVE STUDY "EUROFETUS"

Concern about Congenital Anomalies

Concern about congenital anomalies (CA) rests on the consequence of a defect in fetal health. Whatever the anomaly—structural or functional—the issues will vary from a severe to a minimal physiological, morphological, and psychological detriment of the patient.

- The significance of the study of CA is increasing; although the perinatal mortality rate due to CA has decreased, it is declining far less that the one induced by the other causes of death, such as infectious and nutritional diseases.

[a] This work was supported in part by Concerted Action (XII-E) of the European Union—Direction Générale XII—Comac Health Services Research, Contract No. MR4*-0225-B; the Scientific and Medical Research Fund of the French-speaking Community of Belgium, Contract No. 3.4542.86.

[c] Address correspondence to Dr. S. Levi, Obgyn Diagnostic Ultrasound Unit, Centre Hospitalier Universitaire Brugmann, B.1020 Brussels, Belgium.

- CA are responsible for 25% of perinatal deaths, 50% of deaths in infancy, 30% of deaths during the first week of life, and 50% of severe mental and physical handicaps in children; a review of the literature providing information from eight sources[1]—malformation and perinatal surveys—has confirmed these usually quoted figures: it emerges that the contribution of CA to perinatal mortality ranges from 22 to 34%, with an average of 27%.
- Children affected by CA often require intensive care, repeated surgical treatment, and continuous familial and social support.
- The development of new technologies and increased skills in surgery, intensive care, and others fields—associated with an improved outcome—also have side effects, psychological and economical. CA is a condition hard to endure psychologically and physically by the patient, the parents, and the family, costly to support financially, either by the family or/and the community.
- Nowadays, a need emerges for quantifying precisely and repeatedly the long-term outcome of birth defects, unavoidable for the best CA management, in which changing detection modes, diagnostic procedures, management techniques, and health care policies are constantly taken into account; the required amount of medical care and social assistance is far from precisely known, except for a few anomalies that are frequently studied,[2,3] e.g., spina bifida and Down syndrome. However, more information is appearing on the costs of CA.[4]

Procedures for CA Screening

Several procedures for CA screening are being used. When screening was based only on family history and clinical signs, the large majority of CA were not detected before birth, because only a few CA show clinical signs likely related to the diagnosis; furthermore, they rarely appear before midpregnancy. The antenatal detection tools, which are occasionally diagnostic as well, are either based on invasive or noninvasive procedures.

- Invasive procedures include those invasive only for mothers, i.e., the biochemical evaluations of alpha fetoprotein, β-hCG, and unconjugated estriol from maternal serum; and those invasive for mother and fetuses, i.e., karyotyping, DNA analysis, infection search on fetal material sampled by chorionic biopsy, amniocentesis, cordocentesis. These methods detect a few structural CA and chromosomal abnormalities with a fair sensitivity, whereas when diagnostic they show clearly the chromosomal abnormalities and, until now, a restricted number of genetic defects and diagnoses of infections that may cause fetal anomalies.
- Noninvasive tools, i.e., ultrasound examination, are characterized by a broad spectrum of detectable structural and functional anomalies.

Because of the variety of CA and the limited specificity of the existing tests, none of these methods can detect each and every kind of anomalies; ultrasound, however, is presently the prime technique for detecting a great many CA.

Detection of a CA with ultrasound means that a particular sign—corresponding to a possible CA—is discovered during the examination. The signs may be very simple and correspond to a CA, such as a skull defect, or may draw more attention to the case being examined, such as a shifted cavum septum pellucidum. It warrants referral to expert ultrasound. Depending upon the examiner's knowledge and expertise, the diagnosis of the CA can be determined at the same time—the anomaly, ultrasound detection, *and* the diagnosis.

Diagnosis of a CA can be accurate and refer to a specific, well-recognized anomaly, as usually reported in textbooks. Accuracy is important for substantiating the prognosis.

Factors Influencing the Outcome of CA

With the aim of attenuating the invalidating conditions of CA, the factors influencing the outcome of CA should be investigated. The outcome of CA very much depends upon the effects of CA on the patient; the patient's and gestation ages when diagnosis is made; the diagnostic accuracy and completeness; and the availability of therapeutic management.

Effects of CA on the Patient

The severity of the defect, coupled with the specific prominence of the physiological role played by the affected organ, should explain the effect on the patient's health. The CA classification, mentioned below, helps to categorize the CA in respect of their effect.

Gestational Age When Diagnosis Is Made

The relationship between gestational age and diagnosis depends very much on CA detection, and thus on screening efficiency. Gestational age and CA are linked at many times.

- The law, in the majority of nations, allows pregnancy termination of severely affected fetuses until 22 to 24 weeks. The CA should be ascertained before that period.
- The link between fetal age and CA detection is explained by evolving size and function of affected organs, minimal changes being necessary for CA demonstration. Gastrointestinal tract, cardiac defects, and urogenital CA are frequently detected late in pregnancy.
- The decision to do intrauterine therapy might depend on age because of accessibility, or taking into account the time elapsed before diagnosis, birth, and extrauterine therapy.

Diagnostic Accuracy and Completeness

The outcome might be changed by an accurate and comprehensive diagnosis, because options may change; when a defect is severe but curable, therapy can be predicted for after birth, yet termination may be chosen when an apparently mild anomaly is associated to chromosomal abnormality.

Availability of Therapeutic Management

Is screening useful when no therapy is available? It is scientifically difficult to encourage ignorance deliberately. As explained below, a cesarean section for fetal distress is worthwhile for a normal fetus, yet less indicated for a patient affected by a nontreatable CA.

Programming CA Detection

Which Anomalies?

A classification based on the outcome of the CA is helpful in programming screening, because detection leads to CA management, which depends on the severity of the disease and on the gestational age when detection occurs. The use of "major" and "minor" for qualifying the CA is common for anomalies classification, yet lacks explicit definition. According to Smith,[5] minor anomalies are unusual morphologic features that are of no serious medical or cosmetic consequence to the patient. Major anomalies are considered as producing significant long-term disability and/or death. Not very much space is left for severity and for outcome discrimination between the definitions of major and minor CA. The word minor should not underestimate the significance of the anomaly because often it just means "less severe."

Therefore, we would elect a more comprehensive terminology including six categories of CA, that is,

• lethal anomalies
• noncurable anomalies
• serious anomalies, i.e., curable but frequently necessitating repeated operations
• significant anomalies, corresponding to major but less severe operations, not life-threatening
• mild anomalies, corresponding to minor operations, and
• minor anomalies, i.e., no surgery or prosthesis necessary.

The content of the various categories is defined hereafter:

• Lethal anomalies include the CA responsible for the fetus's or the child's death. Termination—according to the wishes of the parents—cannot be considered as a therapeutic attitude; it only anticipates death. Shortening such an abnormal pregnancy permits starting a new gestation earlier. Antenatal CA diagnosis yields, independently of termination, the avoidance of significant yet hopeless therapeutic attitudes: for example, a cesarean section for fetal distress, which occurs frequently in abnormal fetuses.
• Noncurable major malformations are compatible with life, but frequently associated with a permanent and severe physical, and/or mental handicap. This diagnosis could convey similar attitudes as the lethal CA.
• Serious malformations can benefit from an antenatal diagnosis for reasons different than for the two first-mentioned CA. Serious malformations may benefit from a series of decisions made possible by antenatal diagnosis, for example,
    • intrauterine treatment
    • procedures for health preservation
    • maternal transport as an important option allowing delivery in tertiary units for the immediate management of the newborn baby which enhances the prognosis; indeed, after-birth transportation may reduce the chances of recovery (depending the anomalies), inducing unfavorable conditions for resuscitation, inadequate temperature, and poor expert handling. It is time consuming and with expenditures.

The management of various anomalies, serious and minor, may not be urgent, and antenatal diagnosis might appear unnecessary; these are frequently and paradoxically easily diagnosed antenatally thanks to screening, but not after birth, being symptom-free for months or years. Early diagnosis gives way to a medical follow-up. On the contrary, if unaware of the anomaly, the diagnosis is made after a long time interval, and the chances of satisfactory management and recovery decrease because of the deterioration of the affected structures.

The CA diagnosis made antenatally, curable or not, minor and not, also allows to karyotype the fetus and prepare the parents psychologically before the birth.

For the sake of clarity, only four categories might be used:

- fatal anomalies comprise the two first categories
- serious for those CA necessitating involved surgical procedures
- light for those necessitating light surgical procedures, and
- not significant, for those not requiring significant therapeutic measures.

If the present and standard classification remains unchanged, major should apply to all classes, except the not significant one.

Which Patients?

Any method of CA screening should address the entire population of pregnant women to be efficient, because the paucity of clinical signs leaves the care provider defenseless. Any preliminary selection operated with the aim to reduce the number of patients to be screened and to direct only high-risk[e] pregnant women towards specialized labs would leave about 75% of the affected fetuses undiagnosed. High-risk pregnancies obviously justify special care, but all pregnant women deserve care, and the number of CA to be detected is larger in this particular group.

Examinations

Diagnosis of the full spectrum of (diagnosable) malformations relies upon in-detail examinations, done between 18 and 22 weeks and eventually again at 28 to 32 weeks, by specially trained personnel, using adequate equipment and lasting a sufficient time. The recently suggested scan at 12–14 weeks is very promising and will certainly be included in CA screening programs, but was not yet available when Eurofetus was initiated. These three-stage screening examinations are to replace the usually accepted obstetrical ultrasound.

Efficacy of Routine Obstetrical Ultrasound Examination in CA Diagnosis

The efficacy rests on several factors, such as the detection rate, the compliance of the screening, the spectrum of screened CA—including all systems and tracts, from the major to the minor CA—the experience of the examiner, and how the patient is managed consequent to the detection.

---

[e] The definition of the risk level characterizing the population of pregnant women studied is not clearly established. In our opinion, a population of pregnant women "at low-risk" should only include the group cleared from the women at-risk. The unselected, geographical area-based population, which could be called "at regular-risk," is the population submitted for screening. The prevalence of CA is thus expected to be the one observed in geographical area-based populations ("at regular-risk"), e.g., 2.3%;[6] lower in the "at low-risk," e.g., 1.8%, and higher in the high-risk group, e.g., 4% and more. Mixed population will be difficult to detect, unless clearly stated. Nevertheless, in this paper we apply the "low-risk" usage.

Detection Rate

A large gap exists between the theoretical possibility of CA diagnosis by ultrasound, as proved by the high detection rates shown in a few papers, and by the low detection rate seen in large population surveys. The difference is sound, e.g., the detection rate by ultrasound screening of a population from a geographical area is three times smaller as for hospital population studies. The mean detection rate in private offices should be about five to six times lower.

Compliance of the Screening

From the feasibility study made before Eurofetus was started, it appeared that more than 97% of the patients might be screened, a figure that is confirmed by other studies.[7,8] Once a systematic screening program has been in place for detecting the highest rate of anomalies, it is sound to offer the benefits of screening to the entire population to meet the goal—that of detecting almost all detectable anomalies.

Contents of the Examination

The diagnosis of the full scale of malformations relies on in-depth examinations, done preferably several times during pregnancy because the full range of CA cannot be detected at only one point of gestational age. Ultrasound screening and detection should not be restricted to a defined list of CA. Although some CA undoubtedly will more greatly affect the future life of the patient than others, each CA is important, for reasons explained elsewhere. The prognosis is usually worse when the fetus has more than one anomaly; it is sound to karyotype for any kind of CA, and plan psychological support for the parents when fetal CA is present.

In the Eurofetus project, ultrasound screening was planned to be comprehensive, examining all fetal structures that ultrasound is capable of investigating, which nowadays includes a long list of items. Screening protocols exist in several professional recommendations.[9–13]

Skill and Experience of the Operator

Because screening for CA is a difficult task, it is wise to entrust the ultrasound CA screening to trained people; otherwise too many false negatives would result from the screening. Examining a high number of normal pregnancies—carefully scanned for fetal anatomy—is necessary to recognize the alterations of normal structures, avoiding optimistic interpretation of the possible deviation, which must be referred to expert sonologists for corroboration, or rejection of the suspicion of anomaly. We cannot include highly experienced sonologists in routine screening because such routine procedures should not be a part of their assignment.

The skill of the operators cannot be homogeneously high in hospitals, considering the distribution of the teams embodying the whole range of seniority, experience, skill, education; similarly, differences exist between labs and regions, which allow for a range of variability. Our previous experience and the literature have shown that level II labs can undertake the systematic screening for CA, at least once per pregnancy. The quality of ultrasound should be more homogeneous at level II labs than at level I; level III labs usually could not undertake the routine examination of pregnant women, unless associated with a level II unit.

Quality of Equipment

The range of the quality of the equipment is not so broad, and we roughly distinguish three groups:

- Expensive machines including high technology and very high image definition
- Moderately-priced equipment offering very good image quality, but not as sophisticated as the former ones, and
- Poor quality scanners that can only be used for simple obstetrical ultrasound, i.e., simple biometry, amniotic fluid amount, fetal and placental position, fetal heart beats and body movements. The quality of the equipment is not suitable for CA screening.

Use of only high-quality equipment is important for *diagnosis.*

Management of the Patient after CA Detection

CA detection should activate a series of procedures, starting from ultrasound confirmation, karyotyping, analysis of amniotic fluid components, and any additional examination related to the ultrasound diagnosis. The goal is to make the fetal status clear, with perinatal specialists and geneticists involved in the discussion of diagnosis and prognosis. Finally, information is given to the parents offering them the whole range of appropriate options. Complementary procedures are considered for achieving the diagnostic steps and for possible therapy, as well as its eventual implementation. Thus, the correct management of the diagnosis process will assess the efficiency of the test. If diagnosis is not followed by any kind of useful complementary examination and therapy, including termination of the pregnancy, the test is almost useless.

AIMS OF THE EUROFETUS PROJECT

Evaluation of the Efficiency of Ultrasound Screening for CA Detection

The screening program applies to low-risk populations of pregnant women and ultrasound being performed in hospital ultrasound labs. The centers performing ultrasound on high-risk pregnancies tend nowadays to expand detection programs to all pregnancies. However, the cost-effectiveness ratio of such a practice has never been evaluated on a large scale.

The aim of Eurofetus was the evaluation of screening in centers offering good conditions for fetal examination and already engaged in CA screening, to discuss whether this kind of screening should or should not be generalized to all pregnant women.

The evaluation of the cost-effectiveness ratio of systematic antenatal screening for malformations is particularly important for establishing and supporting health policies. The first item to investigate is the effectiveness and the conditions for optimal ultrasound examination that influence an efficient routine CA search. The parameters of ultrasound efficiency in diagnosing malformations were previously stated, as was the evaluation of the results.

Highlight Areas Where Improvement Can Be Obtained

Screening of CA shows very different sensitivities, depending on the affected system and anomalies. Figures on sensitivity can also vary depending on who is performing the ultrasound. Based on experience gathered from 200–300 examiners, the part attributed to low expertise and to the inherent difficulty in detecting a particular kind of CA will be delineated. Then, targeted education and special training aimed at the less well-detected CA—which are nonetheless important for patient health—should help improve results.[14]

Determine Efficient Timing and Number of Examinations

For the best chances of CA detection, an adequate timing for ultrasound should objectively be fixed from the large, acquired experience, taking into account that there are ideal gestational ages for specific diagnoses when the anomaly becomes sufficiently clear, but they cannot be found too late, as previously explained. For financial reasons only a limited number of ultrasound can be considered. A targeted analysis of the observed timing of diagnosis, and number of ultrasounds needed should help to fix an efficient policy.

Psychological Returns of Detection and Nondetection of CA

It is clear that having a malformed fetus, or a disabled child is a severe psychological injury for the mother, in particular, for both parents and family, in general. Is the trauma influenced by the severity of the defect, and differently when the anomaly is found early, late, or not at all? The quality of the screening clearly influences some of these factors, and besides the emotional stress, sometimes for the entire life of the parents; it is also recognized by courts of justice as having financial importance. Parents, being aware of the financial costs of a quality screening, might be asked if they are ready to pay for it, even when medical insurance exists. Reassurance about the absence of CA may be invaluable, assuming the high accuracy in the level of diagnosis, which produces a very low rate of false negative.

Evaluation of Cost-Effectiveness Ratio of Antenatal Screening of CA

Although relatively infrequent—about 2.5% of births—malformations in children represent an important public health problem because of the severe disabilities as well as the social consequences and financial charges they present for the family and for the community. On the other hand, screening, too, is expensive: a well-performed screening necessitates a qualified examination, with sufficient time allocated for examination, and the use of reliable equipment; more than a single ultrasound might be necessary because the signs of different anomalies are detectable at different gestational ages; and, finally, an efficient screening must address the entire population of pregnant women to be efficient on a public health basis, because a primary selection for high-risk pregnancies by cheap clinical means is unsatisfactory. With financial resources limited, the cost of an efficient screening policy has to be known and compared to the benefit.

The cost-price of the screening includes the ultrasound examinations, the complementary investigations, and the hospital and treatment expenses entailed by the antenatal diagnosis of malformation (correct and false). When no screening is performed, there is a cutback of treatment and cost for the handicaps.

The evaluation might bring arguments to "decide" whether the screening—as applied in the present study—should be generalized to all pregnant women.

RATIONALE OF A EUROPEAN COLLABORATION

Our experience, based on a feasibility study conducted over two years from 1984 to 1986, showed that motivated participants could help to achieve this study. The course of the Eurofetus Concerted Action proved the importance of motivation

- to accept the principle of a collaborative trial,
- to cooperate anonymously to the success of a large scientific study, and
- to help prove particular hypotheses by working on suggested topics.

The centers that accepted participation and those having effectively collected the data did not differ very much. We had to substitute some nations, even outside the area grouping the twelve nations forming the European Union (before extension to fifteen nations). We point out that Denmark, Ireland, Germany, and Greece did not participate and the United Kingdom did so for only a very short period. For some the reason was that their screening organization was too different and could not fit within the study framework; in another no screening is performed. Lacking data from two of the most inhabited nations in Europe we were forced to seek data elsewhere. We found small populations, who were enthusiastic and cooperative. Among these were nations expected to join the European Union soon: Sweden, Finland, Norway, Austria, and also several others such as Poland, Hungary, and Croatia.

Among the twelve members of the European Union, two governmental institutions did provide financial support to their national participating centers, namely, the Fonds de la Recherche Scientifique Médicale (Communauté française de Belgique). The French national leader has obtained support from the Institute National de la Santé et de la Recherche Médicale. The insufficiency of national support undoubtedly put a brake on our undertaking and was partly responsible for creating a longer collecting period than expected.

OUTLINE OF THE CONCERTED ACTION

The participating centers were asked to cooperate by collecting prospectively specific data producing information useful for the Eurofetus study.

The rate of detection and the accuracy of the diagnosis are considered first in the so-called epidemiological study.

Requirements for the Epidemiology Study

We required the recording of

- each ultrasonically suspected (or diagnosed) fetal anomaly, at any age of pregnancy
- the CA found at birth, termination, or neonatal period (usually within one week after birth); the CA not diagnosed during the pregnancy (false negatives), and the validation of detected CA (true positives), or the invalidation of erroneously detected CA (false positives)
- the clinical, surgical and/or pathology findings
- the gestational age when anomaly was detected, as well as the dates of all previous and subsequent ultrasound examinations
- the indication(s) of the ultrasound examinations, in order to clear all referred patients from our database

- the detailed fetal biometry, to draw the possible relationship between fetal size and anomalies
- the data useful to establish the potential utility of antenatal diagnosis of CA—e.g., the suggested and performed complementary examinations, the active measures taken connected with possible change of outcome
- the actual outcome of pregnancies, including termination, late abortion, and relationships with the preceding item
- data on the birth process.

Requirements for the Economics Study

We required the recording of financial costs relating to

- personnel, ultrasound equipment, and documentation demands
- complementary examinations induced by CA detection, when diagnosis was correct or not
- specific obstetrical or/and fetal interventions induced by CA detection, when diagnosis was correct or not
- financial costs related to fetal or neonatal care when CA failed to be detected.

Requirements for the Psychology Study

Questionnaires and interviews of parents who had pregnancy with CA detected and pregnancy with CA not detected were recorded.

DATABASE

The following are the main registered parameters that were required to build the Eurofetus database:

- CA detected, description and gestational age
- precise diagnosis when CA was present
- age of diagnosis
- possible associated signs
- consequences of this diagnosis
- chances of correcting ultrasound diagnoses before birth
- morphological report of each newborn or fetus (at birth or after termination of pregnancy).

We required that the data issued from the participating ultrasound labs from hospital obstetrical departments be sent in two steps to the national leader: first, directly after a fetus with CA was detected; second, after any birth or termination of a pregnancy, with associated CA suspected or *unsuspected* during pregnancy. CA was noted as well to collect the false negatives. The total number of deliveries with antenatal ultrasound also had to be given in order to get information on true negatives and their prevalence. Computing and analysis were done at the end of collecting time when all the data was received (June 1993).

REQUIREMENTS FOR THE LABORATORIES

- The lab should exist as a unit included in an obstetrical department where a significant proportion of normal pregnancies are booked and delivered: ultrasound examination to rule out CA has to be systematically offered to all patients from the hospital antenatal clinic.
- The patients are not selected (neither high- or low-risk), a standard screened population having an expected proportion of high-risk pregnancies; the large majority of the screened pregnant women is expected to deliver in that hospital.
- The majority of screening examination for CA is performed between 18 and 24 weeks of pregnancy.
- Routine recording of patient data is required, including normal and abnormal ultrasound, and normal and abnormal examinations at birth or abortion.

PARTICIPATING LABORATORIES

Fourteen nations and 60 laboratories (see appendix listed at the end of this paper) participated to the study. The systematic participation for the entire period, since acceptance, is acknowledged and we are grateful to their members. Inconstant participation or bewildered data were discarded, but listed as well, with thanks to the people in charge of the labs for having put forth effort helping the project.

The nature of the examination was suggested at the beginning of the trial and its observance is principally connected to the concern and the skills of the operators.

The quality of equipment was not specified as a requirement because the associated labs were using average good-quality equipment, as is usually provided in ob/gyn ultrasound labs in Europe.

CHARACTERISTICS OF THE EUROFETUS DATA

In respect of the diversity of our data sources, the evaluation of the data quality was useful. Our data were compared to another recent data bank concerned with congenital heart defects (CHD).[15] In our sample the CHD were 20.2% of CA and, among the fetuses with isolated anomalies, 18.3% of all abnormal fetuses. Compared with the overall number of estimated screened fetuses of our database (based on 2.3% prevalence of Eurocat[6]), the prevalence of CHD (n=974) is about 61 per 10,000. The incidence of CHD—recorded from eight population-based studies—varies from 48 to 91 per 10,000 live births and an average of 60 per 10,000.[15] The quoted study[15] emphasized the importance of a short collecting period, decreasing the bias due to changes in diagnostic and therapeutic procedures. The expertise of doctors examining newborn babies and the time left for CA recording are important for calculating the prevalence. The first clinical examination is usually the privilege of neonatologists, or of general pediatricians, depending on the center. When comparing the prevalence of CHD, recorded by routine after-birth registration of CA and by pediatric cardiologists, it is shown that the latter perform better: 55 per 10.000 and 64 per 10,000, respectively.[15]

Clinical finding at birth is much more examiner- and technical-dependent for minor CA than for major CA. Ventricular septal defect (VSD) is demonstrative: in the early 1990s, VSD represented 45% of all CHD, but only 30% in 1982.[15] In our sample, 368 (62%) of the 597 minor CHD were VSD, representing 38% of all CHD. This last figure corresponds to the average performance of postnatal control, which is even better than supposed because it relates to all fetuses, and not only live births as in the quoted figures.[15] It is also stressed by Pexieder et al.[15] that the centers with the highest prevalence of CHD also have the highest prevalence of VSD, as well as a very high proportion of small VSD.

Reporting on CHD and associated anomalies might help ascertain the quality of the examination: the percentages of additional extracardiac CA in newborn infants were ranked into a 7–16% group and a 34–45% one. Our data rank the present study among the highest percentage of 44% associated extracardiac anomalies.

More than 40% of major CHD will result in the infant's death during the first year of life, nearly 95% of the left hypoplastic hearts (anomaly representing 12% of our major CHD), 50% of endocardial cushion defect (anomaly representing 14% of our major CHD), 47% of transposition of great arteries (anomaly representing 18% of our major CHD), 25% of total anomalous pulmonary venous return, between 10 and 20% of aortic stenosis, coarctation of aorta and tetralogy of Fallot, and 5% or less for ventricular and atrial septal defects for the larger lesions. A more interventional attitude could result in lower mortality, and ultrasound diagnosis could play a role in outcome, either by termination of the cases with the more desperate prognosis, or by birth in specialized hospitals to allow correct care and highly specialized surgery, as for hypoplastic ventricle.

CONCLUSIONS

The Eurofetus project is unique in terms of the amount of data specifically collected for the study of routine ultrasound screening for fetal anomalies. It was successful because this significant amount of data has allowed us to look inside the various systems and tracts. It offered the possibility to evaluate several aspects related to ultrasound screening of CA, which is a subject of concern for many people. These include patients, families, and professionals—mainly obstetricians, midwives, neonatologists, geneticists, surgeons, and psychologists—to name the most significant, but also economists and politicians. The concern is great because the subject has significant consequences: it involves the unborn child, its entire life and a great part of the life of its family, each a situation that can be impaired because of a birth defect.

The health and well-being of the affected child are threatened, and health care expenses are supported by the family and society. Each year this is a matter that concerns one among 500 persons (2 per 1,000 of the entire population of a nation). The sensitivity of the test is closely related to expertise and technical performance. With both tending to improve with time, it is unavoidable that sensitivity will increase as shown by the trends of the last 10 years.

REFERENCES

1. YOUNG, I.D. 1992. Incidence and genetics of congenital malformations. In Prenatal Diagnosis and Screening. D.J.H. Brock, C.H. Rodeck & M.A. Ferguson-Smith, Eds.: 171–187. Churchill Livingstone. Edinburgh.
2. HENDERSON, J.B. 1982. An economic appraisal of the benefits of screening for open spina bifida. Soc. Sci. Med. 16: 545–560.
3. MOATTI, J.P., C. LE GALES, C. JULIAN, J.L. LANCE & S. AYME. 1990. Cost-benefit analysis of amniocentesis for detection of chromosomal anomalies. Rev. Epidémiol. Santé Publique 39: 309–321.
4. WAITZMAN, N.J., R.M. SCHEFFLER & P.S. ROMANO. 1996. The cost of birth defects. Estimates of the value of prevention. University Press of America. Lanham, MD.
5. SMITH, D.W. 1982. Recognizable Patterns of Human Malformations. 3rd edit. W.B. Saunders. London.

6. EUROCAT WORKING GROUP. 1995. Surveillance of congenital anomalies in Europe 1980–1992 (report 6). European Union Project, Institute of Hygiene and Epidemiology, Brussels.
7. BAKKETEIG, L.S., G. JACOBSEN, C.J. BRODTKORB, S.H. EIK-NES, M.K. ULSTEIN, P. BALSTAD & N.P. JORGENSEN. 1984. Randomised controlled trial of ultrasonographic screening in pregnancy. Lancet 1: 207–210.
8. WALDENSTROM, U., S. NILSSON, O. FALL, O. AXELSSON, G. EKLUND & S. LINDEBERG. 1988. Effects of routine one-stage ultrasound screening in pregnancy: A randomised controlled trial. Lancet 2: 585–588.
9. ISUOG EDUCATION COMMITTEE. 1996. Update on proposed minimum standards for ultrasound training for residents in Ob/Gyn. Ultrasound Obstet. Gynecol. 8: 363–365.
10. Prenatal Care Guidelines of the Federal Republic of Germany issued on October 31, 1979. 1986. In Ultrasound Diagnosis in Obstetrics and Gynecology. M. Hansmann, B.J. Hackeloer, A. Staudach & B. Wittmann, Eds.: 349. Springer Verlag. Berlin.
11. ROYAL COLLEGE OF OBSTETRICIANS AND GYNAECOLOGISTS. 1984. Report of the RCOG Working party on routine ultrasound examination in pregnancy. RCOG. London.
12. CARRERA, J.M. & G.C. DI RENZO. 1993. Recommendations and protocols for prenatal diagnosis. Report of the European Study Group on Prenatal Diagnosis. Barcelona.
13. NATIONAL INSTITUTES OF HEALTH, Department of Health and Human Services, Public Health Service. 1984. Diagnostic ultrasound; imaging in pregnancy. Report of a consensus development conference. National Institutes of Health. Bethesda, Maryland. NIH publication 84-667.
14. LEVI, S., J.P. SCHAAPS, P. DE HAVAY, R. COULON & P. DEFOORT. 1995. End-result of routine ultrasound screening for congenital anomalies. Ultrasound Obstet. Gynecol. 5: 366–371.
15. PEXIEDER, T., D. BLOCH & EUROCAT WORKING PARTY ON CONGENITAL HEART DISEASE. 1995. Eurocat subproject on epidemiology of congenital heart disease—First analysis of the completed study. In Developmental Mechanisms of Heart Disease. E.B. Clark, R.R. Markwald & A. Takao, Eds.: 655–668. Futura Publishing Co. Armonk, NY.

APPENDIX
Eurofetus Collaborating Laboratories

Austria

E. Reinold
Universitäts-Frauenklinik
Dept. Obstet. & Gynecol.
Spitalgasse 23
1090 Wien

M. Haeusler
Dept. Obstet. & Gynecol.
University of Graz
Auenbruggerplatz
8036 Graz

S. Szalay
Dept. Obstet. & Gynecol.
Landesfrauenklinik
St. Veiterstrasse 47
9020 Klagenfurt

Belgium

R. Coulon
Hôpital de la Madeleine
Service de Gyn-Obs.
Rue de l'hôpital
7800 Ath

P. Dehavay
Hôpital civil de Charleroi
Service de Gyn-Obs.
6000 Charleroi

P. Defoort
Akademisch Ziekenhuis
U. V. K.
Dienst Gyn-Obs.
9000 Gent

S. Levi
Hôpital Universitaire
Brugmann
Service de Gyn-Obs.
Place A. Van Gehuchten 4
1020 Bruxelles

J.P. Schaaps
Hôpital de la Citadelle
Service de Gyn-Obs.
4000 Liège

Croatia

A. Kurjak
Dr. J. Kajfes Hospital

Pavieka Miskinina 64
41000 Zagreb

Finland

H. Rosendahl
Central Hospital of Kanta-Häme
13500 Hameenlinna

E. Koistinen
Central Hospital of Pohjois-Karjala
Tikanmäentie 21
80210 Joensuu

France

M. Delcroix
Centre hospitalier St-Philibert
Rue du grand but 115
59160 Lommes

H. Grandjean
INSERM—C.H.U. Hôpital
La Grave
31052 Toulouse Cedex

P. Grosieux
C.H.R.
44000 Angers

G. Magnin
Hôpital de la Miletrie
Av. Jacques Coeur 350
86021 Poitiers

F. Puech
Maternité Salengro
Rue Malpart 10-14
59037 Lille Cedex

Hungary

Z. Papp
Semmelweis University
Medical School
Ob/Gyn Dept.
Baross utca 27
1088 Budapest

Italy

G. P. Mandruzzato
Divisione di Ost. e Gin.
Istituto per l'Infanzia
Via dell'Istria 65/1
34100 Trieste

Dr. Moroder
Ospedale Civile di Bolzano
Divisione di Ost. e Gin.
V.L. Bochler 2
39100 Bolzano

V. Marsoni
Ospedale Civile Treviso
Primario Ost. e Gin.
V. Borgo Cavalli 42
31100 Treviso

G.C. Dolfin
Ospedale Ostretico Gin.
"S.Anna"
Div. di Ost. e Gin.
Corso Spezia 60
10126 Torino

Dr. Ferrazzi
Ospedale "S. Paolo"
Clinica Ost. e Gin.
Via A. di Rudini 8
20142 Milano

M. Campogrande
Ospedale Civile "S. Croce"
V. M. Cappino 26
12100 Cuneo

T. Todros
Centro di ecografia
Via Ventimiglia 3
10126 Torino

Luxembourg

J. Arendt
Centre Hospitalier de
Luxembourg
Rue Barblé 4
Luxembourg

The Netherlands

J. M. J. Van Vugt
Acad. Ziekenhuis der Vrije
Universiteit
P.O. Box 7057
1007 MB Amsterdam

Norway

S. H. Eik-Nes
Kvinnekliniken
Regionsykenhuset
Trondheim

Poland

M. Respondek
Polish Mother Health Center
Sonography Department
Rzgowska 281/289
93-345 Lodz

Portugal

N. Montenegro
Hopital San Joao
Servico de Obstetricia
4200 Porto

J. Carlos Santos
H. Sto. Antonio
Servico de Obstetricia
Largo Abel Salazar
4000 Porto

A. Vieira
Maternidade Julio DINIS
Largo de maternidade
4000 Porto

J. Fagulha
Maternidade Daniel de
Matos
Rue Miguel Torga
3000 Coimbra

J. M. Cruz
H. Viana Do Castelo

Servico de Obstetricia
4900 Viana do Castelo

H. Castro Botas
Hôpital Sta. Maria
F.M.L.
Servico de Obstetrica
Av. prof. Egas Moniz
1600 Lisboa

J. Branco
H. S. Franscisco Xavier
Servico de Obstetrica
Estrade de Forte do Alto de
Duque
1499 Lisboa

J. Correia
Maternidade Alfredo Da
Costa
Servico de Obstetricia
Rue Viriato
1000 Lisboa

Drs. Delgado/Gomes
H.V.N. Gaia
Servico de Obstetricia
Rua Dr. Francisco Sa
Carneiro
4400 Vila Nova de Gaia

Spain

P. de la Fuente
Hospital Universitario
"12 de Octubre"
28041 Madrid

J. Gonzalez Merlo
Hospital Clinic I
Provincial de Barcelona
Catedratico de Obst. y Gin.
Villarroel 170
08036 Barcelona

J. Montalvo Cristobal
Facultad de Medicina de la
Universidad Complutense
Hospital Clinico "San
Carlos"
28040 Madrid

J. M. Carrera Macia
Instituto Dexeus
P° da Bosanova, 67
08017 Barcelona

X. Domingo I Cochs
Hospital General de
Granollers
Servei D'Obstetricia I
Ginecologia

Av. Francesc Ribas, s/n
08400 Granollers

J.M. Troyano Luque
Hospital General y
Clinico de Tenerife
Ofra, La Cuesta
38320 La Laguna
Santa Cruz de Tenerife

F. Gonzalez Gomez
Hospital Clinico "San
Cecilio"
University of Granada
Avda. Dr. Oloriz, s/n
Granada

Ferrer I Morron
Hospital Maternal "Val
d'Hebron"
08023 Barcelona

J. Yanguas
Hospital "Virgen del
Camino"
31008 Pamplona

M. A. Diaz Lopez
Hospital "Virgen de las
Nieves"
Granada

Sweden

P. Malcus
Dept. Obst. Gyn.

Sjukhuset
26281 Angelholm

H. Almström
Dept. Obst. Gyn.
Danderyds Sjukhus
18288 Danderyd

J. Laurin
Dept. Obst. Gyn.
Lasarettet
25187 Helsingborg

P. Buchhave
Dept. Obst. Gyn.
Centrallasarettet
37185 Karlskrona

K. Arstrom
Dept. Obst. Gyn.
Centralsjukhuset
65185 Karlstad

C. Jorgensen
Dept. Obst. Gyn.
Lasarettet
22185 Lund

K. Marsal
Dept. Obst. Gyn.
Allmanna Sjukhuset
21401 Malmö

K. H. Hokegard
Dept. Obst. GynOstra
Sjukhuset
41685 Göteborg

T. Lofstrand
Dept. Obst. Gyn.
Kärnsjukhuset
54185 Skovde

B. Dennefors
Dept. Obst.Gyn.
Sjukhuset
43281 Varberg

B. Sultan
Dept. Obst. Gyn.
Sahlgrenska Sjukhuset
41345 Göteborg

M. Magiste
Dept. Obst. Gyn.
Länssjukhuset
391 85 Kalmar

L. Hakan
Dept. Obst. Gyn.
Sjukhuset
431 80 Molndal

United Kingdom

L. Chitty
King's College Hospital
Denmark Hill
London SE5 8RY

Sensitivity of Routine Ultrasound Screening of Pregnancies in the Eurofetus Database

HÉLÈNE GRANDJEAN,[a] DANIÈLE LARROQUE,[a] SALVATOR LEVI,[b] AND THE EUROFETUS TEAM

[a]INSERM, Hôpital La Grave, Toulouse, France
[b]Brugmann Hospital, Brussels, Belgium

ABSTRACT: In this prospective study, we recorded details on 3,685 fetuses with congenital structural abnormalities from an unselected population of women who underwent routine ultrasound examination during their pregnancies. Overall, 2,262 fetuses were diagnosed as being abnormal before birth (sensitivity = 61.4%). The total number of abnormalities was 4,615, of which 1,733 (37.5%) were major abnormalities. The overall number of detected abnormalities was 2,593 (sensitivity = 56.2%). If only major abnormalities were considered, the sensitivity rose to 73.7%, compared to only 45.7% for the minor abnormalities. Within each severity group, the accuracy of detection varied across systems. For the major abnormalities, it was higher for the central nervous system (88.3%) and urinary tract (84.8%), but lower for heart and great vessels (38.8%). Detection of minor abnormalities was also effective for the urinary tract (89.1%), but not for the heart and great vessels (20.8%) and the musculoskeletal system (18%).

INTRODUCTION

The reliability of screening of congenital malformation by routine sonographic examination has been a matter of debate for some years. The debate has been fueled recently by the publication of contradictory claims.[1-4] In view of the diversity and frequency of malformations, the overall performance of screening can only be evaluated in a large population, which requires the cooperation of several centers.

MATERIALS AND METHODS

Over the study period, from January 1, 1990 to June 30, 1993, the 60 centers participating in the Eurofetus project recorded prospectively all ultrasonographic diagnoses of malformation during pregnancy, along with the undiagnosed malformations noted at birth despite ultrasonographic examination in the center during pregnancy. Pregnant women referred for suspected abnormalities after ultrasonographic examination outside the participating centers were excluded, because the main objective was to evaluate the reliability of routine screening.

Definition of Cases

We defined as congenital abnormalities the various structural abnormalities present at birth, including malformations, deformations, and dysplasias. We excluded the abnormalities without serious medical consequences that cannot be considered as malformations (minor deformity of the nose, ears and face, clicking hip, umbilical or inguinal hernia, undescended testes, hydrocele, phimosis, hypospadias, isolated skin lesions, functional cardiac murmurs, and single umbilical artery). Isolated growth retardation, amniotic fluid abnormalities or hydrops were also excluded. Chromosomal abnormalities are considered in a separate paper.

Data Collection

This prospective study comprised two data files. The first file included the malformations detected during pregnancy, and detailed the abnormalities diagnosed by echography and their course during pregnancy (malformations confirmed or excluded), the consequences of the diagnosis (examinations, management), the outcome of the pregnancy, the malformations at term (on birth or after termination or abortion), and the status of the infant at birth and at 6 days.

The second file included all malformations discovered at birth (or after abortion) and detailed the abnormalities, the dates of ultrasonographic examination carried out during pregnancy, the outcome of the pregnancy, and the status of the infant.

Data Analysis

The data for each patient were compared with those obtained at birth or on autopsy of the stillbirths and terminations.

An ultrasonographic sign was classified as:

- true positive if the abnormality was confirmed on examination at birth, or mentioned in the autopsy report for the stillbirths
- false negative if observed at birth and undetected by echography
- false positive if diagnosed on ultrasonographic examination, but not confirmed by examination at birth or on autopsy for the stillbirths
- false alarm if an abnormality was first suspected and then ruled out by subsequent ultrasonographic examinations and also not found at birth.

We discriminated major from minor malformations. The major malformations included those that were lethal, as well as the incurable or curable severe abnormalities with a high risk of residual handicap. The minor malformations comprised the remainder and were a heterogeneous group of less severe and benign abnormalities.

RESULTS

Abnormalities Observed

In total, we recorded 4,615 malformations in 3,686 infants, or 1.25 abnormality per malformed child. Out of these 3,686 malformed infants, 2,907 (78.9%) had a single abnormality, 484 (13.1%) two abnormalities, and 295 (8.0%) three or more abnormalities.

TABLE 1 lists the distribution of the principal abnormalities per system. Out of the overall study population, most malformations were found in the musculoskeletal system (22.6%), urinary system (20.7%), heart and great vessels (20.7%), and central nervous system (16.0%).

TABLE 1. Distribution of Malformations between Systems

Classification	Malformations	
	n	%
Central nervous system abnormalities	738	16.0
Heart and great vessels abnormalities	953	20.7
Musculoskeletal abnormalities	1043	22.6
Urinary tract abnormalities	954	20.7
Digestive system abnormalities	229	5.0
Cleft lips and palates	316	6.8
Multiple congenital abnormalities	120	2.6
Miscellaneous	262	5.6
Total	4615	100

Detection Sensitivity

The overall detection sensitivity for a malformed infant was 61.4% at a 95% confidence interval (CI 95%) of 59.8–63.0%. It was significantly higher for the infants with several abnormalities than for those with a single abnormality (Odds ratio [OR] : 1.77; CI 95%: 1.49–2.11). TABLE 2 summarizes the sensitivity for ultrasonographic detection as a function of the number of abnormalities per infant. Out of the 4,615 malformations recorded in our series, 2,593 were diagnosed during pregnancy. The overall sensitivity for detection of malformations by echography in this unselected population was thus 56.2% (CI 95%: 54.7–57.7%).

TABLE 3 lists the results for detection as a function of the type of malformation. It can be seen that there were significant differences between the different organs. The malformations most readily detected were those of the urinary tract (88.5%) and central nervous system (88.3%), followed by the multiple congenital abnormalities (75.0%). Heart and great vessels abnormalities were poorly detected (38.8% for major and 20.8% for minor), as were the minor musculoskeletal abnormalities and cleft lips and palates (18%). For all the major abnormalities, the overall percentage detection was 73.7% compared to 45.7% for the minor abnormalities.

TABLE 2. Sensitivity for Ultrasonographic Detection of Malformations as a Function of Number of Malformations per Infant

	Diagnosis Made during Pregnancy	Diagnosis Not Made during Pregnancy	Sensitivity (%)	Odds Ratio (CI 95%)
One malformation	1704	1204	58.6	1
Two malformations	332	151	68.7	1.55
				(1.26–1.92)
Three or more malformations	226	72	75.8	2.22
				(1.67–2.95)
Total	2262	1427	61.4	

TABLE 3. Detection Sensitivity as a Function of the Type of Malformation

Abnormality (ICD 9 codes)		True Positive (n)	False Negative (n)	Total Abnormalities (n)	Sensitivity (%)
Central nervous system[a] (740.0–742.9)		652	86	738	88.3
Heart and great vessels (745.0–747.9)	Major abnormalities	142	224	366	38.8
	Minor abnormalities	122	465	587	20.8
	Total	264	689	953	27.7
Digestive system (750.0–752.9)	Major abnormalities	8	0	8	
	Minor abnormalities	115	106	221	52.0
	Total	123	106	229	53.7
Urinary tract (753.0–753.9)	Major abnormalities	117	21	138	84.8
	Minor abnormalities	727	89	816	89.1
	Total	844	110	954	88.5
Musculoskeletal (754.0–756.9)	Major abnormalities	257	92	349	73.6
	Minor abnormalities	125	569	694	18.0
	Total	382	661	1043	36.6
Cleft lips and palates[b]	(749.0–749.2)	57	259	316	18.0
Multiple congenital abnormalities[a]	(759.4; 759.7; 759.8)	90	30	120	75.0
Other abnormalities	Major abnormalities	11	3	14	78.6
	Minor abnormalities	170	78	248	68.5
	Total	181	81	262	69.1
Total major abnormalities		1277	456	1733	73.7
Total minor abnormalities		1316	1566	2882	45.7
Total		2593	2022	4615	56.2

[a]All are considered as major abnormalities.
[b]All are considered as minor abnormalities.

Age at Diagnosis

For the whole population, the malformations were detected at 25.8 ± 7.5 weeks (24.2 ± 7.2 weeks for the major and 27.6 ± 7.4 weeks for the minor). The type of malformation was found to influence the age of detection. The multiple malformations were detected first (22.3 weeks) followed by those of the musculoskeletal system (23.3 weeks, major or minor) and the major abnormalities of the urinary tract (24.2 weeks). The following malformations were detected later during pregnancy: major or minor heart and great vessels abnormalities (27.4 weeks), cleft lips and palates (28.1 weeks), minor abnormalities of the urinary tract (29.1 weeks), and those of the digestive tract (29.7 weeks).

Overall, 44% of malformations were detected within the first 24 weeks of gestation, this figure rising to 56% for the severe malformations.

Outcome of Malformed Infants

Out of the cases detected during pregnancy, 12% led to a spontaneous abortion or death *in utero* and 27% to an elective termination. For the severe malformations there were 15% spontaneous abortions or deaths *in utero* and 41% terminations. Eighty-three percent of the terminations were carried out before 24 weeks.

TABLE 4 lists the outcomes of the pregnancies for the malformed infants, detected or not, according to the severity of the malformation. Twenty-seven percent of infants with a severe malformation detected prior to birth were born alive compared to 76% for those undetected before birth. There was also a difference, albeit much smaller, for the minor malformations (85 and 95% for those detected before and after birth, respectively).

False Positives and False Alarms

All the diagnoses of malformations made during pregnancy in the participating centers were recorded. Some erroneous diagnoses were made on normal infants, which in some cases were corrected on subsequent ultrasonographic examination during the pregnancy. These cases were recorded as false alarms. In other cases, the error was only found on the birth of a normal child, which was thus recorded as a false positive.

Out of the 2,789 infants considered as malformed during pregnancy, only 2,262 (81.1%) were in fact found to be malformed at birth. There were 271 false alarms (9.7%) and 256 false positives (9.2%).

Out of the 256 false positives, only one led to a termination, which was carried out at 26 weeks. This case was a severe growth retardation with oligoamnios with a diagnosis of bilateral renal agenesis, which was not found on autopsy.

In the overall analysis of the reliability of detection as a function of the type of abnormality, we must add to the 256 false positive cases of normal infants 50 cases of wrongly diagnosed malformations for infants who also had correctly diagnosed malformations. Therefore, we recorded overall 306 false positive diagnoses for 2,593 true positive diagnoses, or a ratio of 1 false positive for 11.8 true positives. The most common malformation in the false positives (146 cases, 48%) was hydronephrosis with 1 false positive for 3.5 true positives. The only other malformations with a high incidence of false positives were those of the digestive tract (25 out of 140 or 1 false positive for 4.9 true positives).

Out of the 271 false alarms, 115 (42%) were for choroid plexus cysts. There was an even distribution of false alarms between the other malformations.

TABLE 4. Outcome of Malformed Infants as a Function of Severity and Ultrasonographic Detection

	Severe Malformation with Ultrasonographic Diagnosis		Minor Malformation with Ultrasonographic Diagnosis	
	Yes	No	Yes	No
Alive infant	349 (28)[a]	243 (76)	805 (86)	929 (95)
Dead infant	883 (72)	75 (24)	138 (14)	45 (5)
Terminations	516 (42)	2 (1)	59 (6)	0
Spontaneous deaths	367 (30)	73 (23)	79 (8)	45 (5)

[a]Numbers in parentheses indicate percentages.

DISCUSSION

This study on a population of 3,683 infants is the largest to date on the assessment of reliability of routine sonography for detection of congenital malformations. In view of the diversity of the malformations, and differences in the performance of sonography for detection of the different abnormalities, reliability can only be evaluated on a large population.

In our study, the overall sensitivity of prenatal ultrasonography in correctly identifying structural defects was 61.4%. The results reported in the literature for detection of malformations in the general population[1-7] range from 35[1] to 78.3%.[7] However, studies cannot readily be compared because there are differences in the criteria for recording malformations, and in small series, there may be chance differences in the types of recorded malformations, which have significant impact on the accuracy of detection. Higher sensitivity may be obtained in centers using technologically advanced equipment on high-risk populations. For example, Sabbagha *et al.*[8] in 1985 reported a 95% sensitivity for ultrasonic-targeted imaging for fetal abnormalities in women at high risk for birth defects, excluding cardiac defects. It is generally considered that, in contrast to predictive value, sensitivity should be similar in any given population and is unaffected by the prevalence of the disease. However, for ultrasonographic detection of malformations, it is quite possible that the existence of risk factors will tend to encourage more extensive examination of the fetus with a concomitantly enhanced efficiency of detection. In practice, screening cannot be restricted to such high-risk populations as congenital malformations that arise in women with no known risk factors.[5]

We excluded the minor abnormalities as yet undetectable by echography, and only included those detectable at birth or on spontaneous or elective abortion. For the abortions and the stillbirths, the malformation was verified at autopsy in 90% of cases. The only malformations recorded were those detected within the first 6 days of life. It is known, however, that a significant number of abnormalities, especially in the heart and digestive tract, only become apparent over the first months of life. The overall detection sensitivity should thus be considered to be an overestimate, although it should be borne in mind that these late detected abnormalities tend to be minor.

With respect to the consequences of antenatal screening for fetal abnormalities, two elements are of particular significance: the severity of the abnormality and the age on detection. In common with other authors, we found that the major malformations were more readily detected than the minor ones. In total, 75% of the major malformations were detected on ultrasonographic examination, which is close to the figures reported by other authors.[3,9] This clearly has an important influence on pregnancy management. In our population, we noted a significantly lower proportion of live births in the group whose malformations were detected antenatally. This was largely due to the higher number of terminations carried out in this group.

The age at which the termination is carried out is also important, because practices vary between countries. In some countries such as France, as soon as an abnormality is considered incurable and particularly severe, at the request of parents, termination is authorized by law at any gestational age. In many other countries including most states of the United States, termination is only allowed in the first 24 weeks. Out of all malformations in our study, the abnormality was only detected in 44% of cases within the first 24 weeks. This percentage rose to 56% for the severe abnormalities, and 83% of terminations were able to be carried out within the first 24 weeks of gestation. Only one study[3] found a higher rate of early detection. Most of the other studies either found a similar level of detection[5] or a lower one than ours.[1,4,9] In most cases, the later diagnoses were not due to any delay in ultrasonographic examination. In our population, 93% of cases benefited from an ultrasonographic examination within the first 24 weeks, and we found no difference between the detected and undetected cases in frequency of examination before 24 weeks. In several cases, the malformations detected after 24 weeks were those with a late expression such as those of the digestive tract. However, in most cases the abnormalities were present at the first ultrasonographic examination and were only revealed on repeated examination.

CONCLUSION

In this study, we evaluated the reliability of antenatal ultrasonographic detection of congenital abnormalities in an unselected population, by studying a large population, which included a large number of malformations. The interest of the results is threefold. First, by giving an indication of the reliability of detection of major malformation and the age at which they can be detected, it allows to assess the impact that routine ultrasonographic screening may have on pregnancy management, especially for severe cases where the parents may request a termination. Second, by underlining the limitations of ultrasonographic diagnosis of fetal abnormalities, it can provide parents with more objective information about the possibilities of antenatal detection. Third, it highlights areas where more effort is required to improve accuracy and reliability of this detection.

REFERENCES

1. EWIGMAN, B., M. LEFÈVRE & J. HESSER. 1990. A randomized trial of routine prenatal ultrasound. Obstet. Gynecol. **76:** 189–194.
2. SAARI-KEMPPAINEN, A., O. KARJALAINEN, P. YLÖSTALO & O.P. HEINONEN. 1990. Ultrasound screening and perinatal mortality: Controlled trial of systematic one-stage screening in pregnancy. Lancet **336:** 387–391.
3. CHITTY, L.S., G.H. HUNT, J. MOORE & M.O. LOBB. 1991. Effectiveness of routine ultrasonography in detecting fetal structural abnormalities in a low risk population. Br. Med. J. **303:** 1165–1169.
4. LEVI, S., J. P. SCHAAPS, P. DE HAVAY, R. COULON & P. DEFOORT. 1995. End-result of routine ultrasound screening for congenital anomalies. Ultrasound Obstet. Gynecol. **5:** 366–371.
5. ROSENDAHL, H. & S. KIVINEN. 1989. Antenatal detection of congenital malformations by routine ultrasonography. Obstet. Gynecol. **73:** 947–951.
6. GONCALVES, F.L., P. JEANTY & J. C. PIPER. 1994. The accuracy of prenatal ultrasonography in detecting congenital anomalies. Am. J. Obstet. Gynecol. **171:** 1606–1612.
7. CARRERA, J. M., M. TORRENTS, C. MORTERA, V. CUSI & A. MUÑOZ. 1995. Routine prenatal ultrasound screening for fetal abnormalities: 22 years' experience. Ultrasound Obstet. Gynecol. **5:** 174–179.
8. SABBAGHA, R.E., Z. SHEIKH, R.K. TAMURA, S. DALCOMPO, J.L. SIMPSON, R. DEPP & A.B. GERBIE. 1985. Predictive value, sensitivity, and specificity of ultrasonic targeted imaging for fetal anomalies in gravid women at high risk for birth defects. Am. J. Obstet. Gynecol. **152:** 822–827.
9. MACQUART-MOULIN, G., C. JULIAN & S. AYME. 1989. Sensibilité de l'échographie obstétricale dans le diagnostic anténatal des anomalies foetales majeures. Rev. Epidémiol. Santé Publique **37:** 197–205.

Sensitivity of Fetal Anomaly Detection as a Function of Time[a]

B. DERVAUX,[b,e] H. LELEU,[b] TH. LEBRUN,[b] S. LEVI,[c] AND H. GRANDJEAN[d]

[b]CRESGE, Department of Health Economics, Catholic University of Lille, 60 bd Vauban, B.P. 109, 59016 Lille Cedex, France
[c]Brugmann Hospital, Bruxelles, Belgium
[d]La Grave Hospital, Toulouse, France

ABSTRACT: In this paper, we show that the ratio of the number of fetal anomalies detected by ultrasounds (US) to the total number of cases is not a consistent estimator of the US sensitivity. As Eddy[1] pointed out, when the disease evolves over time, the sensitivity of a test also varies over time according to the development of the disease. To assess correctly the detection capability of a test, it is therefore necessary to estimate a time continuous function (sensitivity function) instead of a single parameter. From a methodological point of view, by considering the "detectability" time of a fetal anomaly as a random variable and parametrizing its distribution function, we estimate the probability that an anomaly is detected conditional upon the precise timing of actually performed US during pregnancy. We fit this model with Eurofetus data (about 7,300 abnormal fetuses), and we compare estimations for different kinds of anomalies (classification based on the system involved and/or severity of the handicap). To allow for heterogeneity of anomalies regarding the detectability time, we generally adopt mixture models. For instance, we select a bi-gamma distribution for major malformations and estimate that 63% of such anomalies are detectable quite early in pregnancy (conditional mean: 15.2 weeks of amenorrhea (WA) ± 4.2 WA), the others becoming detectable later (30.3 WA ± 6.4 WA). Such results are then integrated in a cost-effectiveness analysis.

INTRODUCTION

To carry out an economic assessment of prenatal screening by ultrasound (US), we need to compare numerous follow-up protocols which differ with regard to the number of examinations performed and the dates at which such examinations are realized. This leads us to study the evolution of the US sensitivity during the pregnancy.

The sensitivity of a test measures its ability to detect pathologic cases among an asymptomatic population. In a static context, the estimation of this parameter seems relatively straightforward: it suffices, for a well-defined population, to compute the ratio of the number of individuals with true positive tests to the total number of individuals with the disease. Nevertheless, this kind of computation is only consistent for a nonprogressive pathology. If the disease evolves with time, as Eddy[1] emphasized, the sensitivity of the test varies according to the state of development of the disease. Accordingly, we need to estimate a time continuous function instead of a single parameter to assess the test capability to detect cases. In such circumstances, the above-defined ratio depends not only on the technical features of the test, but also on the time at which

[a] The Eurofetus Research Program was subsidized by the European Union, Comac Health Services Research, Concerted Action (XII-E), Contract No. MR4-0225-B. S. Levi, project leader.
[e] E-mail: b.dervaux@cresge.fupl.asso.fr

it is performed. Therefore, it is necessary to clearly distinguish between the detection rate (or the seeming sensitivity) and the sensitivity function.

In this paper, we first describe the statistical model developed to estimate the US sensitivity function for fetal anomalies screening. We present some results based on simulated data in order to analyze the behavior of our model. Then, we work with real data collected through the Eurofetus Research Program (follow-up of about 190,000 pregnancies in 14 European countries leading to the diagnosis of 7,331 abnormal fetuses). Finally, we illustrate the usefulness of this model in conducting a cost-effectiveness analysis of prenatal screening by US.

THE MODEL

During pregnancy, the malformation evolves until it reaches a critical state of development, which allows the detection by US. This "detectability" time, noted τ, is a random variable. Indeed, the malformations do not follow a strictly deterministic process. This occurrence or detectability time varies according to the type of malformation (e.g., hydrocephalus, spina bifida and so on), the technical features of the equipment, the skills of the ultrasonographist (see FIG. 1).

The time at which the malformation becomes detectable by US constitutes the key variable of our model. An US performed before τ cannot detect the malformation; an US realized after τ, by contrast, does detect the malformation. In the case of a nondetectable anomaly, τ occurs after the delivery. Evaluating the effectiveness of the obstetrical ultrasound for the detection of fetal malformations is equivalent to adjusting the distribution of the random variable τ on screening data and to estimate the moments of this distribution (mean, variance and so forth).

For the statistical analysis, we proceed in two steps: (1) We parametrize the density function of τ [denoted $f(\tau)$]; and (2) then we estimate the parameters of this function using data on observed events (see below). We also compare different specifications for the density function in order to retain the best one on the basis of some statistical criteria (for instance, value of the log-likelihood function, the Akaike or Schwartz information criteria). The ultrasound sensitivity function corresponds to the cumulative

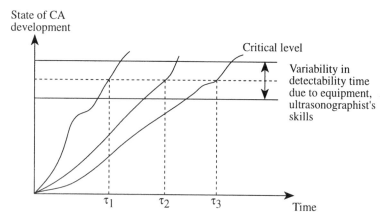

FIGURE 1. CA development and definition of the "detectability" time.

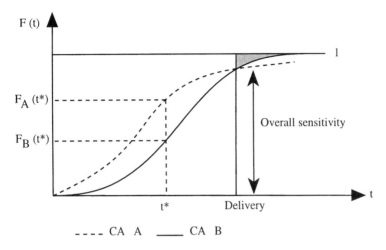

FIGURE 2. Graphical definition of the sensitivity function and of overall sensitivity.

distribution of τ [denoted $F(\tau)$]. This function gives the probability that the US detects the anomaly before any moment in pregnancy. For each anomaly, two situations can be distinguished: (1) The US detects all cases before the delivery. The cumulative distribution equals 1 at the time of the delivery. (2) The US does not detect all cases before the delivery. Then, the value of the cumulative distribution at the time of delivery constitutes a synthetic indicator of the US capability to detect the anomalies. Nevertheless, this indicator does not account for the earliness of the detection. Thus, for two different anomalies, the US can present the same overall sensitivity even though the sensitivity functions have really contrasting shapes (FIG. 2).

To estimate $F(\tau)$, we need information about all the US performed during the pregnancy (recorded in weeks of amenorrhea, WA thereafter), and about the time at which each malformation is actually detected. Thus, we compute the probabilities related to the two following events:

1. The malformation is detected at t_1 (event noted E_1^+), given the last negative US was performed at t_0 (event noted E_0^-; t_0 equals 0 if the malformation is detected at the first US). On a chronological time scale, things look like this:

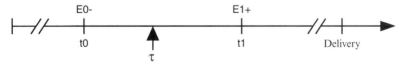

2. The malformation is detected at the time of the delivery, given the last negative US was performed at t_0.

Graphically, as above:

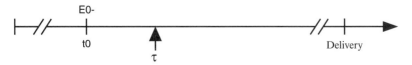

More formally, these two probabilities are written down as:

1. If the malformation is detected:

$$\text{Prob (detected malformation)} \quad \begin{aligned} &= \text{Prob } (t_0 < \tau \le t_1) \\ &= F(t_1) - F(t_0) \end{aligned}$$

2. If the malformation is not detected:

$$\begin{aligned} \text{Prob (not detected malformation)} &= \text{Prob } (\tau > t_0) \\ &= 1 - F(t_0) \end{aligned}$$

Combining these two quantities, we obtain the log-likelihood function:

$$Ln\,L = \sum_{i=1}^{n} \{D_i[Ln(F(t_1) - F(t_0))] + (1 - D_i)[Ln(1 - F(t_0))]\}$$

with $D_i = 1$ if the malformation is detected; $D_i = 0$ otherwise.

For statistical reasons, we work in general on pooled data. We never get enough observations in considering a single anomaly. Thus, we aggregate observations on different anomalies because the associated degree of handicap is equivalent or because the observations are related to the same organ or system. This constitutes a source of heterogeneity. In the data set, some anomalies may have different distributions for τ. To cope with this issue, we use a mixture of densities as specification for τ's density function. Thus, we test for specifications like $f(\tau) = \sum_{j=1}^{k} \alpha_j\, f_j(\tau, \theta_j)$, with α_j, the distribution parameters (evidently, $\sum_{j=1}^{k} \alpha_j = 1$) and f_j, the density function of the detectability time for the jth latent group of malformations (of parameters θ_j). Using mixture models makes both the estimation and the statistical inference much more difficult.

A SIMPLE EXAMPLE

This simple example illustrates the shortcomings of the usual definition of sensitivity in screening for fetal anomalies. Let us assume that, given the state of the art, the detectability time for a given anomaly is distributed as a normal variate with mean and standard deviation fixed at 20 WA and 5 WA, respectively. Then, let us consider a fictive cohort

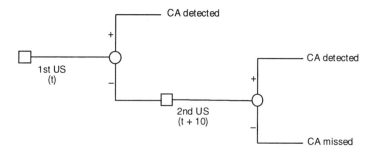

FIGURE 3. A protocol with two ultrasound examinations: (t; t + 10) for all women.

TABLE 1. Number of Ultrasounds and CA Detected with Two Examinations Performed (t; t + 10)

Time of First US	US (*n*)	CA Detected (*n*)	Time of Second US	US (*n*)	CA Detected (*n*)	Missed CA (*n*)
10 WA	10,000	228	20 WA	9,772	4,772	5,000
15 WA	10,000	1,587	25 WA	8,413	6,826	1,587
20 WA	10,000	5,000	30 WA	5,000	4,772	228
25 WA	10,000	8,413	35 WA	1,587	1,574	13
30 WA	10,000	9,772	40 WA	228	228	0
Total	50,000	25,000	Total	25,000	18,172	6,828

of 50,000 pregnant women (or equivalently, in this illustrative example, 50,000 abnormal fetuses). Each woman gets two US during her pregnancy at t and t+10. If the first examination turns out positive, then the follow-up is canceled. Assume further that the first US are uniformly distributed between the 10th and the 30th WA (see FIG. 3 and TABLE 1). At the end, 43,172 anomalies are detected corresponding to a 86.3% sensitivity.

Now let us change at the margin the women's follow-up, but leave the intrinsic characteristics of the test unchanged. There is no change for the first US (performed at time t). But now the second US is performed for half of the women at t+5 and for the remaining ones at t+10 (FIG. 4 and TABLE 2). The total number of detected malformations decrease to 38,965 and the sensitivity reaches only 77.9%.

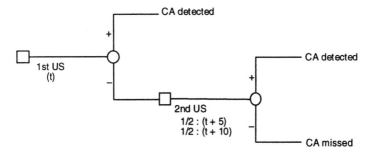

FIGURE 4. A protocol with two ultrasound examinations—(t; t + 5) for half of the women; (t; t + 10) for the other half.

TABLE 2. Number of Ultrasounds and CA Detected with Two Examinations Performed (t; t + 5) or (t; t + 10)

Time of First US	US (*n*)	CA Detected (*n*)	Time of Second US	US (*n*)	CA Detected (*n*)	Missed CA (*n*)
10 WA	10,000	228	15 WA	4,886	680	4,206
			20 WA	4,886	2,386	2,500
15 WA	10,000	1,587	20 WA	4,206	1,706	2,500
			25 WA	4,207	3,413	794
20 WA	10,000	5,000	25 WA	2,500	1,707	793
			30 WA	2,500	2,386	114
25 WA	10,000	8,413	30 WA	793	679	114
			35 WA	794	787	7
30 WA	10,000	9,772	35 WA	114	107	7
			40 WA	114	114	0
Total	50,000	25,000	Total	25,000	13,965	11,035

Using our model, we conclude that the test features do not change with the experimental setup and that we are capable of estimating the true parameters.

A MORE REALISTIC ILLUSTRATION

The previous example was very simple: we supposed a well-shaped distribution for τ, the US were uniformly spread during the pregnancy and the detection power of the test was very high (overall sensitivity was about 1). To move to a more realistic illustration, we need to consider a heterogeneous case (with at least two latent groups), to deal with a bimodal distribution of US during pregnancy, and to admit less favorable situations concerning the detection power of US. The bimodal distribution is necessary to accommodate the observed US distribution within the Eurofetus Research Project sample.

To analyze the behavior of our model, we conduct a Monte Carlo simulation. To simulate data, we proceed as follows: **(1)** We first keep 1,000 couples of dates between 10 and 40 WA. We choose two different shapes for US distributions over time (a uniform distribution as previously and a distribution with two modes [15 and 30 WA]). **(2)** Then we draw 1,000 values for τ from a mixed distribution (linear combination of two normal distributions (see TABLE 3 for the values of the parameters we impose). Depending on the simulated values of τ, by comparison with the dates at which examinations are performed, the malformation is detected either at the first US, or at the second US, or at delivery. As in the first example, when the anomaly is detected, the follow-up is interrupted. We repeat this data generation process 200 times. For each data set, we estimate our model and keep the values of estimated parameters and compute means and standard deviations (TABLE 3). We distinguish between two types of malformations: (1) those detectable during early pregnancy ($\mu_1=17$ WA, $\sigma_1=5$ WA) and (2) those only detectable during late pregnancy if detectable at all ($\mu_2=30$ WA, $\sigma_2=9$ WA). We also consider two models differing in the postulated proportions of malformations of both kinds. Model 1 (denoted M1 in TABLE 3) assumes that 70 and 30% of malformations are of the first and the second type, respectively. In contrast, model 2 (denoted M2) reverses both proportions.

These results show that the model yields reliable estimates independent of the assumed distribution of US. The least reliable estimates are obtain for μ_2 and σ_2. There

TABLE 3. Results of Simulation: US Distribution over Time

Model	True Values		Uniform Distribution		Bimodal Distribution	
			Mean	SD	Mean	SD
M1	α	0.70	0.749	0.078	0.753	0.084
	μ_1	17.0	17.27	0.74	17.21	0.71
	μ_2	30.0	32.46	2.85	32.74	3.47
	σ_1	5.0	4.99	0.57	5.01	0.53
	σ_2	9.0	7.20	2.09	6.56	2.59
M2	α	0.30	0.403	0.134	0.431	0.165
	μ_1	17.0	17.54	1.77	17.71	2.12
	μ_2	30.0	31.96	2.25	32.61	3.84
	σ_1	5.0	4.97	1.05	5.04	1.23
	σ_2	9.0	7.70	1.48	7.06	2.04

is also a slight bias in the estimated proportion of each type of malformations. Clearly, M1 performs better overall than M2.

WORKING WITH REAL DATA SETS

The Eurofetus Project

Because of the low incidence of fetal malformations (2 to 3% of all births), 56 maternity centers in 14 countries[f] take part in the Eurofetus Research Program. The selected centers have extensive experience in the field of pregnancy surveillance by ultrasound (with at least 3,000 examinations performed at the time of their inclusion in the study). They have good-quality equipment available and perform complete ultrasound examinations (precise control of the fetus's anatomy, identification of the major organs, and so forth). The observations refer to pregnant women who do not present a specific risk factor (systematic screening). These women are regularly treated in the referral center; they have at least one ultrasound between the 18th and the 22nd WA. Nevertheless, it appears that the centers did not strictly respect these criteria for inclusion.

The data were collected between January 1, 1990 and June 30, 1993. The data collection was organized as follows: Once a CA is suspected, the center gives notice of the case by filling in a first sheet. This sheet is immediately addressed to the team responsible for the epidemiological part of the study (sheet 1). In the course of the pregnancy, using the same process, the center points out every modification in the diagnosis based on new ultrasound pictures (sheet 2). Finally, after delivery, the center gives a precise description of the child's real state (clinical diagnosis and/or autopsy) (sheet 3). Thus, the information concerning the true positives is contained in sheets 1 and 2. The information concerning the false negatives is in sheet 3. The false positives can be identified by comparing the diagnosis figuring in sheets 1 and 2 with the one established at the end of the pregnancy.

In addition to the evolution of the diagnosis during pregnancy and the final state of the child, the sheets contain information on associated malformations (lateness of intrauterine growth, hydramnios, oligoamnios), on how the pregnancy was terminated, on prescribed supplementary examinations (in particular, establishment of the karyotype), on the ultrasound realization times before the suspicion.

In total, 7,331 cases were collected. After exclusion of incomplete files or of files related to referred patients, we kept records on 4,626 patients. Among them, 3,824 are related to fetuses presenting at least one malformation; 266 are false positives (the 526 remaining files refer to suspicions which have been invalidated during pregnancy, or to isolated chromosomal anomaly cases). These 3,834 fetuses present 4,824 malformations, which correspond to 1.26 malformation per fetus on average. Among the malformations, we distinguish major and minor malformations. Major malformations, if not lethal, lead to a severe handicap and, more often than not, to a therapeutic termination of the pregnancy. Minor malformations constitute a more heterogeneous category concerning the level of the associated handicap. To estimate the ultrasound sensitivity function, we have precise information available about the date of ultrasound as

---

[f] In parentheses, we list number of maternity centers taking part in the program: Austria (3), Belgium (5), Croatia (1), Finland (2), France (5), Italy (7), Luxembourg (1), the Netherlands (1), Norway (1), Poland (1), Portugal (9), Spain (9), Sweden (10), and the United Kingdom (1).

TABLE 4. Selection of the Data

	Lethal	Incurable	Curable	Minor	Total
Tumors	0	0	2	104	122
CNS	**209**	**460**	92	0	767
CHD	23	101	**785**	9	928
Facial anomalies	0	0	0	36	41
Genital organs	0	0	0	38	38
Ear and eye anomalies	0	13	6	4	23
Respiratory system	9	13	6	0	28
Lip and palate clefts	0	0	0	296	296
Gastrointestinal tract	0	20	199	3	230
Urinary tract	156	0	**661**	0	941
Muscle and skeleton system	3	74	268	**676**	1026
Multiple anomalies syndrome	115	0	17	0	132
Total	515	681	2036	1166	4572

well as about the diagnostic time concerning 4,572 malformations (that is to say 95% of the initial sample) (TABLE 4).

SELECTION OF THE DATA

From this sample of 4,572 CA, we keep only data on lethal and incurable malformations of the central nervous system (CNS) (detection rate: 91.6%), major curable congenital heart diseases (CHD) (detection rate: 26.4%), major curable urinary tract malformations (detection rate: 88.8%), and minor CA of the musculoskeletal system (detection rate: 19.8%) (TABLE 4).

For each group, we test for the number of distributions in the mixtures before estimating the model for each kind of malformation. We always accept a linear combination of two gamma distributions and reject adjunction of a third component in the mixture. Our results are presented in TABLES 5 and 6. The first column in TABLE 5 shows the proportion of CA detectable early in pregnancy. This proportion looks very different from one system to another and varies from 14.4% for musculoskeletal CA to 69.8% for CNS malformations. The time at which anomalies become detectable is also

TABLE 5. Maximum Likelihood Estimation

	δ	α_1	β_1	α_2	β_2
CNS	0.698	17.52	12.49	12.14	4.21
Lethal or incurable malformations	(0.115)	(5.94)	(4.77)	(8.21)	(2.34)
CHD	0.282	7.86	3.70	19.76	3.65
Major incurable malformations	(0.073)	(3.60)	(2.21)	(24.48)	(5.06)
Urinary tract	0.516	21.72	12.49	35.25	11.50
Major curable malformations	(0.105)	(9.41)	(6.21)	(12.95)	(3.76)
Muscle and skeleton system	0.144	15.05	9.45	1.20	0.04
Minor malformations	(0.042)	(11.38)	(7.30)	(0.48)	(0.04)

Numbers in parentheses represent standard errors of the estimators.

TABLE 6. Expectancy and Standard Deviation of the Occurrence Time and Overall Sensitivity

	$\mu1\,(\tau)$	$\sigma_1(\tau)$	$\mu_2(\tau)$	$\sigma_2(\tau)$	Overall Sensitivity (%)
CNS	14.03	3.35	28.83	8.28	97.1
Lethal or incurable malformations	(0.70)	(0.33)	(37.61)	(5.49)	
CHD	21.21	7.57	54.08	12.17	35.9
Major incurable malformations	(4.75)	(2.32)	(36.65)	(1.69)	
Urinary tract	17.40	3.73	30.67	5.17	97.9
Major curable malformations	(1.28)	(0.26)	(22.47)	(2.09)	
Muscle and skeleton system	15.92	4.10	286.15	261.64	22.3
Minor malformations	(1.21)	(0.20)	(∞)	(∞)	

Numbers in parentheses represent standard errors of the estimators.

very different among systems. We calculate average occurrence times and associated standard errors in TABLE 6. The estimation for the minor musculoskeletal CA looks less reliable given the low detection rate of such CA.

AN APPLICATION: A COST-EFFECTIVENESS ANALYSIS OF SCREENING FOR MAJOR MALFORMATIONS

In this final section, we illustrate one use of the model by using the estimated sensitivity function in a cost-effectiveness analysis of screening for major malformations. FIGURE 5 presents the ultrasound sensitivity function for major CA and its 95% confidence interval. With all severe malformations, τ's density has the shape of a unimodal

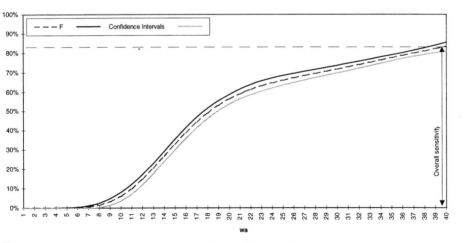

FIGURE 5. Ultrasound sensitivity function—major CA.

TABLE 7. Conditional Mean and Standard Deviation of τ—Major CA

	All Major CA	Type 1 CAs	Type 2 CAs
$E(\tau\|\tau \leq 40$ WA$)$	18.94 WA	15.22 WA	30.29 WA
$\sigma(\tau\|\tau \leq 40$ WA$)$	8.09 WA	4.19 WA	6.40 WA

distribution with a fat tail on the right. To facilitate the interpretation of the central moments, we consider the density, which is conditional to the fact that the detectability time happens before 40 WA. In other words, the malformation is detectable thanks to the ultrasound (TABLE 7).

The objectives of prenatal screening for fetal malformations by ultrasound are threefold. First, US reduces the occurrence of births with incurable major malformations. Second, it directs therapeutic attitudes. The screening allows for the avoidance of some unnecessary actions (e.g., cesarean in case of lethal malformation); sometimes it allows an early medical follow-up of the affected child (e.g., to place a valve *in utero* in case of hydrocephalus); it gives the opportunity to admit the mother into an adequate facility for the delivery; finally, it sometimes makes the prenatal diagnosis easier (e.g., certain urinary tract anomalies are more easily visible before rather than after birth). Third, the screening reassures the pregnant woman about the state of her baby. When a malformation is detected, it allows the parents to accept the loss of a baby who is terminally ill or to better prepare for the arrival of a baby presenting a minor malformation.

The statement of these objectives leads us to select the following three effectiveness indicators: the detection rate, the average detection time (in WA), and the latest detection time (in WA). The first indicator evaluates the screening capacity to detect the fetuses presenting a malformation. The second indicator measures the earliness of detection (for medical and psychological reasons, it is better to detect a malformation at the beginning of the pregnancy rather than at the end). The third indicator refers to the legal provisions forbidding the termination of the pregnancy in certain countries beyond a certain stage. These legislative provisions reflect the society's point of view concerning the coming baby's status. As far as the cost measurement is concerned, we use the number of scheduled ultrasounds and not the number of ultrasounds effectively performed.

Once the ultrasound sensitivity function for fetal malformation screening is known and the effectiveness criterion is determined, we calculate the dates of US examinations which, for a given protocol (one, two, or three ultrasounds per pregnancy), allow to maximize the detection rate and/or to minimize the average detection time. By successively considering all relevant values of the parameters of the problem, we precisely establish the relation between the rate of malformation detection and the average detection time.

The objective is, for a given protocol, to determine the optimal time of examination to maximize the detection rate while keeping the average detection time constant. Or, stated differently, to minimize the average detection time for a given detection rate. The latest detection time does not explicitly appear in the optimization program anymore. Indeed, the hypothesis that the malformation does not regress during the pregnancy makes this indicator redundant compared with the detection rate. Because of the sensitivity function's monotonicity (in a weak sense), the realization date of the latest examination determines the percentile of detected malformations. By considering a protocol with n ultrasounds (whatever n), and by fixing a priori the detection rate γ, we determine the optimal realization dates for the examinations by solving the following program:

$$\underset{t_1,\ldots,t_n}{\text{Min}} \frac{\sum_{i=1}^{n} t_i[F(t_i) - F(t_{i-1})]}{F(t_n)}$$

subject to $F(t_n) = \gamma$

In this problem, we search after the ultrasound realization times which allow to minimize the average detection time under the constraint of a defined detection rate. The average detection time is calculated thanks to the weighting of the ultrasound realization dates by the percentage of detected malformations at each examination $[F(t_i) - F(t_{i-1})]$ represents the increment of the detection rate allowed by the realization of a supplementary ultrasound in t_i].

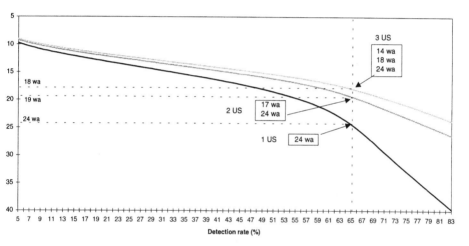

FIGURE 6. Relation between the average detection time and detection rate with respect to number of examinations.

FIGURE 6 presents the optimization results for the severe malformations. It gives the optimal dates of ultrasound examination as well as the average detection time for a detection rate which varies from 5 to 83% (total ultrasound sensitivity for the considered malformations, to be compared with the 73% apparent sensitivity), and for each of the considered protocols (from one to three ultrasounds). To detect 65% of the malformations, it is necessary that the last ultrasound be performed during the 24th WA; if a second examination is allowed, this one must be performed during the 17th week, and from 24.29 WA, the average detection time becomes 19.33 WA. For a protocol with three ultrasounds, the examinations are performed during the 14th, 18th, and 24th week; the average detection time declines to 17.92 WA. In this figure, it is apparent that the detection rate and detection earliness evolve in an opposite way.

REFERENCE

1. EDDY, D. 1980. Screening for Cancer: Theory, Analysis and Design. Prentice-Hall. Englewood Cliffs, NJ.

Detection of Chromosomal Abnormalities, an Outcome of Ultrasound Screening

HÉLÈNE GRANDJEAN,[a] DANIÈLE LARROQUE,[a] SALVATOR LEVI,[b] AND THE EUROFETUS TEAM

[a]INSERM, Hôpital La Grave, Toulouse, France
[b]Brugmann Hospital, Brussels, Belgium

ABSTRACT: Chromosomal abnormalities were recorded from all the fetuses of women who benefited from sonographic examinations in the Eurofetus centers, excluding those for whom karyotyping was motivated by age or personal history. Among the 378 chromosomal abnormalities recorded, 210 were detected before birth (sensitivity = 55.6%). Down syndrome (trisomy 21) represented 197 cases, of which 68 were detected before birth (sensitivity = 34.5%). Eighty-two of the cases of Down syndrome had associated structural abnormalities; the sensitivity in these cases increased to 57%. Among the 115 cases of Down syndrome without structural abnormalities, 21 (18.3%) had associated abnormal ultrasound findings that led to prenatal detection. Sensitivity of prenatal detection was 58.1% for trisomy 13 and 79% for trisomy 18. For the abnormalities detected before birth, spontaneous fetal death occurred in 27% of cases, and an early termination of pregnancy was decided in 53% of cases.

INTRODUCTION

Chromosomal abnormalities are commonly associated with structural malformations and/or abnormalities in development of the fetus and annexes. Such deformations can in principle be detected by routine echographic examination. Furthermore, sonography can be employed to guide fetal biopsy for detection of chromosomal abnormalities at any gestational age. Generalization of sonographic monitoring of pregnancy should thus lead to improvements in the antenatal detection of chromosomal abnormalities. We evaluated here the performance of echography from the data in the Eurofetus multicenter prospective survey.

MATERIALS AND METHODS

Over the study period, from January 1, 1990 to June 30, 1993, we recorded prospectively all cases of fetal chromosomal abnormalities in patients booked in the 60 centers participating in the Eurofetus survey, apart from those referred for karyotyping because of maternal risk factors (age, biochemical findings, personal or family history). We also excluded patients referred for abnormal echographic findings, as well as those who gave birth to an infant bearing an abnormality but who had not benefited from echographic examination in the participating centers. Overall, 378 infants with chromosomal abnormalities were analyzed.

RESULTS

Out of the 378 cases with chromosomal abnormalities, 210 were diagnosed during pregnancy, giving an overall detection sensitivity of 55.6% (95% confidence interval [CI

95%]: 50.6–60.6%). Out of these 210 cases, 168 (80%) were diagnosed with one or more structural malformations detected during pregnancy, and 12 with retarded growth, associated in some cases with abnormal volume of amniotic fluid. In the remaining 31, echography detected minor morphological defects, which were not considered to be true malformations, but which were an index of a potential chromosomal abnormality (increase in nuchal skinfold, shortened limbs, facial dysmorphia, hydrops, dilatation of cerebral ventricles).

Out of the 168 infants undiagnosed before birth, 20 (12%) had been recognized as being malformed on antenatal echographic examination but had not benefited from karyotyping, 47 (28%) had one or more structural malformations that had not been detected, 22 (13%) had intrauterine growth retardation and/or a abnormal volume of amniotic fluid, which had been noted on echographic examination but without motivating karyotyping, and 78 (47%) had no prior signs. All the latter cases apart from two were trisomy 21. In total, 93% of the cases of trisomies 13 and 18 presented structural abnormalities versus only 41% for trisomy 21. The detection sensitivity depended on the type of chromosomal abnormality (TABLE 1). Among the trisomies, trisomy 18 was the best detected (79%) followed by trisomy 13 (58.1%), whereas trisomy 21 was only detected in 34.5% of cases.

The diagnoses were made on average at 20.0 ± 7.1 weeks; the only abnormality detected at a much earlier age was Turner syndrome (15.6 ± 2.3 weeks) due to its frequent association with hygroma colli detectable during the first trimester (20 cases out of 26). All the cases of Turner syndrome were detected before 24 weeks, compared to 68% for the other chromosomal abnormalities.

The outcome of the infants depended on whether the chromosomal abnormality was detected before or after birth. Out of the detected cases, 27% died *in utero,* 53% led to an elective termination, 12% died in labor or in the first six postnatal days, and 8% were alive six days after birth. The outcomes as a function of the type of chromosomal abnormality are listed in TABLE 2. All the detected cases of trisomies 13 and 18 died either *in utero* or before the sixth postnatal day. Ten of the undetected cases were alive after day 6, although most of these infants died within the following two months. An overall survival rate of 95% was noted for the undetected cases of trisomy 21, versus

TABLE 1. Sensitivity for Detection of Chromosomal Abnormalities by Echographic Screening

	ICD 9 Codes	Cases (*n*)	Abnormalities Detected (*n*)	Sensitivity (%)
Down syndrome (trisomy 21)	7580	197	68	34.5
Edwards syndrome (trisomy 13)	7581	31	18	58.1
Patau's syndrome (trisomy 18)	7582	81	64	79.0
Turner syndrome (X0)	7586	29	26	89.7
Other abnormalities	7585, 7587, 7588, 7589	40	34	85.0
Total		378	210	55.6

TABLE 2. Outcome of Infants with Chromosomal Abnormalities as a Function of Age at Diagnosis

		Alive Infants		Total Deaths		Induced Terminations	
		n	%	*n*	%	*n*	%
T21	Diagnosed	14	21	54	79	37	54
	Not diagnosed	122	95	7	5	0	0
T13	Diagnosed	0	0	18	100	10	56
	Not diagnosed	5	38	8	62	1	8
T18	Diagnosed	0	0	64	100	27	42
	Not diagnosed	5	29	12	71	1	6
XO	Diagnosed	0	0	26	100	20	77
	Not diagnosed	3	100	0	0		0
Other	Diagnosed	4	12	30	88	16	47
	Not diagnosed	2	33	4	67	0	0
Total	Diagnosed	18	9	192	91	110	53
	Not diagnosed	137	82	31	18	2	1

21% for the detected cases, the diagnosis only being made before 24 weeks in 2 out of these 14 cases.

Overall, 7.1% (CI 95%: 6.4–7.9%) of the structural malformations recorded in the survey were associated with a chromosomal abnormality. The frequency of association with a chromosomal abnormality depended on the type of malformation. It was only 2.9% for the urinary tract malformations, but rose to 9.7% for the cardiac malformations and 43.8% for the endocardial cushion defect, which is associated with trisomy 21 in a majority of cases (90%). The frequency was also high for hygroma colli (46.5%) and for the multiple malformations (33.7%) and omphalocele (17.1%).

DISCUSSION

Analysis of the detection of chromosomal abnormalities in the Eurofetus survey gives an indication of the value of ultrasound screening in the identification of chromosomal abnormalities, especially when associated to morphological abnormalities. Most of the reported studies on the association of malformations with chromosomal abnormalities have been carried out on rather small series[1-5] apart from that of Nicolaïdes et al.[6] The frequency of the chromosomal abnormalities associated with malformations ranged from 14 to 25% depending on the series.[1-6] In our series, the frequency of chromosomal abnormalities associated with echographic abnormalities was found to be 7.1%, which is much lower than the previously reported figures. Several possibilities may account for this difference. First, the chromosomal abnormalities referred to the total number of structural abnormalities recorded in the Eurofetus database whether they had been detected before or after birth and whether or not they had motivated karyotyping. In the reported studies on the association between structural abnormalities and chromosomal abnormalities, only the cases in which karyotyping was carried out were considered, which thus excluded the structural abnormalities not thought to be associated with any chromosomal abnomality. A high proportion of in-

TABLE 3. Frequency of Association of Chromosomal Abnormalities with Structural Malformations

| | Chromosomal Abnormalities | | | | | | Structural Abnormalities | |
	T21 (*n*)	T13 (*n*)	T18 (*n*)	XO (*n*)	Other (*n*)	Total (*n*)	(*n*)	(% association)
Central nervous system	5	9	10	1	13	38	738	5.1
Heart and vessels	39	9	28	8	8	86	953	9.0
Cleft lip and palates	3	9	2	0	4	18	316	5.7
Digestive system	12	1	3	0	0	16	229	7.0
Urinary tract	9	4	5	1	9	28	954	2.9
Musculoskeletal system	5	11	33	0	8	57	1043	5.5
Hygroma colli	16	1	8	20	2	47	101	46.5
Multiple congenital abnormalities	3	8	16	2	4	33	98	33.7
Miscellaneous	2	2		1	1	6		
Total	94	54	105	27	49	329	4615	7.1

fants with structural abnormalities in our study were not subjected to karyotyping during pregnancy: this included most of the infants who were not identified as malformed during pregnancy, as well as 20% of the live born who were diagnosed during pregnancy. It is unlikely that any cases of trisomy were missed in the live births because they are readily identifiable. However, there was probably a significant number of infants with minor chromosomal abnormalities who were either never detected or detected at a much later time. In addition, some of the infants who died *in utero*, for whom karyotyping was not performed, may well have harbored a chromosomal abnormality.

The wide range of structural abnormalities associated with chromosomal abnormalities in our series and the frequency of the associations support the current practice of proposing karyotyping to all pregnant women bearing a child with an echographically detectable abnormality.

Overall, we found a detection sensitivity of chromosomal abnormalities of 55.6%, a better result than those observed by Stoll *et al.*[7] A proportion of the undetected cases (20 out of 168, or 12%) were those in which a structural abnormality had been detected on echographic examination but without motivating karyotyping. Adding the 47 with malformations whose diagnosis was missed at echographic examination, we can estimate that antenatal sonography could reveal three-quarters of chromosomal abnormalities and nearly all cases of trisomies 13 and 18. On the other hand, a significant proportion of cases of trisomy 21, 60% in our series, did not present with any associated structural abnormalities. Improvement in detection thus hinges on utilization of indirect signs such as shortened limbs and thickened nuchal skinfold. In our study, 16% of the cases of trisomy 21 were diagnosed with the help of these markers.

REFERENCES

1. GAGNON, S., W. FRASER, B. FOUQUETTE, A. BASTIDE, M. BUREAU, J.Y. FONTAINE & C. HUOT. 1992. Nature and frequency of chromosomal abnormalities in pregnancies with ab-

normal ultrasound findings: An analysis of 117 cases with review of the literature. Prenatal Diagn. **12:** 9–18.

2. TWINNING, P. & J. ZUCCOLLO. 1993. The ultrasound markers of chromosomal disease: A retrospective study. Br. J. Radiol. **66:** 408–414.

3. DEN HOLLANDER, N.S., T.E. COHEN OVERBEEK, R. HEYDANUS, P.A. STEWART, H. BRANDENBURG, F.L. LOS, M.G. JAHODA & J.W. WLADIMIROFF. 1994. Cordocentesis for rapid karyotyping in fetuses with congenital anomalies or severe IUGR. Eur. J. Obstet. Gynecol. Reprod. Biol. **53:** 183–187.

4. MEAGHER, S., R. RENSHAW, A. SMITH & J. MILLIGAN. 1994. Chromosomal abnormalities detected after an abnormal ultrasound in pregnancy. Clin. Exp. Obstet. Gynecol. **21:** 215–220.

5. CLAUSSEN, U., R. ULMER, E. BEINDER & H.J.L. VOIGT. 1994. Six years' experience with rapid karyotyping in prenatal diagnosis: Correlations between phenotype detected by ultrasound and fetal karyotype. Prenatal Diagn. **14:** 113–121.

6. NICOLAIDES, K.H., R.J. SNIJDERS, C.M. GOSDEN, C. BERRY & S. CAMPBEL. 1992. Ultrasonographic markers of fetal chromosomal abnormalities. Lancet **340:** 704–707.

7. STOLL, C., B. DOTT, Y. ALEMBIK & M.P. ROTH. 1993. Evaluation of routine prenatal ultrasound examination in detecting fetal chromosomal abnormalities in a low risk population. Hum. Genet. **91:** 37–41.

Reduced Costs of Congenital Anomalies from Fetal Ultrasound: Are They Sufficient to Justify Routine Screening in the United States?

NORMAN J. WAITZMAN[a,c] AND PATRICK S. ROMANO[b]

[a]*Department of Economics, University of Utah, Salt Lake City, Utah, USA*
[b]*Departments of Medicine and Pediatrics, University of California, Davis, Davis, California, USA*

ABSTRACT: No comprehensive benefit-to-cost analysis has been performed to date on a policy of routine ultrasound screening for fetal anomalies in the United States. We performed a preliminary benefit-to-cost analysis drawing upon our previous research on the cost of birth defects in the United States and upon the literature regarding (1) the sensitivity of ultrasound in detecting congenital anomalies, (2) the rate at which pregnancies are terminated upon detection of fetal anomalies, (3) the number of ultrasounds performed per pregnancy under a routine screening policy, and (4) the average cost of an ultrasound. We assumed a 100% subsequent replacement rate of terminated pregnancies with a normal child, an assumption most favorable to routine screening. The benefit-to-cost ratio ranged from .33 to 3, suggesting that a routine screening policy for fetal anomalies is of uncertain net societal benefit. Routine screening may be justified, however, based on standards that elude the methods for establishing societal benefits adopted in this analysis.

INTRODUCTION

The medical care environment internationally has become much more sensitized to cost over the past decade with the ongoing fiscal crisis in public budgets and soaring medical care costs. Recognition is rapidly growing that although ever more can be done to contribute to health status in the delivery of medical care, current fiscal constraints increasingly impress upon providers to justify interventions in terms of underlying costs. This is part of the impetus behind the recent proliferation of federally supported medical outcome studies in the United States and the call for developing more practice guidelines drawing upon the evidence from such studies.

The controversy over routine ultrasound screening during pregnancy has emerged within this fiscal context. Ultrasound screening in the United States is currently performed on a widespread basis, but not universally. Data from natality records in 1995 show that ultrasound was performed in the course of pregnancy for at least 61% of live births in the U.S.,[1] up from 58% in 1992 and 48% in 1989.[2] The National Institutes of Health Consensus Conference on Ultrasound Imaging in Pregnancy in 1984 concluded that targeted screening was justified for several indications, but that the potential benefits of routine screening did not outweigh the risks.[3] A more recent assessment by the U.S. Preventive Services Task Force largely reaffirmed those guidelines.[4] The literature demonstrates that ultrasound screening may produce a wide array of benefits in the

[c]Address correspondence to Norman J. Waitzman, Ph.D., Department of Economics, University of Utah, 1645 E Central Campus Dr.-Front, Salt Lake City, UT 84112-9300. E-mail: waitzman@econ.sbs.utah.edu

management and outcomes of pregnancy,[4-5] including the detection of many structural congenital anomalies within the first 24 weeks when termination of pregnancy (TOP) in the United States is still a viable option. Some researchers have conjectured that, given the large cost of birth defects, routine ultrasound may be economically justified strictly on the basis of the costs that would be averted by terminating affected pregnancies.[5]

No study to date has systematically addressed how the reduction in birth defect costs through routine ultrasound compares to the costs of screening. Until now, a major impediment to such a study has been the paucity of comprehensive research on the cost of birth defects. We recently undertook the most comprehensive study to date of the societal costs associated with 17 of the most significant congenital anomalies and cerebral palsy,[6,7] and found that the total annual cost of birth defects to the nation was about $8 billion in 1992. Our cost study serves as the foundation for the preliminary assessment of the benefit-to-cost relationship for routine screening provided here.

METHODOLOGY

This benefit-to-cost assessment of routine ultrasound screening focuses strictly on the cost savings associated with reducing congenital anomalies by terminating pregnancies. Clearly, there are other potential benefits to routine ultrasound screening which a full analysis would address, including cost-reducing changes in the clinical management of pregnancies when a birth defect is detected. Of course, such interventions could also increase cost if the associated benefit is relatively small or if they require intensive resource utilization. The evidence in this area is mixed and incomplete. The theoretical benefits of antenatal maternal transport to centers with neonatal intensive care and surgical capabilities are largely unproven. A meta-analysis showed no significant effects of ultrasound on perinatal morbidity.[8] Certain resource-intensive interventions, such as fetal surgery, are relatively rare and in the experimental stage. TOP is certainly the most prevalent change in management resulting from screening in 1997.

Incremental Analysis

In considering the practice of routine screening, the analysis would ideally be based on the incremental benefit-to-cost relationship in newly screening pregnant women who currently are not screened in the United States, rather than on the average benefit-to-cost relationship for all ultrasound screening performed when adopted as universal practice. Although we attempt to construct an incremental framework, the demands of such an analysis pose certain methodological and data problems, which we discuss in more detail below. In any case, we assume that a policy of routine screening would not change the average number of fetal ultrasounds performed in the population that is already screened. This assumption may be conservative in terms of the actual costs associated with a routine screening policy, because reimbursement policies for multiple screens for certain current indications may be relaxed further upon the adoption of such a policy.

Formal Conceptualization of Benefit and Cost

The benefit-cost relationship upon which the analysis was based can be summarized in two simple equations, one for the benefit (BENEFIT), the other for cost (COST).

The benefit is the total cost of birth defects that would be recouped through early detection by fetal ultrasound and depends, in addition to the cost of birth defects, upon the sensitivity of ultrasound in detecting fetal anomalies, and upon the behavioral response of women to information provided by screening. This relationship can be formalized as

$$\text{BENEFIT} = \Sigma_i \ \text{TC}_i[(\text{pSCR}_i \times \text{pDET}_i \times \text{pTOP}_i) - \text{pFDEATH}_i] \qquad (1)$$

where, for each birth defect, i, TC is the total cost associated with the defect; pSCR is the probability of being screened under a routine policy; pDET is the probability of detection of the defect through routine ultrasound in the first 24 weeks of pregnancy when TOP is still a viable option in most states, minus the probability of detection through other routinely administered screening; pTOP is the probability that a woman will elect to terminate the pregnancy based upon information from screening; and pFDEATH is the probability that pregnancies terminated upon detection of fetal anomalies would have resulted in fetal death or stillbirth in any case.

Our estimates of the cost of newborns with birth defects (TC_i) did not include maternity costs. For each aborted fetus that would have otherwise resulted in a live birth, an additional term should be incorporated equal to either the average cost of an abortion or the difference in the average cost of a normal delivery and the average cost of an abortion depending upon whether the child is "replaced," as discussed below. For those cases that would have resulted in fetal death had the fetus not been aborted, the difference between the average cost of an abortion and a fetal death should be subtracted from the benefit equation. If the term in parentheses above, (pSCR × pDET × pTOP − pFDEATH), is set equal to Z, then a revised benefit equation recognizing these refinements can be rewritten as

$$\text{BENEFIT} = \Sigma_i \ \text{TC}_i(Z_i) + \Sigma_i \ [(Z_i \times \$\text{DEL}_i) - \$\text{AB}_i] - \Sigma_i \ [(\text{pFDEATH}_i \times \$\text{AB}_i) - \$\text{FDEATH}_i] \qquad (2)$$

where $\$\text{DEL}_i$ is equal to the number of infants born with a particular birth defect multiplied by the average cost of a normal delivery in the case of zero "replacement," zero otherwise; $\$\text{AB}_i$ is the total cost of all TOPs performed for fetuses with the defect, and $\$\text{FDEATH}_i$ is the total costs associated with fetal deaths that would have taken place had the fetuses with the defect not been aborted. The terms $\$\text{DEL}$, $\$\text{AB}$, and $\$\text{FDEATH}$ would appropriately include an estimate of the value of maternal time devoted to the pregnancy for each respective outcome. The preliminary analysis provided below ignored the issue of fetal deaths (pFDEATH, and therefore $\$\text{FDEATH}$), given the absence of reliable data. The incorporation of cost differentials between normal deliveries and termination of pregnancy summarized in the second term of equation 2, had little impact on the analysis, as discussed below. The analysis therefore effectively adopted equation 1 without significantly altering the findings.

Turning to the cost side of the ledger, the central cost is the number of ultrasounds performed multiplied by the average cost of each ultrasound. There may be additional costs generated by other tests that are performed as a result of the ultrasound. Formally,

$$\text{COST} = \#\text{PREG} \times [\#\text{ULT/PREG} \times (\$\text{ULT} + \text{OTHCOST})] \qquad (3)$$

where COST is the total cost of routine ultrasound screening; #PREG is the number of pregnancies in the population to be newly routinely screened; #ULT/PREG is the average number of ultrasounds per pregnancy that results from routine screening in that population; $ULT is the average cost of an ultrasound, which ideally would include the average time cost to the patient for screening in addition to the value of resources used by providers; and OTHCOST, which is the average cost per ultrasound of other tests and procedures, such as fetal echocardiograms and amniocentesis, which are prescribed based upon ultrasound findings. We ignore OTHCOST in the preliminary analysis below, which makes our estimate of the cost of screening conservative.

The cost equation, as well as our analysis, also ignores the issue of aborting normal fetuses as a result of false positive screening results. False positives are relatively rare and generally arise in the case of relatively minor defects unlikely to be aborted.[5,9] Furthermore, the TOP based on false information certainly carries with it emotional costs, but these are not readily captured under the human capital approach that we adopted.

Estimation of Components

Estimation of Benefit Components (TC_i)

We conducted the most comprehensive study to date on the lifetime costs associated with 17 birth defects and cerebral palsy.[7] Cerebral palsy is only manifest after birth and is not detectable through fetal ultrasound, so it was excluded from the current analysis. The birth conditions for which we estimated costs are listed in TABLE 1 along with summary cost information. Societal costs were estimated for each condition based on the human capital approach, which regards expenditures for medical care and education as "investments" in human capital that are partly justified based on enhanced future economic returns, or productivity, similar to investments in physical capital. Resources, such as medical care, used or "invested" beyond the average per capita expenditure, are "direct" costs associated with an illness or injury, whereas the reduction in future returns or productivity due to heightened morbidity or premature mortality are "indirect" costs.

We estimated the lifetime direct costs of medical care, special education, and developmental services; and indirect costs associated with heightened morbidity and premature mortality for the cohort of children born with any of the listed defects in California in 1988. The estimates, based on the incidence approach, lend themselves to the analysis of prevention strategies. A detailed description of methods and data sources used for the analysis is provided elsewhere.[7] The direct and indirect cost figures provided in columns 1 and 2 in TABLE 1 reflect the 1988 California cohort estimates projected to the nation in 1992 based upon compensation differences between California relative to the rest of the country, and upon changes in medical care and employee compensation indices between 1988 and 1992. All costs beyond the first year of life were discounted back to the year of birth at a 5% rate, reflecting the economic assumption that current consumption is valued higher than future consumption.

Several additional adjustments were made to the cost estimates for the economic analysis of routine ultrasound screening. All estimates were standardized to a rate per 100,000 pregnancies (#PREG) subject to routine screening. The estimates of incidence per 100,000 pregnancies given in the first column of TABLE 2 were derived from data provided by the California Birth Defects Monitoring Program (CBDMP), one of the largest active surveillance programs for birth defects worldwide. These data were adjusted to estimate the birth prevalence of unduplicated cases (column 2, TABLE 2) based as well on information from CBDMP. Cases of multiple defects were assigned to the defect category with the highest average cost, assuming that multiple defect cases cost at least as much as the average case in that category.

Adjustments also were made to incorporate an underlying counterfactual regarding

TABLE 1. Cost of Birth Defects in the United States

Condition	Direct Costs[a]	Indirect Costs[b]	Total Costs	Cost per Case
Spina bifida	247,965	241,324	489,289	294
Truncus arteriosus	108,180	101,496	209,676	505
Transposition/DORV	170,735	343,794	514,529	267
Tetralogy of Fallot	189,096	171,390	360,486	262
Single ventricle	62,530	110,101	172,631	344
Cleft lip or palate	117,613	578,888	696,501	101
TE fistula	61,588	103,444	165,002	145
Atresia, small intestine	63,156	46,905	110,061	75
Colorectal atresia	57,213	162,049	219,262	123
Renal agenesis	24,713	399,466	424,159	250
Urinary obstruction	46,294	296,929	343,223	84
Upper-limb reduction	35,417	134,619	170,036	99
Lower-limb reduction	28,411	138,656	167,067	199
Diaphragmatic hernia	62,772	301,576	364,348	250
Gastroschisis	54,520	54,243	108,763	108
Omphalocele	27,871	104,133	132,004	176
Down syndrome	667,684	1,180,068	1,847,752	451
Cerebral palsy	1,296,426	1,129,355	2,425,781	503
Total	2,991,818	5,038,854	8,030,672	N/A

NOTE: Cost expressed in 1,000s of 1992 dollars. Figures are based on lifetime direct and indirect cost estimates for the 1988 birth cohort in California adjusted for differences in births and costs between California and the nation, as well as for cost inflation between 1988 and 1992. Costs beyond the first year of life were discounted back to the year of birth at a 5% discount rate. Column totals are less than column sums because total cost estimates reflect a downward adjustment in order to avoid double counting due to multiple conditions per case.
[a] Medical care, special education, and developmental services.
[b] Lost productivity due to premature mortality and heightened morbidity.
(From Waitzman et al.[7])

a "replacement child." Cost estimates of a routine screening program depend, first, on the extent to which a pregnancy is assumed to be an independent event versus one that is tied to a potential replacement pregnancy, and second, on the actual rate, timing, and outcome of such replacement. If the pregnancy is regarded as an independent event, then an assumption of zero replacement is appropriate. In the event of such zero replacement, only the direct costs of birth defects are averted through TOP. Because individuals born with birth defects have some household and labor market productivity, there are indirect costs with TOP relative to a child born with birth defects equal to the value of that productivity.

The TC associated with each birth defect under the assumption of zero replacement is therefore the net difference between the value of the average lifetime productivity of individuals with that defect minus the lifetime direct costs expended on those individuals, including what would be expended on normal children. We recalculated our cost estimates under a zero replacement assumption, and found that, with the exception of children born with Down syndrome and one cardiac anomaly, TOP is a net *cost* to society in lost productivity rather than a net benefit. The assumption of zero replacement, therefore, militates against a routine ultrasound policy to detect birth defects based strictly upon reducing net societal costs.

If the pregnancy is regarded instead as a tied rather than an independent event, there is a certain probability that parents who elect to terminate a pregnancy based on the

TABLE 2. Incidence of Birth Defects and Cost of Unduplicated Cases Assuming 100% Replacement with Normal Children One Year after TOP

Condition	Cases per 100,000 Live Births	Non-multiple Cases per 100,000	Cost per Case[a]	Total Cost per 100,000 Cases
Spina bifida	42.4	42.4	295.3	12,520
Truncus arteriosus	10.6	8.9	506.3	4,503
Transposition/DORV	49.3	41.3	267.5	11,038
Tetralogy of Fallot	35.0	29.2	263.0	7,677
Single ventricle	12.8	11.1	344.7	3,825
Cleft lip or palate	177.0	159.0	101.6	16,149
TE fistula	29.0	22.7	145.3	3,291
Atresia, small intestine	37.6	21.8	74.8	1,631
Colorectal atresia	45.4	26.5	122.9	3,253
Renal agenesis	43.3	39	249.9	9.977
Urinary obstruction	104.1	99.8	84.5	8,436
Upper-limb reduction	43.9	34.2	98.9	3,378
Lower-limb reduction	21.5	16.8	199.8	3,355
Diaphragmatic hernia	37.1	33.7	250.5	8,448
Gastroschisis	25.5	20.5	108.7	2,223
Omphalocele	19.1	15.4	176.4	2,709
Down syndrome	104.6	104.6	451.9	47,269
Total				**149,682**

NOTE: Cost expressed in 1,000s of 1992 dollars.

[a] Cost per case differs slightly from those reported in TABLE 1 because the estimates reported there assumed prevention of birth defects, that is, simultaneous replacement with a normal child. The figures reported in TABLE 2 assume 100% replacement with a normal child one year after TOP. Costs and productivity associated with the normal child are therefore discounted by one extra year which, in this case, has the net effect of slightly increasing cost estimates. These are maximum estimates. A longer average delay and a lower average rate of replacement would reduce the per case estimates below those reported in TABLE 1.

(From Waitzman et al.[7])

diagnosis of a structural anomaly will subsequently decide to conceive again and produce a "replacement" child.[10] To the extent that such replacement children are born without major anomalies, both the direct and indirect costs associated with birth defects would appropriately be counted as a potential benefit to be recouped through TOP. This replacement scenario is most favorable to routine screening; to provide a "most favorable" estimate of the benefit from such screening, we assume a 100% replacement rate.

Our cost estimates were discounted present lifetime estimates of prevention and therefore implicitly assumed simultaneous replacement with normal children. The added time between TOP and replacement therefore required certain adjustments to our estimates. The delayed birth of the replacement child created lower discounted present values both for resources the individual consumes and produces relative to an earlier birth of a child with a birth defect. Hence, the net direct costs of children born with birth defects are higher, and the indirect costs lower, the longer the period between TOP and replacement. Cost per case figures in TABLE 2, based on the assumption of a one-year average delay for replacement, therefore are slightly higher than those reported in TABLE 1, based on simultaneous replacement. Longer delays would have produced smaller cost per case estimates.

Of course, there is likely to be a certain level of "replacement" as well for children with birth defects who die in the perinatal period. Moreover, parents who have children who survive with major congenital anomalies may decide to have additional children based upon their experience. The actual relative rate of replacement and the timing and actual outcomes of subsequent pregnancies are important in determining the actual extent to which the upper bound limit provided by our 100% replacement assumption is achieved.

Multiplying the cost per case estimates in column 3 of TABLE 2 by the estimates of unduplicated cases per 100,000 pregnancies in column 2 yields the total costs that would be averted per 100,000 pregnancies in the final column of the table. The sum of the figures in the column yields $149.7 million, the maximum benefit of screening per 100,000 pregnancies if 100% of the listed anomalies were detected through fetal ultrasound screening and subsequently terminated and replaced by normal children one year after TOP.

Estimation of Benefit Components (pSCR)

We assumed 100% compliance with screening so as to assess the benefit among the screened population.

Estimation of Benefit Components (pDET)

The sensitivity of ultrasound in detecting congenital anomalies varies widely depending upon the age of the fetus, the skills and training of the person performing the exam, the time devoted to the exam, the type of anomaly, and the organ system affected, among other factors. In the largest randomized control trial to date in the United States on routine screening, the Routine Antenatal Diagnostic Imaging with Ultrasound (RADIUS) trial, 16.6% of anomalies were detected prior to 24 weeks' gestation in the routinely screened group compared to 4.9% in the control group, a net detection rate of 11.7%.[11] Recent reviews of the literature show gross sensitivities ranging from 16.6% in the RADIUS study to 40–60% in several studies conducted in New Zealand and Europe to as high as 74.4% in one study conducted in the United Kingdom.[5,12,13] Preliminary data from the Eurofetus study show a gross sensitivity of about 44% within 24 weeks.[14] Overall sensitivities are much higher for central nervous system anomalies than for cardiac, skeletal, and craniofacial anomalies.[12] The lower overall sensitivity in the RADIUS trial than in European series is largely attributable to the relative prevalence of anomalies in the population and the broader definition of "major anomalies" in RADIUS. We chose a range of net sensitivity of detection for the current analysis of 20 to 50%, with the lower bound being above the average sensitivity from the RADIUS trial, and with the upper bound approximating the net sensitivity of the best performance in most European trials.

We applied this range across all defects, even though the sensitivity of ultrasound screening is far greater for central nervous system defects such as spina bifida than for congenital heart defects or Down syndrome. The fact that some of the most costly defects fit both into the high- and low-sensitivity range mitigates the need for greater refinement in the application of sensitivity rates to particular defects. Furthermore, central nervous system defects are more amenable to detection through maternal alpha fetoprotein screening (MSAFP) than are heart defects, so the net sensitivity of ultrasound in detecting central nervous system defects is substantially less than the gross sensitivity.

Estimation of Benefit Components (pTOP)

There are no reliable, comprehensive data on elective TOP in the U.S. based on detection of congenital anomalies through ultrasound screening. Recent data on termination of pregnancies in France show that 34% of pregnancies with congenital anomalies were terminated.[15] Preliminary results from the Eurofetus project show a similar rate of termination.[14] In the French study, the termination rate varied across defects as one might expect, with certain central nervous system defects having the highest rates of TOP. Eighty percent of pregnancies where anencephaly was detected were terminated, for example, while a corresponding 60% of pregnancies with spina bifida were terminated.[15] Data published recently by the Centers for Disease Control on rates of termination for spina bifida across all pregnancies in several states showed that California had the highest termination rate for the defect among the states analyzed, at 29%, or about half the rate in France.[16] California has a universal MSFAP program, which likely explains in part why its termination rate for spina bifida is higher than that in other states. Even if California's TOP rate for spina bifida was increased by 50% to reflect the fact that only about two-thirds of pregnant women participate, a termination rate of 45% would still be substantially below the rate in France. In other words, due in part to cultural factors, the rate of TOP in the U.S. with routine screening may be less than that in France. Furthermore, in the RADIUS trial, 29% of pregnancies with detected anomalies were terminated prior to 24 weeks' gestation.[11] We applied an average TOP rate range of 25 to 40% in our analysis, with the lower bound reflecting the above evidence on TOP from the RADIUS trial as well as the above suggestions that the rate of TOP in the U.S. may be significantly below that in France. The 40% upper limit is based on European experience in case the rather limited available information on TOP in the U.S. is very misleading.

Estimation of Cost Components (#ULT/PREG)

It is difficult to assess the number of ultrasounds that would be newly performed under a routine screening policy. Routine screening may not even add one additional screen per pregnancy if the routine screen in the second trimester under the policy substitutes for one currently performed in the first or third trimester. One ultrasound screen was routinely performed per pregnancy in the RADIUS trial during the second trimester whereas 0.2 screens per pregnancy were performed in the control group, a minimum net increase of 0.8 in the screened group. Given a similar net increase in a Swedish trial of routine screening,[17] we adopted 0.8 screens as the minimum additional screens from a routine ultrasound policy.

In the Helsinki trial, there were 0.07 additional follow-up screens for a low-risk population receiving one routine screen in the second trimester.[18] We therefore adopt 1.07 scans as an upper limit estimate of screens per pregnancy under a routine screening policy where there is no substitution of the routine scan for others performed.

Estimation of Cost Components ($ULT)

The Resource-Based Relative Value Scale (RBRVS) was constructed by Medicare in 1992 to reimburse physicians under Medicare, based on the actual value of resources used for each type of visit and procedure. This cost-based valuation was used to establish the lower limit for the average cost of an ultrasound ($ULT) in our analysis. Based on the 1992 schedule of relative value units (RVUs), a basic fetal ultrasound

(CPT 76805) consumed 3.82 total RVUs.[19] To maintain the comparison to birth defect costs, which are provided in 1992 dollars, we multiplied the total RVUs by the appropriate conversion factor in 1992 of $31 to arrive at an estimate of $118.50 for the average cost of a fetal ultrasound in the U.S. Reimbursement from commercial insurers in the U.S. tends to be significantly higher than Medicare payment. A 1991 study reporting on the results of a survey of experts in obstetric ultrasonography found that the mean charges were $209 (SD=$67) for screening and $263 (SD=$94) for targeted scans.[9] An upper limit of $210 per scan was therefore considered reasonable as the average cost per scan in our analysis. Indeed, ultrasound cost and sensitivity are not independent of each other. The detection rate in tertiary centers is significantly higher than that in other venues, but the costs are likely significantly higher as well.

RESULTS

Results from applying the ranges for the relevant variables affecting the benefits and costs of routine ultrasound are provided in TABLE 3. The estimated benefit per 100,000 pregnancies ranged between $7.5 million and $29.9 million. The low end of the range reflects the "low-low" assumptions of a 20% net ultrasound sensitivity rate and a 25% TOP rate, whereas the high end of the benefit range reflects the "high-high" assumptions of a 50% net detection rate and a 40% TOP rate.

The estimated total cost per 100,000 routinely screened pregnancies, also reported in TABLE 3, ranged from $9.5 million to $22.5 million. The low end of the range reflects the "low-low" assumptions of $118.50 cost per scan and 0.8 additional scans per pregnancy, whereas the high end of the range reflects the "high-high" assumptions of $210 per scan and 1.07 additional scans per pregnancy.

TABLE 4 provides the benefit-to-cost ratios under various assumptions, including the "high-high" benefit : "low-low" cost scenario most favorable to the intervention. The ratios are slightly below those generated by dividing the corresponding entries in TABLE 3 because they reflect an additional $626 estimated cost per TOP related to professional

TABLE 3. Total Benefits and Total Costs of Routine Ultrasound per 100,000 Pregnancies Assuming 100% Replacement with a Normal Child for Terminated Pregnancies

| Assumption | Benefit Assessment | | | Cost Assessment | | |
	pDET[a]	pTOP[b]	Total Benefit[c] ($ millions)	#ULT[d]	$ULT[e]	Total Cost[f] ($ millions)
High	.50	.40	29.9 (HH)	1.07	$210	22.5 (HH)
Low	.20	.25	7.5 (LL)	0.8	$118.5	9.5 (LL)

[a] Probability of congenital anomalies detected in the first 24 weeks of gestation.
[b] Probability of pregnancies electively terminated based upon results of screening.
[c] Total benefit represents the proportion of the $149.7 million recouped under the assumptions of high pDET and high pTOP (HH), and under the assumption of low pDET and low pTOP (LL).
[d] Incremental number of ultrasounds performed per pregnancy under a routine ultrasound policy to detect congenital anomalies.
[e] Cost per ultrasound.
[f] Total cost under the assumptions of high #ULT and high $ULT (H/H) and of low #ULT and low $ULT (LL).

fees for abortion (CPT 59841),[20] adjusted to 1992 using the medical care component of the consumer price index. The benefit-to-cost ratio for the most favorable scenario is 3.01, suggesting that the benefits associated with routine screening are about three times the benefits. Under the "low-low" benefit : "high-high" cost assumptions, the algorithm least favorable to the intervention, the benefit-to-cost ratio is 0.33, with costs exceeding benefits by a factor of three. Other assumptions provided in the table yield benefit-to-cost ratios between these extremes.

DISCUSSION

Only under the most favorable assumptions does our preliminary analysis find that the costs associated with a routine ultrasound policy were exceeded by the benefits associated with reduced costs of birth defects through TOP. Given the literature showing higher levels of sensitivity achieved mainly through more comprehensive screening done by better trained personnel, the detection rate and average cost are likely directly correlated. In other words, the "high-high" : "low-low" algorithm most favorable to routine ultrasound is probably unrealistic because it combines an upper bound detection rate with a lower bound estimate of cost. A more realistic upper limit estimate to the benefit-to-cost ratio is 1.73, where a $210 ultrasound cost estimate is integrated alongside the high, 50% detection rate estimate.

Given a benefit-to-cost ratio evenly distributed around one, and a most likely upper-bound estimate of 1.73, our preliminary assessment of routine ultrasound leans against the adoption of the policy based strictly on the parameters of this analysis. This conclusion is particularly reinforced when one relaxes the unrealistic assumption of 100% replacement of TOPs upon detection of anomalies with normal children. Some literature suggests that the replacement rate may be as low as 68%,[21] a rate that would push the likely upper-bound benefit-to-cost ratio estimate below one.

Certain of the critical factors that have contributed to the results are also unlikely to change substantially more in favor of routine ultrasound screening. The rate of termination is closely linked to cultural and socioeconomic factors that are not readily altered through changes in technology or medical policy. The lower limit, 0.8 average number of ultrasounds per pregnancy, is probably not amenable to much further reduction. The $118.50 minimum cost of ultrasound from Medicare reimbursement is already well below that of average commercial reimbursement, as noted above. However, cost-reducing technological change could perhaps reduce the cost of screening. That

TABLE 4. Benefit-to-Cost Ratio of Routine Ultrasound Policy Based on Various Cost and Benefit Assumptions and 100% Replacement of TOPs with a Normal Child

		Benefit Assumptions[a]	
		HH	LL
Cost assumptions[b]	LL	3.01	0.75
	HH	1.31	0.33

[a] Benefit assumptions, as in TABLE 3, with HH comprising pDET=.5 and pTOP=.4 and with LL comprising pDET=.2 and pTOP=.25.

[b] Cost assumptions, as in TABLE 3, with HH comprising #ULT=1.07 and $ULT=$210; and with LL comprising #ULT=0.8 and $ULT=$118.50. Costs estimates also included the average $626 cost of an abortion for all TOPs, so the reported benefit-to-cost ratios are slightly below those using the cost estimates provided in TABLE 3.

leaves the detection rate as the major factor subject to change, one that is not likely independent of cost under current technology, as noted above. A large increase in the upper-bound detection rate to 75%—well over twice the rate achieved in tertiary centers in the RADIUS study, without accompanying cost increases—could substantially alter the benefit-to-cost ratio in favor of routine screening.

Benefit Increasing Limitations

There are certain limitations to our analysis, some of which bias the results against routine screening. The cost of birth defects included in the analysis were for a subset of 17 conditions. These included many, but not all, of the major anomalies that can be detected through ultrasound screening. Anencephaly, for example, a central nervous system defect that is subject to a very high rate of detection and subsequent termination was not included. On the other hand, most anencephalic infants die very soon after birth and incur relatively low direct medical costs that would be averted through TOP. Other defects left out of our analysis, such as hypoplastic left heart, would likely add more significantly to the benefit of routine ultrasound if incorporated.

Our cost estimates for birth defects also did not include an estimate of lost parental productivity due to the extra time spent caring for infants and children with birth defects. Estimates of such lost productivity for certain birth defects, such as spina bifida, have been relatively high,[10] and their incorporation would have increased the estimated benefit of routine ultrasound.

Cost Increasing Limitations

Other limitations to our analysis make our estimates of the benefit-to-cost ratios in Table 4 too high. As mentioned earlier, we ignored the cost of false positives that result in TOP because of the lack of reliable data and because of the difficulties under the human capital approach of assessing the associated costs. We also ignored the costs of other tests and procedures (OTHCOST in equation 3), such as additional fetal echocardiograms, that would be ordered based on results from routine screening. We did not attempt to assess the extent to which pregnancies that were electively terminated based on screening would have resulted in fetal deaths in any case (%FDEATH) nor the associated reduction in costs in such cases as summarized in the final term of equation 2. Of course, the average costs associated with such fetal deaths could also be higher than the average costs associated with TOP.

Finally, we assumed that terminated pregnancies would be replaced at a rate of 100% one year after termination. This is clearly an unrealistic assumption. Lower replacement rates generate disproportionate reductions in the benefit of ultrasound screening, because the value of lifetime productivity of individuals with birth defects exceeds, on average, the medical care and other direct costs expended to treat them.

Limitations of Uncertain Effect

There are still other limitations to our analysis for which the impact on the analysis is uncertain. The estimates of incidence in Table 2, as well as the cost figures, were for all live births rather than for the population that would newly be screened as a result of a policy of routine ultrasound. One might argue that the actual incidence of birth defects, and hence cost, is higher among those not currently screened because, without the information provided through ultrasound, they are less likely to terminate pregnancies with major congenital anomalies. On the other hand, it could be argued that those who are unscreened are a lower-risk population, as there were fewer indications for an ultrasound to be performed.

As mentioned earlier, the analysis focused on TOP only and not on changes in management of pregnancy due to early detection of congenital anomalies. Some research has indicated that the benefits from changes in management have proven to be uncertain,[4,8] whereas some interventions, such as fetal surgery, are very costly.

Routine Ultrasound a Bad Idea?

Given that routine ultrasound does not demonstrate a clear net benefit under the preliminary analysis provided here, does that mean that a policy of routine screening is a bad one? Not necessarily. First, there are certain limitations to our analysis which reduce estimated benefits, as noted above. But more importantly, there are other standards that are likely to be important in establishing such a policy, besides just the societal savings from averting birth defects through TOP.

One such standard is the so-called willingness-to-pay assessment, where the value of an intervention or service is based upon individual preferences regarding reduction in risk rather than upon the use or loss of societal resources because of certain events that form the basis of the human capital approach. The reassurance that ultrasound may bring to a woman who has a fetus with no major detected anomalies, for example, has a value under the willingness-to-pay approach that would elude the human capital approach. Given that fetal ultrasound screening is not a typical commodity that can be purchased off of the shelf, but is instead a procedure that is often paid through insurance and performed based upon certain indications in the United States, the market does not directly reflect willingness-to-pay. Eliciting what women are willing to pay therefore poses some difficulties, but some research indicates that such willingness-to-pay likely exceeds the cost of fetal ultrasound screening.[22] In a competitive environment, health maintenance organizations offer routine screening in the absence of a strict economic rationale, reflecting a concern that women will elect to enroll with other plans that do offer such screening.[23] This serves as indirect market evidence of "willingness-to-pay."

There are also ethical implications with respect to the provision of routine ultrasound.[5] The extent to which women are well informed about the capabilities and limitations of fetal ultrasound screening, and the extent to which providers are aware of the values and preferences of individual patients, play an important role in the ethical arguments for routine screening. Indeed, given the absence of a strong economic justification for a routine screening policy, the routine provision of information to pregnant women, as part of a dialogue between providers and patients regarding fetal ultrasound, may be the most prudent way to proceed in eliciting the societal value of the procedure.

REFERENCES

1. VENTURA, S. J., J. A. MARTIN, S. C. CURTIN, et al. 1997. Report of final natality statistics, 1995. Monthly Vital Statistics Report. Vol. 45, no. 11 (Suppl.). National Center for Health Statistics. Hyattsville, MD.

2. VENTURA, S. J., J. A. MARTIN, S. M. TAFFEL, et al. 1994. Advance report of final natality statistics, 1992. Monthly vital statistics report. Vol. 43, no. 5 (Suppl.). National Center for Health Statistics. Hyattsville, MD.

3. NATIONAL INSTITUTES OF HEALTH CONSENSUS DEVELOPMENT CONFERENCE. 1984. The use of diagnostic ultrasound imaging during pregnancy. JAMA 252: 669–672.

4. U.S. PREVENTIVE SERVICES TASK FORCE. 1996. Guide to Clinical Preventive Services, 2nd edit. Williams & Wilkins. Baltimore, MD.

5. SKUPSKI, D. W., F. A. CHERVENAK & L. B. McCULLOUGH. 1995. Routine obstetric ultrasound. Int. J. Gynecol Obstet. 50: 233–242.

6. WAITZMAN, N. J., P. S. ROMANO & R. M. SCHEFFLER. 1994. Estimates of the economic costs of birth defects. Inquiry 31: 188–205.

7. WAITZMAN, N. J., R. M. SCHEFFLER & P. S. ROMANO. 1996. The Cost of Birth Defects: The Value of Prevention. University Press of America. Lanham, MD.

8. BUCHER, H. C. & J. G. SCHMIDT. 1993. Does routine ultrasound scanning improve outcome in pregnancy? Meta-analysis of various outcome measures. Br. Med. J. 307: 13–17.

9. PITKIN, R. M. 1991. Screening and detection of congenital malformation. Am. J. Obstet. Gynecol. 164: 1045–1048.

10. LIPSCOMB, J. 1986. Human capital, willingness-to-pay, and cost-effectiveness analysis of screening for birth defects in North Carolina. Presented at the annual meeting of the American Economic Association, New Orleans, LA.

11. EWIGMAN, B. G., J. P. CRANE, F. D. FRIGOLETTO, et al. 1993. Effect of prenatal ultrasound screening on perinatal outcome. N. Engl. J. Med. 329: 821–827.

12. ANDERSON, N., O. BOSWELL & G. DUFF. 1995. Prenatal sonography for the detection of fetal anomalies: Results of a prospective study and comparison with prior series. Am. J. Radiol. 165: 943–950.

13. GOMEZ, K. J. & J. A. COPEL. 1993. Ultrasound screening for fetal structural anomalies. Curr. Opin. Obstet. Gynecol. 5: 204–210.

14. GRANDJEAN, H. 1998. Sensitivity of routine ultrasound screening of pregnancies in the Eurofetus database. Ann. N.Y. Acad. Sci. This volume.

15. STOLL, C., B. DOTT, Y. ALEMBIK & M. P. ROTH. 1995. Evaluation of routine prenatal diagnosis by a registry of congenital anomalies. Prenatal Diagn. 15: 791–800.

16. CRAGAN, J. D., H. E. ROBERTS, L. D. EDMONDS, et al. 1995. Surveillance for anencephaly and spina bifida and the impact of prenatal diagnosis—United States, 1985–1994. MMWR CDC Surveillance Summaries 44 (4): 1–13.

17. WALDENSTROM, U., O. AXELSSON, S. NILSSON, G. EKLUND, O. FALL, S. LINDEBERG & Y. SJODIN. 1988. Effects of routine one-stage ultrasound screening in pregnancy: A randomised controlled trial. Lancet 2: 585–588.

18. SAARI-KEMPPAINEN, A., O. KARJALAINEN, P. YLOSTALO & O. P. HEINONEN. 1994. Fetal anomalies in a controlled one-stage ultrasound screening trial. A report from the Helsinki Ultrasound Trial. J. Perinat. Med. 22: 279–289.

19. U.S. CONGRESS. 1991. Addendum B: Relative value units (RVUs) and related information. Federal Register 58 (227): 59720.

20. KIRCHNER, M. 1990. Where do your fees fit in? Med. Economics 67 (19): 92–93.

21. BRANDENBURG, H., W. DeKONING, M. G. JAHODA, et al. 1992. Reproductive behaviour and prenatal diagnosis following genetic termination of pregnancy in women of advanced maternal age. Prenatal Diagn. 12: 1031–1035.

22. BERWICK, D. M. & M. C. WEINSTEIN. 1985. What do patients value? Willingness to pay for ultrasound in normal pregnancy. Med. Care 23: 881–893.

23. BUECHLER, E. J. 1998. Managed care and ultrasound for the diagnosis of fetal anomalies. Ann. N.Y. Acad. Sci. This volume.

Can Decision Analysis Help Us Decide Whether Ultrasound Screening for Fetal Anomalies Is Worth It?

PATRICK S. ROMANO[a,c] AND NORMAN J. WAITZMAN[b]

[a]*Departments of Medicine and Pediatrics, University of California, Davis, California, USA*

[b]*Department of Economics, University of Utah, Salt Lake City, Utah 84112-9300, USA*

ABSTRACT: Decision analysis is a widely used tool to improve clinical decision making when randomized controlled trials are infeasible, underpowered, or lack generalizability. We performed an exploratory decision analysis of routine second trimester ultrasound to detect fetal anomalies, focusing on the assumptions that would have the greatest impact. Six outcome categories were considered: (1) abnormal ultrasound, anomalous child, (2) abnormal ultrasound, elective abortion of anomalous fetus, (3) abnormal ultrasound, healthy child, (4) abnormal ultrasound, elective abortion of healthy fetus, (5) normal ultrasound, healthy child, and (6) normal ultrasound, anomalous child. Live birth and fetal death rates for nine sonographically detectable anomalies were obtained from the California Birth Defects Monitoring Program. The sensitivity and specificity of ultrasound were estimated through meta-analysis of recent series. Plausible ranges for the probabilities of cesarean delivery and elective abortion, by anomaly, were determined through review of the literature. Standard gamble, willingness-to-pay, and human capital estimates of utility were rescaled for comparability. We found that routine ultrasound appears to be the preferred strategy for most women. This choice is sensitive primarily to the specificity of ultrasound and women's willingness-to-pay for the reassurance of a normal ultrasound.

In 1984, a Consensus Development Panel convened by the National Institutes of Health reviewed the available evidence and concluded that "ultrasound examination during pregnancy should be performed for a specific medical indication" because the data "do not allow a recommendation for routine screening."[1] Since that recommendation was published, one randomized controlled trial (RCT) from Helsinki reported lower perinatal mortality among women randomized to receive a routine ultrasound between 16 and 20 weeks of gestation,[2] whereas a larger trial from the United States reported no significant difference in perinatal morbidity or mortality when women were randomized to receive sonograms between 18 and 20 weeks and again between 31 and 33 weeks.[3] Although the latter trial has aroused considerable controversy,[4-6] the U.S. Preventive Services Task Force concluded that "there is currently insufficient evidence to recommend for or against a single routine midtrimester ultrasound in low-risk pregnant women."[7] A similar position has been taken by the American College of Obstetricians and Gynecologists;[8] the Canadian Task Force on the Periodic Health Examination found "fair evidence to support the inclusion of a single routine ultrasound examination in the management of women with no clinical indication."[9]

[c]Address correspondence to Patrick S. Romano, MD, MPH, University of California, Davis, Primary Care Center, Room 3107, 2221 Stockton Boulevard, Sacramento, CA 95817. E-mail: psromano@ucdavis.edu

154

These recommendations have been the subject of intense worldwide debate. This debate has focused on the highly variable quality of ultrasonography in both the Helsinki and RADIUS trials,[10,11] the arguable merits of perinatal mortality and morbidity as primary outcome variables,[4] and respect for the autonomy of the pregnant woman.[12] The dilemma for decision makers in government agencies and managed care organizations is that these considerations are difficult to balance against the lack of definitive evidence from RCTs. RCTs remain the gold standard for evaluating the efficacy of screening tests, because they are less susceptible to selection and confounding bias than cohort or case control studies. The U.S. Preventive Services Task Force, for example, weighed RCTs more heavily than other evidence in developing its recommendations.

It seems unlikely that more RCTs will be organized to evaluate the benefits of routine prenatal ultrasound in the United States. RCTs are too difficult to organize, too time-consuming, and too costly. Yet the Helsinki and RADIUS trials, among others, suggest that the benefits of routine prenatal ultrasound to detect fetal anomalies may be sensitive to several factors:

- *Quality of ultrasound.* The overall sensitivity of second trimester ultrasound in detecting major fetal malformations was higher at academic centers than in other settings, in both the Helsinki (75 versus 35%)[13] and RADIUS (35 versus 13%)[14] trials. Hence, the benefits of screening may depend heavily on the skills of the ultrasonographer.
- *Frequency of relevant outcomes.* A given reduction in the relative risk of adverse outcomes may vary widely in absolute magnitude across populations, depending on their baseline risk. All of the published RCTs have lacked power to detect differences that may be clinically meaningful. For example, RADIUS could not exclude the possibility of a 12% reduction in perinatal morbidity and mortality (RR=1.01, 95% CI 0.88–1.17). Meta-analyzing Helsinki and RADIUS with four other RCTs,[15–18] a 35% reduction in perinatal mortality cannot be excluded (weighted OR=0.87, 95% CI 0.65–1.15). The benefits of screening may be too small to detect in RCTs, but may still be clinically meaningful.
- *Changing technology.* None of the published RCTs reflects recent technologic advances such as 3-dimensional ultrasound, Doppler imaging of the uterine artery, fetal surgery, and "genetic ultrasound" to identify markers for Down syndrome. These advances may significantly enhance the benefits of screening ultrasound.
- *Value of information and personal decision making.* Hard outcomes such as perinatal morbidity and mortality do not capture all of the benefits of prenatal ultrasound. Screened women in RADIUS had a lower risk of tocolysis and a lower risk of postdates induction, compared with unscreened women. Screened women terminated more pregnancies than unscreened women in both trials, although the difference was statistically significant only in Helsinki. Termination rates for prenatally detected spina bifida vary considerably across populations,[19] although the reported difference between Helsinki and RADIUS in the termination rate for anomalous fetuses detected by screening (61 versus 29%) is a spurious result of how malformations were defined. The benefits of screening may be difficult to value (e.g., avoidance of unnecessary interventions), and may depend on beliefs and attitudes that determine whether women continue or terminate affected pregnancies.

When published RCTs have uncertain applicability to women in a particular community or cultural group, decision analysis and cost-effectiveness analysis may be useful tools.[20] These methods allow the analyst to examine systematically all components of the decision-making process, explicitly incorporating the probability of each possible outcome and patient preferences or utilities. The analyst can then select the choice with the highest expected utility, but he or she can also evaluate the sensitivity of that choice to different assumptions. For example, the hypothesized termination rate can be altered to determine whether routine ultrasound is still preferred in communities where relatively few anomalous fetuses are aborted.

Decision analysis has been applied to prenatal diagnostic testing for chromosomal abnormalities. Pauker and Pauker showed that decision analysis could be used to help prospective parents decide whether to undergo amniocentesis, based on their age-specific risk of trisomy 21 and their own estimates of the "costs" of spontaneous and elective abortion, relative to the "cost" of having an affected child.[21,22] Heckerling and Verp showed that amniocentesis is preferred over chorionic villus sampling (CVS) for a 35-year-old pregnant woman, unless the perceived utility of first-trimester elective abortion far exceeds that of second-trimester abortion or the anxiety "cost" of waiting until the second trimester is unusually high.[23] Their model predicted actual decisions for 60% of the women studied.[24] Decision analysis has also been applied to antenatal diagnosis of cystic fibrosis[25] and congenital heart disease.[26] Although women's willingness to pay for ultrasound has been studied,[27] this choice has never been comprehensively evaluated using decision analysis.

We undertook an exploratory decision analysis, using data from the California Birth Defects Monitoring Program (CBDMP) and our own previous studies of the cost of birth defects[28] to identify the key parameters that affect whether a pregnant woman (or a group of women with similar characteristics) should undergo second trimester ultrasonography to detect fetal anomalies. Given financial and time constraints, we did not collect primary data. Therefore, our results are tentative. Our primary objective was simply to determine which of the factors mentioned above (e.g., sensitivity and specificity of ultrasound, frequency of relevant outcomes, pregnancy termination rates) would be most likely to affect the optimal choice and therefore most important to measure accurately in future studies.

ESTIMATING UTILITIES

Utility is a measure of the strength of a patient's preference for a given health outcome. It provides a quantitative tool for scaling qualitatively different health states, such as having a child with spina bifida and miscarrying a normal fetus. The four most common approaches for assessing utilities are:

- *Direct rating scale.* The most desirable health state (e.g., birth of a normal child) is placed at one end of a horizontal or vertical line and assigned a utility of one. The least desirable health state (e.g., death of mother and fetus) is placed at the other end and assigned a utility of zero. Study participants are asked to locate specific health states on this line, between the two extremes.
- *Standard gamble.* Study participants are offered a choice between a certain outcome with unknown utility and a gamble that may lead either to an ideal outcome (with probability p) or to the worst possible outcome (with probability $1-p$). The probability p is varied until the respondent is indifferent between the two alternatives.
- *Time trade-off.* This is a simpler approach in which study participants are asked how much of their life expectancy they would be willing to give up to trade a specific health state for an optimal state with a utility of one.
- *Willingness to pay.* Study participants are asked how much money, or what proportion of their family income, they would be willing to pay to trade a specific health state for an optimal state with a utility of one.

We comprehensively reviewed the medical and health services literature to identify articles on patient preferences or utilities related to outcomes of prenatal ultrasound.

Standard gamble estimates were favored because the standard gamble best embodies the construct of decision making under uncertainty, offers adequate intrarater and test-retest reliability, and generates the highest or most conservative utility estimates.[29] We also favored studies of pregnant women undergoing prenatal diagnosis, because our aim was to maximize the expected utility of pregnant women rather than the expected utility of families or of society as a whole.[30] We assumed that consequences involving spouses and older children[31] would be expressed through the pregnant women's preferences.

Prenatal ultrasound for the purpose of detecting fetal anomalies was assumed to have four possible outcomes: an abnormal result with an anomalous fetus (true positive), an abnormal result with a normal fetus (false positive), a normal result with an anomalous fetus (false negative), and a normal result with a normal fetus (true negative). Any true positive or false positive result could lead to continuation or termination of pregnancy; continuation of pregnancy could lead to either fetal death or live birth by either vaginal or cesarean delivery. Each of these outcomes required a separate utility estimate. To simplify the analysis, we focused on ultrasound and did not consider the potential roles of maternal serum alpha fetoprotein (MSAFP) screening and amniocentesis in detecting neural tube and abdominal wall defects.

Because the birth of a child with a congenital anomaly may not be the worst possible outcome for a pregnant woman, all utility estimates were anchored at zero by the death of both mother and fetus and at one by the birth of a healthy child. Only one published utility estimate for any fetal anomaly was anchored in this manner: 0.80 for the birth of a child with Down syndrome.[32] (This estimate is slightly higher than a subsequent estimate of 0.69–0.75 reported by the same group).[33]

Based on the arguable principle that willingness to pay to avoid a birth defect should be proportional to the human capital cost of that defect, we then used human capital estimates derived from multiple data sources in California[34] to estimate utilities for other major anomalies detectable by ultrasound. These anomalies included spina bifida, anencephaly, conotruncal heart anomalies, gastroschisis, omphalocele, diaphragmatic hernia, bilateral renal agenesis, urinary tract obstruction with hydrophrosis, and limb reduction defects. The estimates for spina bifida were stratified by neurologic level using cost data from North Carolina,[35] which were rescaled for comparability to California using birth prevalence data from Washington.[36] Our cost of illness study did not include hydrocephalus, hydranencephaly, iniencephaly, or holoprosencephaly; we postulated that maternal utility with these defects would equal that with transposition of the great vessels (which has similar mortality during the first year of life). Although the list in TABLE 1 does not include all sonographically detectable anomalies, only a few of the remaining anomalies (e.g., cystic hygroma or cystadenomatoid lung malformation with hydrops, hypoplastic left heart, large encephalocele)[37] would justify abortion or fetal therapy.

The utility of second trimester therapeutic abortion was estimated from a study of 468 women who received genetic counseling, primarily because of advanced maternal age.[38] We rescaled this estimate to the top and bottom anchors described above; the resulting estimate of 0.9284 is consistent with Kuppermann's path state estimates of 0.93–0.96 with, and 0.86–0.88 without, subsequent birth of a healthy child.[32,33] The long-term emotional distress that follows prenatal diagnosis and termination of pregnancy is well recognized.[39,40] The utility of aborting a normal fetus after a false positive ultrasound was estimated at 0.8312 by rescaling the results from a survey of 62 population genetics students, medical students, and obstetric residents.[23]

The utility of late fetal death was approximated by the reported utility of second trimester miscarriage after amniocentesis (0.9700);[23] this estimate may be too high if maternal attachment to the fetus increases in the third trimester, but it may be too low

TABLE 1. Human Capital Cost and Utility of Major Fetal Anomalies Detectable by Second Trimester Ultrasound

Anomaly	Cost per Case (1988, thousand $)	True Positive Mean Utility (maximum = 1)	False Positive Mean Utility (maximum = 1)	False Negative Mean Utility (maximum = 1)
Down syndrome[a]	409.91	0.80000	0.99893	0.79000
Spina bifida (aggregate)[b]	258.30	0.87397	0.99933	0.86767
Thoracic/high lumbar	243.61	0.83726	0.99913	0.82912
Low lumbar	178.63	0.88067	0.99936	0.87470
Sacral	133.12	0.91107	0.99952	0.90662
Spina bifida[c]				
Prelabor cesarean delivery	235.66	0.88502	0.99939	0.87927
Vaginal or other delivery	267.71	0.86938	0.99930	0.86285
Anencephaly	329.89	0.83904	0.99914	0.83099
Conotruncal heart (aggregate)	261.48	0.87242	0.99932	0.86604
Truncus arteriosus	440.73	0.78496	0.99885	0.77421
Transposition/DORV	236.52	0.88460	0.99938	0.87883
Tetralogy of Fallot	226.90	0.88929	0.99941	0.88375
Single ventricle	305.47	0.85096	0.99920	0.84351
Bilateral renal agenesis	352.29	0.82811	0.99908	0.81952
Hydronephrosis	76.72	0.96257	0.99980	0.96070
Limb reduction (aggregate)	121.03	0.94095	0.99968	0.93800
Upper limb	90.99	0.95560	0.99976	0.95338
Lower limb	182.68	0.91087	0.99952	0.90641
Diaphragmatic hernia	227.13	0.88918	0.99941	0.88364
Abdominal wall (aggregate)	121.98	0.94049	0.99968	0.93751
Gastroschisis	94.29	0.95399	0.99975	0.95169
Omphalocele	158.89	0.92248	0.99959	0.91860
Abdominal wall[d]				
Prenatal diagnosis	116.60	0.94311	0.99970	0.94027
Antenatal diagnosis	123.32	0.93983	0.99968	0.93682
Hydrocephalus (aggregate)[e]	236.52	0.84201	0.99916	0.83411
Cesarean delivery	330.66	0.77912	0.99882	0.76808
Vaginal delivery	218.03	0.85436	0.99922	0.84708

[a] Down syndrome utilities were not actually used in the decision model, as we assumed that Down syndrome fetuses would be detected only if they had a structural anomaly. The Down syndrome utility estimate was used to scale all other utility estimates.

[b] The aggregate cost estimate for spina bifida[34] was stratified by neurologic level using cost data from North Carolina,[35] which were rescaled for comparability to California using birth prevalence data from Washington.[36]

[c] Costs for spina bifida cases born after prelabor cesarean delivery (or after other types of delivery) were estimated by reweighting level-specific costs to reflect the distribution of neurologic deficits reported after elective cesarean delivery.[36]

[d] Costs for abdominal wall defects diagnosed before (or after) birth were estimated based on several assumptions: (1) Infants inborn at referral centers have 30% fewer hospital days in the first year of life than those born elsewhere; (2) this results in a 27% drop in total medical costs per capita; (3) 20% of pregnant women currently receive prenatal care at referral centers (with 80% prenatal detection of abdominal wall defects), whereas 80% receive care at community hospitals (with 20% prenatal detection and referral of abdominal wall defects); and (4) among prenatally diagnosed cases, 80% should be inborn at referral centers.

[e] Costs for hydrocephalus cases born after cesarean (or vaginal) delivery were estimated by adjusting our cost estimates for a similarly burdensome condition (transposition of the great vessels) to reflect either 80% (vaginal) or 32% (cesarean) mortality in the first year of life.

because harmful commissions (e.g., postprocedural miscarriage) are often considered more immoral than equally harmful omissions (e.g., spontaneous fetal loss).[41] Indeed, Kuppermann *et al.* found that the path state utility of miscarriage after CVS was almost equal to that of elective abortion for Down syndrome.[32] Another consideration is that the expressed preferences of women undergoing prenatal diagnosis may correlate poorly with the assessments of women experiencing fetal loss. For example, women surveyed 8 weeks after spontaneous fetal loss in the second or third trimester actually reported *more* grief in one study than those surveyed after abortion of a malformed fetus.[42] In another study, women reported more depressive symptoms and posttraumatic stress after spontaneous fetal loss than after abortion of a malformed fetus, but these differences disappeared at 7 weeks and remained absent over the next year.[43] Two other studies reported no clear differences between women who experienced spontaneous perinatal loss and those who elected termination for fetal anomalies;[44] however, there was a trend toward higher depression scores and poorer adjustment 16–20 months after abortion.[45] The confusion in this area led us to test a wide range of utility values in our sensitivity analyses (TABLE 2).

Pregnant women are willing to pay for information about fetal health.[27,46] Prenatal ultrasound may promote bonding with the fetus[47] and may reduce maternal anxiety,[48] depression, and hostility.[49] We estimated the average utility benefit of knowing that one's fetus is sonographically normal by inflating and rescaling Berwick's 1984 willingness-to-pay estimate of $363.[27] This information is even more valuable to pregnant women with a history of previous pregnancy loss[50] or an elevated MSAFP value,[51] but the sizes of these subpopulations are unknown. We assumed that women with a false positive diagnosis of a minor anomaly, such as choroid plexus cyst or clubfoot,[52] lose this utility benefit.[53]

The disutility of a false positive ultrasound (without abortion) was estimated to equal the disutility of the corresponding anomaly, but only until further evaluation establishes the correct diagnosis.[54,55] This period was assumed to average 15 weeks, if half of the false positive diagnoses are corrected at 30 weeks and the remainder are corrected at term, of an average life expectancy of 54 years[56] (at the median maternal age at birth, 26.3 years).[57] The disutility of a false negative ultrasound (without abortion)

TABLE 2. Other Utility Estimates Used in Decision Analysis

Health State	Baseline Utility (maximum=1)	Sensitivity Analysis: Lower Bound	Sensitivity Analysis: Upper Bound
Cesarean delivery	0.9990	0.95	1.00
Elective abortion of anomalous fetus	0.9284	0.7	1.0
Elective abortion of normal fetus (false positive)	0.8312	0.5	1.0
Fetal death (after 20 weeks gestation)	0.9700	0.7	1.0
No normal ultrasound	0.999792	0.99	1.00
Minor false positive finding	0.999792	0.99	1.00
False negative ultrasound (multiply by disutility of defect missed)	1.05	0.95	2.00
False positive ultrasound (mean duration of misinformation in weeks)	15	10	20

was estimated to equal the disutility of the corresponding anomaly, inflated by 5% to reflect parental bitterness over the missed diagnosis. Because this assumption is based on minimal data,[58] we also tested the possibility that higher utility ("blissful ignorance") during pregnancy totally compensates for the postpartum shock of a false negative ultrasound.

We found no published estimates of the utility of cesarean delivery. However, the maternal mortality rate after cesarean delivery is at least 0.22 per 1,000 women,[59] or seven times the rate after vaginal delivery.[60] Hemorrhage and infection also occur more often after cesarean delivery.[61] Mothers are less satisfied with their birth experience after cesarean than after vaginal delivery.[62] Recent studies have found long-term psychosocial consequences of cesarean delivery, including a lower likelihood of breast-feeding and subsequent childbearing, less positive feelings for the newborn at 6 weeks,[63] lower levels of stimulation and play at 1–5 months,[62] and greater fatigue at 2 months to 4 years.[64] For these reasons, we assumed that the average utility of cesarean delivery is 0.999 times the corresponding utility of vaginal delivery.

For spina bifida, we used recent data from the University of Washington to estimate the utility gain due to improved motor function with prelabor cesarean delivery.[36] Microcephalic fetuses without other major anomalies probably have lower mortality with cesarean delivery, but the magnitude of this benefit is difficult to estimate because nonviable fetuses tend to be selected for vaginal delivery. We reestimated the human capital costs of hydrocephalus, assuming 80% mortality after vaginal delivery and 35% mortality after cesarean delivery, based on four recent series.[65–68] Direct costs for surviving infants were assumed to be independent of the mode of delivery.

The perinatal management of fetuses with abdominal wall defects is controversial. Based on meta-analysis of the available literature, we assumed that vaginal and cesarean delivery have equal utility.[69–86] However, four of five published studies have shown that prenatally transferred (inborn) patients spend 25 to 30% fewer days in the hospital than postnatally transferred (outborn) patients, presumably because of complications that result from delayed repair.[85–89] We adjusted the inpatient component of direct medical costs accordingly, and used the resulting estimates of total human capital costs to derive separate maternal utilities for inborn and outborn cases. Prenatal transfer may improve the preoperative condition of infants with hypoplastic left heart, but it is unclear whether improved outcomes result.[90] There is little evidence of improved outcomes after prenatal diagnosis of other anomalies, although such benefits may exist for diaphragmatic hernia[91] and duodenal atresia.[92]

High-volume hospitals probably have lower mortality after congenital heart disease repair than low-volume hospitals,[93] but there is no system in place to refer affected fetuses selectively to high-volume centers. Recent data from New York,[94] California, and Massachusetts[95] suggest that closing pediatric cardiac surgery programs with less than 100 cases per year could lower risk-adjusted mortality by about 30% for 20–35% of affected infants.

Several components of a pregnant woman's utility function were not estimated because of lack of information. We did not posit any utility benefit from prenatal diagnosis of anomalies, except by changes in medical management (e.g., the mode or setting of delivery) or by termination of pregnancy. Information about the presence of an anomaly may have utility in helping a woman prepare for the birth of an affected child,[95] but any such benefit could be outweighed by the disutility of having to consider termination, additional anxiety and stress during the pregnancy, and regrets after the delivery. In addition, some sonographic findings may lead to amniocentesis (e.g., omphalocele), which may in turn cause fetal loss. We assumed that the utility benefits of screening accrue only to women who choose to be screened; women who refuse ultrasound are excluded. Finally, we assumed that screening has no effect on present or future fertility,[96] although one study suggests a modest positive effect.[97] We presume that our utility estimates, based on published studies, were implicitly weighted by the participants' *expectation* of whether a spontaneous or therapeutic abortion would be followed by the birth of a replacement child.

ESTIMATING PROBABILITIES

The sensitivity and specificity of second trimester ultrasound in detecting fetal anomalies were estimated by meta-analysis of six recently published series,[98–103] plus the Helsinki[13] and RADIUS[14] trials described above. The MEDLINE bibliographic database and recent literature summaries were used to identify candidate studies. Our inclusion criteria for this meta-analysis were (1) performance of general sonographic examinations between 16 and 24 weeks of gestation; (2) a low-risk, community-based sample involving at least 2,000 fetuses; (3) nearly complete follow-up of both normal and abnormal sonograms, using medical records to ascertain anomalies; (4) description of all false positive findings; and (5) detailed reporting of specific anomalies detected during *routine* second trimester examinations. Because sonographic methods have improved dramatically over the past 25 years, we excluded studies of sonograms performed before 1983.[104] We also excluded studies of sonography performed for specific clinical indications, such as a family history of congenital anomalies, an abnormal MSAFP value, or a suspected abnormality on first-stage ultrasound. Studies of targeted sonography for specific anomalies (e.g., cardiac, chromosomal) were excluded. As a result, detection of Down syndrome using markers such as nuchal edema and limb shortening was not included in the analysis.

The final meta-analysis included over 82,094 fetuses; three studies reported the number of scans rather than the number of fetuses scanned. TABLE 3 shows the aggregate sensitivity and specificity for each anomaly. The overall sensitivity was high (over 75%) for anencephaly and abdominal wall defects; intermediate (45–75%) for renal agenesis, spina bifida, and hydrocephalus; and poor (less than 45%) for hydronephrosis, limb reduction defects, diaphragmatic hernia, and cardiac anomalies. About 0.22% of fetal sonograms had minor false positive findings. In general, the two RCTs and the series by Levi *et al.* reported the lowest sensitivities, which may best represent community practice. These three studies were aggregated separately to establish the lower bound for sensitivity analysis.

The probability of each major anomaly was estimated using data from 1984 through 1992 from the CBDMP, which is one of the world's largest active surveillance programs for birth defects (TABLE 4). The CBDMP data system includes all live-born and stillborn (>20 weeks of gestation) infants in selected California counties. From February 1, 1989 through January 31, 1991, the CBDMP also ascertained all electively terminated fetuses with neural tube defects.[105] This ascertainment was probably nearly complete because of California's statewide MSAFP screening program, which includes reporting from ultrasound and cytogenetics laboratories. These data were combined with similar data from Arkansas, Atlanta, Iowa, and South Carolina to estimate the second trimester prevalence of anencephaly and spina bifida.[106] For other anomalies, the second trimester prevalence was estimated by adding the stillbirth and live-birth rates from CBDMP, and adjusting that total upward to account for prenatal detection and elective termination. The overall fetal death rate in the United States is 7.3 per 1,000 viable fetuses (at 20 weeks of gestation).[56]

The proportion of detected anomalies leading to termination varies substantially by region.[19] We obtained our baseline estimates from the largest published series to report termination rates after prenatal detection for all structural anomalies.[107] These esti-

TABLE 3. Sensitivity and Specificity of Routine Second Trimester Ultrasound

Anomaly	Baseline Sensitivity (%)[a]	Lower-bound Sensitivity (%)[b]	Upper-bound Sensitivity (%)	Baseline Specificity (%)[a]	Lower-bound Specificity (%)[c]	Upper-bound Specificity (%)
Spina bifida	62.1	36.7	100.0	100.000	99.990	100
Anencephaly	100.0	100.0	100.0	100.000	100.000	100
Cardiac	16.7	8.2	100.0	99.997	99.990	100
Renal agenesis	54.3	36.4	100.0	100.000	99.990	100
Hydronephrosis	33.1	18.2	100.0	99.984	99.900	100
Limb reduction	39.1	16.7	100.0	99.999	99.990	100
Diaphragmatic hernia	40.7	14.3	100.0	99.999	99.990	100
Abdominal wall	79.5	56.2	100.0	99.999	99.990	100
Hydrocephalus	50.0	31.2	100.0	99.988	99.900	100

[a] Baseline sensitivity and specificity estimates are based on meta-analysis of published series meeting specific criteria described in the text.[13,14,98-103]

[b] Lower-bound sensitivity estimates are based on meta-analysis of three series in which the majority of scans were performed outside specialized centers.[13,14,100]

[c] Lower-bound specificity estimates are extrapolated from studies that reported relatively high false positive rates.[13,103]

TABLE 4. Other Probability Estimates Used in Decision Analysis, including Prevalence Rates, Elective Termination Rates, Fetal Death Rates, and Cesarean Delivery Rates

Anomaly	Prevalence (per 100,000 fetuses)[a]	Baseline Probability of Termination[b,107]	Lower-bound Probability of Termination[b]	Upper-bound Probability of Termination[b]	Probability of Fetal Death[c]	Probability of Cesarean Delivery[c]
Spina bifida	53.21	0.627	0.455[109]	1.000[108]		0.840[d]
Anencephaly	39.67	1.000	0.667[9]	1.000[108]		0.000
Cardiac		0.266	0.082[11]	0.551[113]		0.208
Renal agenesis		0.424	0.424[07]	1.000[108]		0.000
Hydronephrosis		0.045	0.000[109]	0.455[108]		0.208
Limb reduction		0.533	0.333[12]	1.000[108]		0.208
Diaphragmatic hernia		0.463	0.250[109]	0.500[108]		0.208
Abdominal wall		0.528	0.000[109]	0.702[112]		0.255[e]
Hydrocephalus		0.697	0.667[109]	1.000[108]		0.720[f]
Minor false positive	21.9	0.000	0.000	0.000		0.208

[a] Total prevalence includes live births, fetal deaths after 20 weeks of gestation, and elective terminations. All three components have been reported for spina bifida and anencephaly.[106] For other anomalies, live births and fetal deaths were ascertained from the California Birth Defects Monitoring Program (CBDMP) and elective terminations were estimated from recent series.[107,118]

[b] Probability of elective termination for fetal anomalies detected before the legal gestational age limit for termination.

[c] Probability of fetal death after 20 weeks of gestation, including stillbirths at term, from the CBDMP.

[d] Probability of cesarean delivery *before the onset of labor* among prenatally diagnosed cases at centers where physicians routinely recommend such management.[36] The comparable value among cases diagnosed at birth is 10%.

[e] Probability of cesarean delivery among prenatally diagnosed cases at centers where physicians routinely recommend vaginal delivery for abdominal wall defects.[71,72,76–78] The comparable value among cases diagnosed at birth is the same.

[f] Probability of cesarean delivery in four series of prenatally diagnosed cases.[65–68] The comparable value among cases diagnosed at birth, from an older series, is 56%.[114]

mates may not apply to the United States, because France has no legal restrictions on third trimester abortion for fetal anomalies. We therefore used smaller series from Hungary[108] and Michigan[109] to establish upper and lower bounds for defect-specific termination rates. Corroborating estimates were obtained from several other sources; termination rates are generally lower in American series[109,110] than in European series.[111,112]

Finally, we estimated the probability of cesarean delivery for prenatally diagnosed cases of each anomaly. We assumed that cesarean delivery would rarely, if ever, be used for fetuses known to have anencephaly or bilateral renal agenesis. Given the evidence supporting elective cesarean delivery of infants with spina bifida[36] and hydrocephalus,[65–68] we assumed cesarean rates of 84% (before the onset of labor) and 72%, respectively. Abdominal wall defects were ascribed a rate of 25.5% based on five studies showing increased risk of fetal distress or dystocia.[71,72,76–78] All other prenatally diagnosed anomalies were ascribed a cesarean rate equal to that of the general population (20.8%).[113] Because of the risk of dystocia or malpresentation, we posited intermediate values for the probability of cesarean delivery among women carrying fetuses with undiagnosed spina bifida (10% before the onset of labor),[36] hydrocephalus (56%),[114] or abdominal wall defects (25.5%).[71,72,76–78]

ANALYTIC METHODS

All analyses were performed using Decision Maker Version 6.2 and Corel QuattroPro. One-way sensitivity analyses were performed, based on plausible ranges of every probability and utility estimate in the model. Threshold analyses were performed when appropriate to identify the threshold probability or utility value beyond which ultrasound would no longer be preferred. Two-way and multiway sensitivity analyses were performed on specific combinations of variables that appeared likely to influence the results. Both individual-level and population-level models were developed; elective termination was considered a choice in the individual model, but a chance event in the population model. In the former analysis, we assumed that the average woman terminates her pregnancy if the expected utility of termination exceeds the expected utility of continuation.

PRELIMINARY RESULTS

Under our baseline assumptions for the population of low-risk pregnant women, the expected utility of undergoing routine ultrasonography to detect fetal anomalies in the second trimester is 0.9991, whereas the expected utility of not undergoing ultrasonography is 0.9989. This difference is small because fetal anomalies are relatively rare, but it is consistent and clinically significant. For the average pregnant woman, as an individual, the decision analysis also favors routine ultrasonography (EU=0.9991 versus 0.9989). The expected utility of termination exceeds that of continuation for spina bifida, anencephaly, bilateral renal agenesis, cardiac anomalies, and diaphragmatic hernia. The expected utility of continuation exceeds that of termination for abdominal wall defects, hydronephrosis, and limb reduction defects; hydrocephalus is a close call. These findings are generally consistent with observed termination rates.

In one-way sensitivity analyses, these results were minimally sensitive to plausible values of the defect-specific elective abortion rate, the defect-specific sensitivity and specificity of ultrasound, the prevalence of fetal anomalies, the overall cesarean rate, and the disutilities of cesarean delivery, fetal death, minor false positive findings, terminating a normal pregnancy because of major false positive findings, false negative findings, and being unaware of a congenital anomaly because sonography was not performed. As described below, the benefit of routine ultrasound is highly dependent on the pregnant woman's willingness-to-pay for the knowledge that her fetus is sonographically normal. The disutility of aborting an anomalous fetus is an important variable in the population model but not in the individual model (because a woman can avoid this disutility by continuing her pregnancy).

In two-way and multiway sensitivity analyses, two interesting patterns were observed. If the specificity of ultrasound is actually 99.9% for hydrocephalus and hydronephrosis (consistent with the lowest values recently reported)[13,103] and 99.99% for all other anomalies (except anencephaly), the utility of aborting a normal fetus becomes an important variable. If that utility is somewhat lower than our baseline estimate (e.g., 0.743 instead of 0.831), no ultrasound becomes the preferred strategy. If willingness-to-pay for a normal sonogram result is less than about $240 (in 1988 U.S. dollars), no ultrasound again becomes the preferred strategy when specificities are relatively low. The prevalence of birth defects has an enhanced effect on the model at low specificity values, because the false positive rate is inversely related to prevalence.

Second, if we set the utility of true negative scans equal to one, ignoring their psychological value to pregnant women, routine ultrasound shows a very small benefit and the decision becomes a close call. The benefit of ultrasound completely disappears if the disutility of a false negative scan is more than 1.2 to 1.3 times the disutility of the corresponding anomaly, if the utility of electively aborting an anomalous fetus is less than 0.85 to 0.90, or if the probability of abortion is extremely low (e.g., less than 20% for craniospinal anomalies and zero for all others).

DISCUSSION

As this paper demonstrates, decision analysis is an exceedingly complex enterprise. It may be a useful tool to evaluate the expected benefit of routine second trimester ultrasonography to detect fetal anomalies, in the absence of convincing data from RCTs that reflect current technology and practice. However, the decision framework is exceedingly complex because of the number of potential findings of ultrasound and the wide array of implications. Most diagnostic tests have two or at most three (e.g., normal, abnormal, borderline) possible results. Even in our simplified analysis with aggregated categories of fetal anomalies, prenatal ultrasound has at least 11 possible results related to the fetus alone. Key probability and utility estimates are essentially unknown, and are likely to vary considerably from woman to woman and from nation to nation.

Given these caveats, however, routine second trimester ultrasound appears likely to be the preferred strategy for most women. The results of our decision analysis are notably insensitive to the parameters most likely to vary by site: the sensitivity of ultrasound, the proportion of anomalous fetuses electively aborted, and the disutility of false negative and false positive findings. However, there are plausible scenarios under which no ultrasound may have higher expected utility than ultrasound. These scenarios generally involve specificity estimates at the lower end of what has been reported in the literature, and relatively low willingness-to-pay for the reassurance of a normal ultrasound. Although these threshold values differ from our literature-based "best estimates," they are well within the range of plausibility. Because fetal anomalies are relatively rare, the accuracy of ultrasound in normal pregnancies and the utility of true negative or false positive information to prospective parents are dominant variables in the decision model.

As noted earlier, these findings are preliminary. We focused exclusively on ultrasound in low-risk women to detect fetal anomalies. Therefore, our analysis did not include such benefits as detecting twin gestations and uteroplacental abnormalities, identifying gender, and dating pregnancies more accurately with concomitant avoidance of tocolysis and artificial induction of labor. Our analysis did not include new uses of ultrasound such as screening for markers of aneuploidy (e.g., nuchal edema, echogenic bowel, limb shortening), or new technologies such as 3-dimensional ultrasound.[115] We focused on the most important anomalies potentially detectable by ultrasound; including less frequent or more minor anomalies in the analysis might further increase the benefit of routine ultrasound. This benefit would also increase if ultrasound enhances fertility by reducing parental concern about the risk of birth defects, or if our human capital approach underestimates parental willingness-to-pay to avoid having an affected child.

However, our decision analysis might overestimate the benefit of routine ultrasound if sensitivities and specificities in the community are lower than those reported in the literature, or if false positive and false negative findings cause more lasting distress than we have hypothesized. Equivocally positive findings, which are disproved by follow-up testing,[116] cause significant maternal anxiety and may even lead to spontaneous abortion (after amniocentesis), but are not enumerated in most published studies. Our alternative to ultrasound was no screening; ultrasound may have less benefit relative to MSAFP screening or other alternatives. Most importantly, our analysis may be biased by the irrational confidence that many women place in the results of ultrasonography. Pregnant women's willingness-to-pay in Berwick and Weinstein's study might have been substantially less if they have been informed that a normal sonogram would lower their likelihood of having an affected child by as little as 17%.[14]

We conclude that the complexity of the decision regarding routine second trimester ultrasound, the role of cultural values and local factors (e.g., test specificity), the largely unknown consequences of false negative and false positive findings, and the dominant influence of such variables as willingness-to-pay for normal results argue against firm international policies. Ultrasound screening for fetal anomalies appears to be "worth it" for the great majority of pregnant women in developed nations, according to both this analysis and empirical observations of women's behavior.[117] However, it is prudent to be cautious about establishing screening policies based on maternal perceptions that have not been fully corroborated by randomized controlled trials. Additional research is necessary to quantify and minimize the potentially adverse consequences of routine second trimester ultrasound.

REFERENCES

1. CONSENSUS CONFERENCE. 1984. The use of diagnostic ultrasound imaging during pregnancy. JAMA 252: 669–672.
2. SAARI-KEMPPAINEN, A., O. KARJALAINEN, P. YLOSTALO & O.P. HEINONEN. 1990. Ultrasound screening and perinatal mortality: Controlled trial of systematic one-stage screening in pregnancy. The Helsinki Ultrasound Trial. Lancet 336: 387–391.
3. EWIGMAN, B.G., J.P. CRANE, F.D. FRIGOLETTO, M.L. LEFEVRE, R.P. BAIN, D. MCNELLIS & THE RADIUS STUDY GROUP. 1993. N. Engl. J. Med. 329: 821–827.
4. SKUPSKI, D.W., F.A. CHERVENAK & L.B. MCCULLOUGH. 1995. Routine obstetric ultrasound. Int. J. Gynecol. Obstet. 50: 233–242.
5. BERKOWITZ, R.W. 1993. Should every pregnant woman undergo ultrasonography? (editorial). N. Engl. J. Med. 329: 874–875.
6. ROMERO, R. 1993. Routine obstetric ultrasound (editorial). Ultrasound Obstet. Gynecol. 3: 303–307.
7. U.S. PREVENTIVE SERVICES TASK FORCE. 1996. Guide to Clinical Preventive Services, 2nd edit. Williams & Wilkins. Baltimore, MD.

8. AMERICAN COLLEGE OF OBSTETRICIANS AND GYNECOLOGISTS. 1993. Ultrasonography in pregnancy, Tech. Bull. no. 187. American College of Obstetricians and Gynecologists. Washington, DC.

9. CANADIAN TASK FORCE ON THE PERIODIC HEALTH EXAMINATION. 1992. Periodic health examination, 1992 update. 2. Routine prenatal ultrasound screening. CMAJ **147:** 627–633.

10. DEVORE, G.R. 1994. The routine antenatal diagnostic imaging with ultrasound study: Another perspective. Obstet. Gynecol. **84:** 622–626.

11. GONCALVES, L.F. & R. ROMERO. 1993. A critical appraisal of the RADIUS study. Fetus **3(6):** 7–18.

12. CHERVENAK, F.A. & L.B. MCCULLOUGH. 1992. Ethical issues in obstetric sonography. Clin. Obstet. Gynecol. **35:** 758–762.

13. SAARI-KEMPPAINEN, A., O. KARJALAINEN, P. YLOSTALO & O.P. HEINONEN. 1994. Fetal anomalies in a controlled one-stage ultrasound screening trial. A report from the Helsinki Ultrasound Trial. J. Perinat. Med. **22:** 279–289.

14. CRANE, J.P., M.L. LEFEVRE, R.C. WINBORN, J.K. EVANS, B.G. EWIGMAN, R.P. BAIN, F.D. FRIGOLETTO, D. MCNELLIS, & THE RADIUS STUDY GROUP. 1994. A randomized trial of prenatal ultrasonographic screening: Impact on the detection, management, and outcome of anomalous fetuses. Am. J. Obstet. Gynecol. **171:** 392–399.

15. WALDENSTROM, U., O. AXELSSON, S. NILSSON, G. EKLUND, O. FALL, S. LINDEBERG & Y. SJODIN. 1988. Effects of routine one-stage ultrasound screening in pregnancy: A randomised controlled trial. Lancet **2:** 585–588.

16. BAKKETEIG, L.S., S.H. EIK-NES, G. JACOBSEN, M.K. ULSTEIN, C.J. BRODTKORB, P. BALSTAD, B.C. ERIKSEN & N.P. JORGENSEN. 1984. Randomised controlled trial of ultrasonographic screening in pregnancy. Lancet **2:** 207–211.

17. EWIGMAN, B., M. LEFEVRE & J. HESSER. 1990. A randomized trial of routine prenatal ultrasound. Obstet. Gynecol. **76:** 189–194.

18. EIK-NES, S.H., O. OKLAND, J.C. AURE & M. ULSTEIN. 1984. Ultrasound screening in pregnancy: A randomised controlled trial. Lancet **1:** 1347.

19. EUROCAT WORKING GROUP. 1991. Prevalence of neural tube defects in 20 regions of Europe and the impact of prenatal diagnosis, 1980–1986. J. Epidemiol. Community Health **45:** 52–58.

20. KASSIRER, J.P., A.J. MOSKOWITZ, J. LAU & S.G. PAUKER. 1987. Decision analysis: A progress report. Ann. Intern. Med. **106:** 275–291.

21. PAUKER, S.P. & S.G. PAUKER. 1979. The amniocentesis decision: An explicit guide for parents. Birth Defects Orig. Artic. Ser. **15:** 289–324.

22. PAUKER, S.P. & S.G. PAUKER. 1977. Prenatal diagnosis: A directive approach to genetic counseling using decision analysis. Yale J. Biol. Med. **50:** 275–289.

23. HECKERLING, P.S. & M.S. VERP. 1991. Amniocentesis or chorionic villus sampling for prenatal genetic testing: A decision analysis. J. Clin. Epidemiol. **44:** 657–670.

24. HECKERLING, P.S., M.S. VERP & T.A. HADRO. 1994. Preferences of pregnant women for amniocentesis or chorionic villus sampling for prenatal testing: Comparison of patients' choices and those of a decision-analytic model. J. Clin. Epidemiol. **47:** 1215–1228.

25. CAIRNS, J., P. SHACKLEY & V. HUNDLEY. 1996. Decision making with respect to diagnostic testing: A method of valuing the benefits of antenatal screening. Med. Decision Making **16:** 161–168.

26. BUSKENS, E., E.W. STEYERBERG, J. HESS, J.W. WLADIMIROFF & D.E. GROBBEE. 1997. Routine prenatal screening for congenital heart disease: What can be expected? A decision-analytic approach. Am. J. Public Health **87:** 962–967.

27. BERWICK, D.M. & M.C. WEINSTEIN. 1985. What do patients value? Willingness to pay for ultrasound in normal pregnancy. Med. Care **23:** 881–893.

28. WAITZMAN, N.J., P.S. ROMANO & R.M. SCHEFFLER. 1994. Estimates of the economic costs of birth defects. Inquiry **31:** 188–205.

29. FROBERG, D.G. & R.L. KANE. 1989. Methodology for measuring health-state preferences. 2. Scaling methods. J. Clin. Epidemiol. **42:** 459–471.

30. TORRANCE, G.W. 1986. Measurement of health state utilities for economic appraisal. J. Health Econ. **5:** 1–30.

31. FURLONG, R.M. & R.B. BLACK. 1984. Pregnancy termination for genetic indications: The impact on families. Soc. Work Health Care **10:** 17–34.

32. KUPPERMANN, M., S. SHIBOSKI, D. FEENY, E.P. ELKIN & A.E. WASHINGTON. 1997. Can preference scores for discrete states be used to derive preference scores for an entire path of events? An application to prenatal diagnosis. Med. Decision Making **17:** 42–55.

33. KUPPERMANN, M., D. FEENY, E. GATES, S.F. POSNER, B. BLUMBERG & A.E. WASHINGTON. 1996. Preferences of women facing a prenatal diagnostic choice: Implications for genetic testing guidelines. 1996 Annual Meeting Abstracts. Society for Medical Decision Making.

34. WAITZMAN, N.J., R.M. SCHEFFLER & P.S. ROMANO. 1996. The Cost of Birth Defects. Estimates of the Value of Prevention. University Press of America. Lanham, MD.

35. LIPSCOMB, J. 1986. Human Capital, Willingness-To-Pay, and Cost-Effectiveness Analyses of Screening for Birth Defects in North Carolina. Duke University. Durham, NC.

36. LUTHY, D.A., T. WARDINSKY, D.B. SHURTLEFF, K.A. HOLLENBACH, D.E. HICKOK, D.A. NYBERG & T.J. BENEDETTI. 1991. Cesarean section before the onset of labor and subsequent motor function in infants with meningomyelocele diagnosed antenatally. N. Engl. J. Med. **324:** 662–666.

37. SANDERS, R.C. 1990. Prenatal ultrasonic detection of anomalies with a lethal or disastrous outcome. Radiol. Clin. North Am. **28:** 163–177.

38. PAUKER, S.P. & S.G. PAUKER. 1987. The amniocentesis decision: Ten years of decision analytic experience. Birth Defects Orig. Artic. Ser. **23:** 151–169.

39. WHITE-VAN MOURIK, M.C.A., J.M. CONNOR & M.A. FERGUSON-SMITH. 1992. The psychosocial sequelae of a second-trimester termination of pregnancy for fetal abnormality. Prenatal Diagn. **12:** 189–204.

40. LLOYD, J. & K.M. LAURENCE. 1985. Sequelae and support after termination of pregnancy for fetal malformation. Br. Med. J. **290:** 907–909.

41. SPRANCA, M., E. MINK & J. BARON. 1991. Omission and commission in judgment and choice. J. Exp. Soc. Psychol. **27:** 76–105.

42. LORENZEN, J. & W. HOLZGREVE. 1995. Helping parents to grieve after second trimester termination of pregnancy for fetopathic reasons. Fetal Diagn. Ther. **10:** 147–156.

43. SALVESEN, K.A., L. OYEN, N. SCHMIDT, U.F. MALT & S.H. EIK-NES. 1997. Comparison of long-term psychological responses of women after pregnancy termination due to fetal anomalies and after perinatal loss. Ultrasound Obstet. Gynecol. **9:** 80–85.

44. ZEANAH, C.H., J.V. DAILEY, M.J. ROSENBLATT & D.N. SALLER. 1993. Do women grieve after terminating pregnancies because of fetal anomalies? A controlled investigation. Obstet. Gynecol. **82:** 270–275.

45. LILFORD, R.J., P. STRATTON, S. GODSIL & A. PRASAD. 1994. A randomised trial of routine versus selective counselling in perinatal bereavement from congenital disease. Br. J. Obstet. Gynecol. **101:** 291–296.

46. DONALDSON, C., P. SHACKLEY, M. ABDALLA & Z. MIEDZYBRODZKA. 1995. Willingness to pay for antenatal carrier screening for cystic fibrosis. Health Econ. **4:** 439–452.

47. LANGER, M., M. RINGLER & E. REINOLD. 1988. Psychological effects of ultrasound examinations: Changes in body perception and child image in pregnancy. J. Psychosom. Obstet. Gynecol. **8:** 199–208.

48. ZLOTOGORSKI, Z., O. TADMOR, E. DUNIEC, R. RABINOWITZ & Y. DIAMANT. 1996. The effect of the amount of feedback on anxiety levels during ultrasound scanning. J. Clin. Ultrasound **24:** 21–24.

49. MICHELACCI, L., G.A. FAVA, S. GRANDI, L. BOVICELLI, C. ORLANDI & G. TROMBINI. 1988. Psychological reactions to ultrasound examination during pregnancy. Psychother. Psychosom. **50:** 1–4.

50. HUNFELD, J.A.M., G. AGTERBERG, J.W. WLADIMIROFF & J. PASSCHIER. 1996. Quality of life and anxiety in pregnancies after late pregnancy loss: A case-control study. Prenatal Diagn. **16:** 783–790.

51. HUNTER, M.S., M.M. TSOI, M. PEARCE, P. CHUDLEIGH & S. CAMPBELL. 1987. Ultrasound scanning in women with raised serum alpha fetoprotein: Long-term psychological effects. J. Psychosom. Obstet. Gynecol. **6:** 25–31.

52. BAR-HAVA, I., M. BRONSHTEIN, R. ORVIETO, Y. SHALEV, S. STAL & Z. BEN-RAFAEL. 1997.

Caution: Prenatal clubfoot can be both a transient and a late-onset phenomenon. Prenatal Diagn. **17:** 457–460.

53. ANGIER, N. 1996. Ultrasound and fury: One mother's ordeal. New York Times. Nov. 26, 1996: B7, B10.

54. MARTEAU, T.M., R. COOK, J. KIDD, S. MICHIE, M. JOHNSTON, J. SLACK & R.W. SHAW. 1992. The psychological effects of false-positive results in prenatal screening for fetal abnormality: A prospective study. Prenatal Diagn. **12:** 205–214.

55. BURTON, B.K., R. G. DILLARD & E.N. CLARK. 1985. The psychological impact of false positive elevations of maternal serum alpha-fetoprotein. Am. J. Obstet. Gynecol. **151:** 77–82.

56. NATIONAL CENTER FOR HEALTH STATISTICS. 1996. Vital Statistics of the United States, 1991. Vol. 2. Mortality, part A. Public Health Service. Washington, DC.

57. NATIONAL CENTER FOR HEALTH STATISTICS. 1995. Vital Statistics of the United States, 1992. Vol. 1. Natality. Public Health Service. Washington, DC.

58. MCNEIL, T.F. 1997. Anomalies and the mental health professional. Ann. N.Y. Acad. Sci. This volume.

59. FRANCOME, C. & W. SAVAGE. 1993. Caesarean section in Britain and the United States 12% or 24%: Is either the right rate? Soc. Sci. & Med. **37:** 1199–1218.

60. LILFORD, R.J., H.A. VAN COEVERDEN DE GROOT, P.J. MOORE & P. BINGHAM. 1990. The relative risks of caesarean section (intrapartum and elective) and vaginal delivery: A detailed analysis to exclude the effects of medical disorders and other acute pre-existing physiological disturbances. Br. J. Obstet. Gynecol. **97:** 883–892.

61. JOFFE, M., J. CHAPPLE, C. PATERSON & R.W. BEARD. 1994. What is the optimal cesarean section rate? An outcome based study of existing variation. J. Epidemiol. Community Health **48:** 406–411.

62. DIMATTEO, M.R., S.C. MORTON, H.S. LEPPER, T.M. DAMUSH, M.F. CARNEY, M. PEARSON & K.L. KAHN. 1996. Cesarean childbirth and psychosocial outcomes: A meta-analysis. Health Psychol. **15:** 303–314.

63. GREEN, J.M., V.A. COUPLAND & J.V. KITZINGER. 1988. Great Expectations: A Prospective Study of Women's Expectations and Experiences of Childbirth. University of Cambridge, Childcare and Developmental Group. Cambridge, England.

64. GAREL, M., N. LELONG, A. MARCHAND & M. KAMINSKI. 1990. Psychosocial consequences of caesarean childbirth: A four-year follow-up study. Early Hum. Dev. **21:** 105–114.

65. COCHRANE, D.D., S.T. MYLES, C. NIMROD, D.K. STILL, R.G. SUGARMAN & B.K. WITTMANN. 1985. Intrauterine hydrocephalus and ventriculomegaly: Associated anomalies and fetal outcome. Can. J. Neurol. Sci. **12:** 51–59.

66. CHERVENAK, F.A., R.L. BERKOWITZ, M. TORTORA & J.C. HOBBINS. 1985. The management of fetal hydrocephalus. Am. J. Obstet. Gynecol. **151:** 933–942.

67. VINTZILEOS, A.M., W.A. CAMPBELL, P.J. WEINBAUM & D.J. NOCHIMSON. 1987. Perinatal management and outcome of fetal ventriculomegaly. Obstet. Gynecol. **69:** 5–11.

68. GLICK, P.L., M.R. HARRISON, D.K. NAKAYAMA, M.S.B. EDWARDS, R.A. FILLY, D.H. CHINN, P.W. CALLEN, S.L. WILSON & M.S. GOLBUS. 1984. Management of ventriculomegaly in the fetus. J. Pediatr. **105:** 97–105.

69. SAKALA, E.P., L.N. ERHARD & J.J. WHITE. 1993. Elective cesarean section improves outcomes of neonates with gastroschisis. Am. J. Obstet. Gynecol. **169:** 1050–1053.

70. HADDOCK, G., C.F. DAVIS & P.A. RAINE. 1996. Gastroschisis in the decade of prenatal diagnosis: 1983–1993. Eur. J. Pediatr. Surg. **6:** 18–22.

71. ADRA, A.M., H.J. LANDY, J. NAHMIAS & O. GOMEZ-MARIN. 1996. The fetus with gastroschisis: Impact of route of delivery and prenatal ultrasonography. Am. J. Obstet. Gynecol. **174:** 540–546.

72. SERMER, M., R.J. BENZIE, L. PITSON, M. CARR & M. SKIDMORE. 1987. Prenatal diagnosis and management of congenital defects of the anterior abdominal wall. Am. J. Obstet. Gynecol. **156:** 308–312.

73. LEWIS, D.F., C.V. TOWERS, T.J. GARITE, D.N. JACKSON, M.P. NAGEOTTE & C.A. MAJOR. 1990. Fetal gastroschisis and omphalocele: Is cesarean section the best mode of delivery? Am. J. Obstet. Gynecol. **163:** 773–775.

74. SIPES, S.L., C.P. WEINER, D.R. SIPES 2d, S.S. GRANT & R.A. WILLIAMSON. 1990. Gas-

troschisis and omphalocele: Does either antenatal diagnosis or route of delivery make a difference in perinatal outcome? Obstet. Gynecol. **76:** 195–199.

75. LENKE, R.R. & E.I. HATCH, JR. 1986. Fetal gastroschisis: A preliminary report advocating the use of cesarean section. Obstet. Gynecol. **67:** 395–398.

76. MORETTI, M., A. KHOURY, J. RODRIGUEZ, T. LOBE, D. SHAVER & B. SIBAI. 1990. The effect of mode of delivery on the perinatal outcome in fetuses with abdominal wall defects. Am. J. Obstet. Gynecol. **163:** 833–838.

77. MERCER, S., B. MERCER, M.E.G. D'ALTON & P. SOUCY. 1988. Gastroschisis: Ultrasonographic diagnosis, perinatal embryology, surgical and obstetric treatment and outcomes. Can. J. Surg. **31:** 25–26.

78. KIRK, E.P. & R.M. WAH. 1983. Obstetric management of the fetus with omphalocele or gastroschisis: A review and report of one hundred twelve cases. Am. J. Obstet. Gynecol. **146:** 512–518.

79. SWIFT, R.I., M.P. SINGH, D.A. ZIDERMAN, M. SILVERMAN, M.A. ELDER & M.G. ELDER. 1992. A new regime in the management of gastroschisis. J. Pediatr. Surg. **27:** 61–63.

80. BETHEL, C.A.I., J.H. SEASHORE & R.J. TOULOUKIAN. 1989. Cesarean section does not improve outcome in gastroschisis. J. Pediatr. Surg. **24:** 1–4.

81. MORROW, R.J., M.J. WHITTLE, M.B. MCNAY, P.A.M. RAINE, A.A.M. GIBSON & J. CROSSLEY. 1993. Prenatal diagnosis and management of anterior abdominal wall defects in the west of Scotland. Prenatal Diagn. **13:** 111–115.

82. CHESCHEIR, N.C., R.G. AZIZKHAN, J.W. SEEDS, S.R. LACEY & W.J. WATSON. 1991. Counseling and care for the pregnancy complicated by gastroschisis. Am. J. Perinatol. **8:** 323–329.

83. BOND, S.J., M.R. HARRISON, R.A. FILLY, P.W. CALLEN, R.A. ANDERSON & M.S. GOLBUS. 1988. Severity of intestinal damage in gastroschisis: Correlation with prenatal sonographic findings. J. Pediatr. Surg. **23:** 520–525.

84. NOVOTNY, D.A., R.L. KLEIN & C.R. BOECKMAN. 1993. Gastroschisis: An 18-year review. J. Pediatr. Surg. **28:** 650–652.

85. QUIRK, J.G., JR., J. FORTNEY, H.B. COLLINS II, J. WEST, S.J. HASSAD & C. WAGNER. 1996. Outcomes of newborns with gastroschisis: The effects of mode of delivery, site of delivery, and interval from birth to surgery. Am. J. Obstet. Gynecol. **174:** 1134–1138.

86. STRINGER, M.D., R.J. BRERETON & V.M. WRIGHT. 1991. Controversies in the management of gastroschisis: A study of 40 patients. Arch. Dis. Child. **66:** 34–36.

87. COUGHLIN, J.P., D.E.M. DRUCKER, M.R. JEWELL, M.J. EVANS & M.D. KLEIN. 1993. Delivery room repair of gastroschisis. Surgery **114:** 822–827.

88. DILLON, E. & M. RENWICK. 1995. The antenatal diagnosis and management of abdominal wall defects: The Northern Region experience. Clin. Radiol. **50:** 855–859.

89. STOODLEY, N., A. SHARMA, H. NOBLETT & D. JAMES. 1993. Influence of place of delivery on outcome in babies with gastroschisis. Arch. Dis. Child. **68:** 321–323.

90. CHANG, A.C., J.C. HUHTA, G.Y. YOON, D.C. WOOD, G. TULZER, A. COHEN, M. MENNUTI & W.I. NORWOOD. 1991. Diagnosis, transport, and outcome in fetuses with left ventricular outflow tract obstruction. J. Thorac. Cardiovasc. Surg. **102:** 841–848.

91. SHARLAND, G.K., S.M. LOCKHART, A.J. HEWARD & L.D. ALLAN. 1992. Prognosis in fetal diaphragmatic hernia. Am. J. Obstet. Gynecol. **166:** 9–13.

92. ROMERO, R., A. GHIDINI, K. COSTIGAN, R. TOULOUKIAN & J.C. HOBBINS. 1988. Prenatal diagnosis of duodenal atresia: Does it make any difference? Obstet. Gynecol. **71:** 739–741.

93. NORWOOD, W.I., A.R. DOBELL, M.D. FREED, J.W. KIRKLIN, E.H. BLACKSTONE, AND THE CONGENITAL SURGEONS HEART SOCIETY. 1988. Intermediate results of the arterial switch repair. A 20-institution study. J. Thorac. Cardiovasc. Surg. **96:** 854–863.

94. HANNAN, E.L., M. RACZ, R.E. KAVEY, J.M. QUAEGEBUR & R. WILLIAMS. Pediatric cardiac surgery: The effect of hospital and surgeon volume on in-hospital mortality. Pediatrics. In press.

95. JENKINS, K.J., J. W. NEWBURGER, J.E. LOCK, R.B. DAVIS, G.A. COFFMAN & L.I. IEZZONI. 1995. In-hospital mortality for surgical repair of congenital heart defects: Preliminary observations of variation by hospital caseload. Pediatrics **95:** 323–330.

96. MOONEY, G. & M. LANGE. 1993. Ante-natal screening: What constitutes "benefit"? Soc. Sci. & Med. **37:** 873–878.

97. FEENY, D.H. & G.W. TORRANCE. 1989. Incorporating utility-based quality-of-life assessment measures in clinical trials. Two examples. Med. Care **27:** S190–204.

98. LAURENCE, K.M. & J. MORRIS. 1981. The effect of the introduction of prenatal diagnosis on the reproductive history of women at increased risk from neural tube defects. Prenatal Diagn. **1:** 51–60.

99. LUCK, C.A. 1992. Value of routine ultrasound scanning at 19 weeks: A four year study of 8849 deliveries. Br. Med. J. **304:** 1474–1478.

100. CHITTY, L.S., G.H. HUNT, J. MOORE & M.O. LOBB. 1991. Effectiveness of routine ultrasonography in detecting fetal structural abnormalities in a low risk population. Br. Med. J. **303:** 1165–1169.

101. LEVI, S., J.P. SCHNAPPS, P. DEHAVAY, R. COULON & P. DEFOORT. 1995. End-result of routine ultrasound screening for congenital anomalies: The Belgian Multicentric Study 1984–92. Ultrasound Obstet. Gynecol. **5:** 366–371.

102. BROCKS, V. & J. BANG. 1991. Routine examination by ultrasound for the detection of fetal malformations in a low risk population. Fetal Diagn. Ther. **6:** 37–45.

103. SHIRLEY, I.M., F. BOTTOMLEY & V.P. ROBINSON. 1992. Routine radiographer screening for fetal abnormalities by ultrasound in an unselected low risk population. Br. J. Radiol. **65:** 564–569.

104. ANDERSON, N., O. BOSWELL & G. DUFF. 1995. Prenatal sonography for the detection of fetal anomalies: Results of a prospective study and comparison with prior series. Am. J. Roentgenol. **165:** 943–950.

105. CARRERA, J.M., M. TORRENTS, C. MORTERA, V. CUSI & A. MUNOZ. 1995. Routine prenatal ultrasound screening for fetal abnormalities: 22 years' experience. Ultrasound Obstet. Gynecol. **5:** 174–179.

106. VELIE, E.M. & G.M. SHAW. 1996. Impact of prenatal diagnosis and elective termination on prevalence and risk estimates of neural tube defects in California, 1989–1991. Am. J. Epidemiol. **144:** 473–479.

107. CRAGAN, J.D., H.E. ROBERTS, L.D. EDMONDS, M.J. KHOURY, R.S. KIRBY, G.M. SHAW, E.M. VELIE, R.D. MERZ, M.B. FORRESTER, R.A. WILLIAMSON, et al. 1995. Surveillance for anencephaly and spina bifida and the impact of prenatal diagnosis—United States, 1985–1994. MMWR CDC Surveillance Summaries **44(4):** 1–13.

108. STOLL, C., B. DOTT, Y. ALEMBIK & M.P. ROTH. 1995. Evaluation of routine prenatal diagnosis by a registry of congenital anomalies. Prenatal Diagn. **15:** 791–800.

109. PAPP, Z., E. TOTH-PAL, C. PAPP, Z. TOTH, M. SZABO, L. VERESS & O. TOROK. 1995. Impact of prenatal mid-trimester screening on the prevalence of fetal structural anomalies: A prospective epidemiological study. Ultrasound Obstet. Gynecol. **6:** 320–326.

110. PRYDE, P.G., N.B. ISADA, M. HALLAK, M.P. JOHNSON, A.E. ODGERS & M.I. EVANS. 1992. Determinants of parental decision to abort or continue after non-aneuploid ultrasound-detected fetal abnormalities. Obstet. Gynecol. **80:** 52–56.

111. MONTANA, E., M. J. KHOURY, J. D. CRAGAN, S. SHARMA, P. DHAR & D. FYFE. 1996. Trends and outcomes after prenatal diagnosis of congenital cardiac malformations by echocardiography in a well-defined birth population, Atlanta, Georgia, 1990–1994. J. Am. Coll. Cardiol. **28:** 1805–1809.

112. LE-HA, C., D.H. STONE & W.H. GILMOUR. 1995. Impact of prenatal screening and diagnosis on the epidemiology of structural congenital anomalies. J. Med. Screening **2:** 67–70.

113. ALLAN, L.D., G.K. SHARLAND, A. MILBURN, S.M. LOCKHART, A.M.M. GROVES, R.H. ANDERSON, A.C. COOK & N.L.K. FAGG. 1994. Prospective diagnosis of 1,006 consecutive cases of congenital heart disease in the fetus. J. Am. Coll. Cardiol. **23:** 1452–1458.

114. VENTURA, S.J., J.A. MARTIN, S.C. CURTIN & T.J. MATHEWS. 1997. Report of final natality statistics, 1995. Monthly Vital Statistics Rep. **45(Supp. 2):** 2.

115. MCCULLOUGH, D.C. & L.A. BALZER-MARTIN. 1982. Current prognosis in overt neonatal hydrocephalus. J. Neurosurg. **57:** 378–383.

116. MERZ, E., F. BAHLMANN & G. WEBER. 1995. Volume scanning in the evaluation of fetal malformations: A new dimension in prenatal diagnosis. Ultrasound Obstet. Gynecol. **5:** 222–227.

117. LEIVO, T., R. TUOMINEN, A. SAARI-KEMPPAINEN, P. YLOSTALO P, O. KARJALAINEN &

O.P. HEINONEN. 1996. Cost-effectiveness of one-stage ultrasound screening in pregnancy: A report from the Helsinki ultrasound trial. Ultrasound Obstet. Gynecol. **7:** 309–314.

118. BUECHLER, E.J. 1997. Managed care and ultrasound for the diagnosis of fetal anomalies. Ann. N.Y. Acad. Sci. This volume.

119. JULIAN-REYNIER, C., N. PHILIP, C. SCHEINER, Y. AURRAN, F. CHABAL, A. MARON, A. GOMBERT & S. AYME. 1994. Impact of prenatal diagnosis by ultrasound on the prevalence of congenital anomalies at birth in southern France. J. Epidemiol. Community Health **48:** 290–296.

Routine Ultrasound Scanning for Congenital Abnormalities

NICHOLAS J. WALD[a] AND ANNE KENNARD

Department of Environmental and Preventive Medicine, Wolfson Institute of Preventive Medicine, St. Bartholomew's and the Royal London School of Medicine and Dentistry, Charterhouse Square, London EC1M 6BQ, United Kingdom

ABSTRACT: Screening has been defined as "the systematic application of a test or enquiry, to identify individuals at sufficient risk of a specific disorder to benefit from further investigation or direct preventive action, among persons who have not sought medical attention on account of symptoms of that disorder" (Wald, N.J. 1994. J. Med. Screen. 1: 76). The purpose of screening is to benefit the individuals being screened. The early detection of abnormalities should not be an end in itself, and the value of a screening approach needs to be determined before it is introduced into practice. Ultrasound as a means of screening for fetal abnormalities has not been adequately assessed even though it is widely used in this way. To assess its value it is helpful to classify abnormalities that can be detected on the basis of the clinical usefulness of doing so. To this end we propose four categories similar to those independently suggested by the Royal College of Obstetricians and Gynaecologists Working Party on Ultrasound Screening for Fetal Abnormalities. Four groups were specified: (A) major abnormalities—death inevitable, (B) abnormalities associated with long-term handicap, (C) abnormalities potentially amenable to intrauterine treatment, and (D) fetal conditions that require immediate postnatal investigation and/or treatment. For each abnormality, the screening detection *and* false-positives need to be estimated together with the medical and financial costs of screening, particularly those arising from findings of uncertain or little medical consequence that may lead to worry and further unnecessary obstetric intervention.

INTRODUCTION

Antenatal ultrasound anomaly scanning has become widespread in many parts of the world. A recent survey[1] reported that 82% of maternity units in the United Kingdom now offer such a scan, usually at about 18 weeks of pregnancy. Many firmly believe that such scanning is useful whereas others remain unconvinced. It is acknowledged that in certain pregnancies scanning can identify abnormalities, but it is also recognized that it can cause harm by prompting unnecessary medical intervention.

The reason for the uncertainty over the application of the technology is that it is a complex subject to evaluate. The main difficulty in this respect is that it is, as currently offered, a nonspecific investigation in which the ultrasound examiner looks for a wide range of structural abnormalities as well as other findings that might be markers of a medical disorder. Over 100 different abnormalities can be identified using an ultrasound scan examination. This capability explains both the attraction of the procedure and the problems in its evaluation. There are few areas in medicine where a test involves examining everything that can be seen or measured. For example, when a blood sample is taken, we do not test for everything that can be measured, even though the cost of extra tests may be small. It is recognized that abnormal values can occur more often by chance than because of genuine disease, and many diseases identified have no effective treatment.

[a]E-mail: n.j.wald@mds.qmw.ac.uk

SCREENING OR DIAGNOSIS

When a test is used routinely in a large population there is a tendency to describe it as a screening test. The purpose behind the use of a test determines whether it is a screening test or a diagnostic test. If the *intention* is to identify a high-risk group who would benefit from a diagnostic test, it is a screening test. If it is being used to make a diagnosis, which if positive will be followed by the offer of a remedy, then it is being used as a diagnostic test. The distinction between screening and diagnosis rests more on the reason for performing the test than on whether it is performed on everyone or only on a few. For example, using ultrasound to identify the cranial signs associated with spina bifida is screening; confirming that spina bifida is present is diagnosis. Using ultrasound to identify markers, for example, of Down syndrome, and then offering an amniocentesis and a karyotype if such markers are present is screening; to identify a structural abnormality directly is diagnosis. We limit the scope of our paper to the use of ultrasound in the diagnosis of fetal abnormality.

NEED TO DEFINE PURPOSE

There is a need to specify those abnormalities to be detected, recognizing the purpose in doing so, and then to assess the efficacy of this relative to the harm and cost. The potential benefit of antenatal ultrasound scanning for congenital abnormalities is to be gained in relation to four groups of abnormalities, defined according to the clinical action that may be taken. The categories we had derived were similar to those specified independently by the Royal College of Obstetricians and Gynaecologists Working Party on Ultrasound Screening for Fetal Abnormalities, and we here use the same order of categories, namely:

A. abnormalities in which a termination of pregnancy avoids continuing with a pregnancy in which fetal or neonatal death is inevitable
B. those associated with serious disability for which termination of pregnancy is justifiable
C. those for which *in utero* treatment reduces morbidity
D. those for which immediate postnatal treatment reduces morbidity.

The definition of these potentially beneficial outcomes allows the establishment of criteria needed to define a true-positive. A true-positive in this context means that the specified pathological condition is identified (for example, spina bifida), and a specific effective intervention would be offered that can alter prognosis. There is no purpose in making a diagnosis of other abnormalities.

In effect this means the disorder should fall into one of the four categories given above. A false-positive can then be defined by exclusion, namely, an identified ultrasound abnormality that is either not confirmed, or is confirmed but for which no effective intervention exists.

EVALUATION OF TEST PERFORMANCE

To determine the performance of a test, three parameters need to be estimated: the detection rate (proportion of affected individuals with positive results), the false-positive rate (proportion of unaffected individuals with positive results), and the odds of being affected given a positive result (OAPR, the ratio of the number of true-positives to the number of false-positives). The OAPR is the positive predictive value expressed as an odds. The critical parameters are the detection rate and the false-positive rate, which are both independent of the prevalence of the disease in the population being scanned. The OAPR is determined by the detection rate, false-positive rate, and the prevalence of the disorder. The difficulty in reviewing the literature in this area is that many studies publish estimates of detection rates without giving the corresponding false-positive rates. More important, many studies present only an OAPR. This arises because in clinical practice it is usual to scan a population and only follow up women with positive ultrasound findings. This, in effect, yields the OAPR which, by itself, is unhelpful in evaluating the test. A further difficulty is that most of the disorders of importance are rare, so the numbers in any particular study are small and unreliable. There is also uncertainty over the definition of the disorder; sometimes it is the ultrasound finding itself, for example, pyelectasis, which may or may not reflect the presence of a disorder of clinical importance, and sometimes the disorder itself, for example, spina bifida.

ILLUSTRATION OF THE IMPORTANCE OF ESTABLISHING THE DEFINITION OF TRUE- AND FALSE-POSITIVES

TABLE 1 shows a hypothetical example in which 10,000 women were scanned. In this group there were 50 pregnancies with congenital heart defects, of which 20 were detected. Of the 50 congenital heart defects, four were sufficiently serious to justify either a termination of pregnancy or special immediate postnatal treatment (two of which were among the detected). In addition, there was one case in which diagnosis of congenital heart disease was made but on subsequent review was not present. If only the first criterion for a true-positive (namely, having congenital heart disease) is used to define a positive, the detection rate is 40% (20 out of 50) and the false-positive rate is 0.01% or 1 out of 10,000. If both criteria are used (namely, having congenital heart disease which merits termination or special early treatment) and there are only two true-positives, the detection rate increases to 50% (2 out of 4), whereas 18 of the previous true-positives become false-positives. These, together with the previous one, yield 19 false-positives in total; a false-positive rate of 0.19% instead of 0.01%. The OAPR using only the first criterion is 20:1 whereas the OAPR using both criteria is about 1:10.

A similar exercise can be done on real data from the US RADIUS study.[2] This was a randomized trial of about 15,000 women who were allocated into two groups: the

TABLE 1. Hypothetical Example of the Results of an Ultrasound Screening Program for Heart Defects Using Two Different Criteria for a True-Positive Result
[Number of pregnancies scanned: 10,000; heart defects: 50 (4 major); true-positives: 20 (2 major); false-positives: 1.]

	Specified Disorder	Specified Disorder with a Remedy
True-positives	20 (40%)	2 (50%)
False-positives	1 (0.01%)	19 (0.19%)
OAPR	20:1	2:19
		~1:10

OAPR, the odds of being affected given a positive result.

TABLE 2. Results from the RADIUS Study Relating to the Detection of Fetal Abnormality in the "Screened" Group and Adjusted according to Different Criteria for True- and False-Positives[a]

	Reported (any abnormality)	Adjusted (abnormalities for which termination is offered)	New Approach	Excess Relative to Control Group
True-positives detected before 24 weeks	31 (17%)	9	9	5
False-positives	6 (0.08%)	28 (0.4%)	~0	0
OAPR	5:1 (i.e., 31:6)	1:3 (i.e., 9:28)	9:0	5:0
"Success"	31/7,685 (4.0/1,000)	9/7,685 (1.2/1,000)	9/7,685 (1.2/1,000)	5/7,685 (0.7/1,000)
"Failure"	6/7,685 (0.8/1,000)	28/7,685 (3.6/1,000)	0/7,685 (<0.1/1,000)	0/7,685 (<0.1/1,000)

OAPR, the odds of being affected given a positive result.
[a] 7,685 pregnancies in screened group; 187 reported to have an abnormality.
(Based on Crane et al.[2])

women in one group received a routine scan; in the other they received an ultrasound scan only when clinically indicated (control group). TABLE 2 shows the results relating to the 7,685 pregnancies in the "screened" group and the 187 with a variety of congenital abnormalities in this group. The reported detection rate before 24 weeks of pregnancy was 17% (31 out of 187) with a false-positive rate of 0.08% (based on six cases in which an abnormality was suspected but later not confirmed and did not lead to an invasive intervention). The reported results yield an OAPR of about 5:1. If the same data are reexamined using the definitions proposed and restricting outcomes to those for which the effective intervention is a termination of pregnancy, there are only nine true-positives and 28 false-positives, an OAPR of 1:3 (the detection rate cannot be specified because the total number of affected pregnancies in the "screened" group for which the offer of a termination of pregnancy would be indicated was not reported, although it may have been close to 100%). An OAPR of 1:3 is clearly unsatisfactory when the remedy is a termination of pregnancy.

If it is accepted that an ultrasound finding that does not warrant the recommendation of definitive medical or surgical intervention is a negative, then the 28 pregnancies in TABLE 2 classified as false-positives become true-negatives. The OAPR is then 9:0. Clinical action has been limited to those cases that require intervention without causing distress to other women by advising them of an abnormality for which there is no effective intervention. The last column in TABLE 2 shows the excess relative to the control group in the RADIUS study. There were four terminations in the control group and therefore an estimated five extra terminations in the "screened" group which otherwise would not have been identified. The table also shows the rate of finding abnormalities sought for expressed as a prevalence, that is, prevalence of "successes" and, in the same way, the prevalence of failures. TABLE 2 illustrates our proposition that it is the approach to routine ultrasound scanning that needs to be reviewed and, in particular, the definition of a true-positive. It means looking at it from the perspective of offering an ultrasound scan and reporting the result as positive or negative on the basis of whether an intervention is offered, as well as if an abnormality is found.

OBSERVATIONS ON THE RADIUS STUDY

The RADIUS study, judged to be a large randomized trial (over 15,000 women), reported that routine scanning had no effect on perinatal outcome (5% of the "screened" group had adverse perinatal outcomes compared with 4.9% in the control group), no effect on preterm deliveries, and that the detection of congenital anomalies had no effect on birth weight. The overall conclusion was that "screening ultrasonography did not improve perinatal outcome as compared with selective ultrasonography on the basis of clinical judgement."[2] The data produced from the RADIUS study is undoubtedly of value, but the negative conclusion is probably not justified in the light of the data published. For example, the number of terminations associated with serious disorders in the screened group was nine compared with four in the control group, a result that was correctly reported as being not statistically significant. However, if the same effect had been observed in a study that was 10 times larger, there would have been 90 terminations versus 40 terminations, a result that would have been statistically significant. It would be equivalent to avoiding the births of 0.7 per 1,000 pregnancies destined to die *in utero* or shortly after birth, or lead to viable severe disability. This would be comparable with the effect of other screening programs for fetal abnormalities. The study was too small to say that there was no worthwhile benefit. Similarly, the study reported that the survival among infants with acute life-threatening anomalies was 21 out of 28 (75%) in the screened group compared with 11 out of 21 (52%) in the control group. This difference could, however, be due to more patients with less severe abnormalities being identified in the screened group, thus inflating the denominator. The preferred analysis would be to compare mortality in the two groups. There were seven deaths in the screened group and 10 in the control group—a result that could be due to chance or, if real, would require a trial over 10 times larger to be statistically significant. The results are, however, useful in suggesting that the expected benefit due to early postnatal treatment can only be small. The RADIUS study has provided a reasonably objective indication of the magnitude of the expected benefits that might arise from routine scanning. They are less than some may have expected, but large enough to compare with alternative similar strategies such as serum screening.

EXAMPLE OF THE ESTIMATION OF DETECTION RATE FOR A SPECIFIC DISORDER

TABLE 3 shows a summary of the studies of routine ultrasound anomaly scanning in which spina bifida pregnancies were identified. Data are limited to reports published after 1988 and data collected after 1986. One hundred and twenty affected pregnancies were identified out of 141, a detection rate of 85%. Within this population of over 160,000, no false-positives were reported. This highlights a further difficulty. Because the test is being used as a diagnostic procedure followed by the offer of a termination of pregnancy (usually accepted), it may become impossible to determine whether an aborted fetus was unaffected, if the process of abortion damages the fetus too much. There is probably no solution to the problem of not being able to recognize false-positive diagnoses. Nonetheless, for each disorder to be diagnosed by ultrasound,

TABLE 3. Summary of Routine Ultrasound Anomaly Scanning in which Pregnancies with Spina Bifida Were Identified (Excluding Reports Published before 1989 and Data Collected before 1987)

Study	Study Period	Pregnancies with Spina Bifida		Pregnancies Scanned (approx. n)
		Detected (n)	Total (n)	
Chitty et al.[3]	1988–1989	5	5	8,000
Constantine & McCormack[4]	1988–1989	4	5	5,000
Crane et al.[2]	1987–1991	3	4	7,000
Goncalves et al.[5]	1987–1991	19	21	600
Levi et al.[6]	1990–1992	9	11	9,000
Luck[7]	1988–1991	3	3	9,000
Papp et al.[8]	1988–1989	40	44	52,000
Roberts et al.[9]	1988–1989	14	16	11,000
Shirley et al.[10]	1989–1990	3	3	6,000
Stoll et al.[11]	1989–1992	20	29	56,000
Total		120	141	160,000

Detection rate = 120/141 (85%)

False-positive rate = 0/160,000 (0%)[a]

[a]No spina bifida false-positives reported.

the kind of analysis illustrated in TABLE 3 for spina bifida is needed before the test can be fully validated.

APPROPRIATENESS OF STUDY DESIGN

A randomized trial is not always the appropriate study design. The assumption that evidence from such a study is more compelling than evidence from other sources should not automatically be made. It usually provides the best evidence in circumstances where bias could have influenced the result. If this is impossible, or extremely unlikely, it is an inefficient design because it reduces statistical power through some individuals not receiving the intervention. TABLE 4 shows the study design that we think is appropriate for the four different categories of women having an ultrasound antenatal diagnosis of a congenital abnormality. For category A, as described earlier, in which a termination of pregnancy is the only available remedy, a randomized trial is inappropriate because the results are not materially subject to bias. It is also probably unnecessary for category C (where fetal surgery may be the outcome). In category D, where immediate postnatal treatment may improve prognosis compared with routine care, a trial is probably necessary to provide an unbiased answer, but the numbers needed for such a trial would be so large (probably 100,000 or more) that it is unlikely that such a study will be a practical option. TABLE 4 gives an approximate indication of the birth prevalence of disorders amenable to each of the three. This is based on tentative estimates of detectable abnormalities that are fatal (such as anencephaly), or would result in a viable but seriously disabled individual (such as one with spina bifida), and conditions such as abdominal wall defects, for which early surgery may be beneficial. These estimates are probably generous and should be regarded as maximal estimates. In total, the overall maximum rate of pregnancies that stand to benefit is about 0.5%.

TABLE 4. Study Designs Appropriate for Evaluating Ultrasound Scanning for the Four Different Categories of Fetal Disorders[a]

Group[b]	Remedy	RCT of Routine Scanning	Nonrandomized Study of Routine Scanning	Approx. Birth Prevalence of Ultrasound Detectable Amenable to Remedy	Approx. Size of Study Needed	Is Such a Study a Practical Option?
A + B	Termination	No	Yes	3/1000	70,000	Yes
C	Fetal surgery	No	Yes	<1/10000	>100,000	No
D	Immediate postnatal treatment	Yes	No	2/1000	100,000	Unlikely

[a] Overall rate of pregnancies that stand to benefit: ~ 5/1,000 or 0.5%.
A: Abnormalities in which a termination of pregnancy avoids continuing with a pregnancy in which fetal or neonatal death is inevitable.
B: Abnormalities associated with serious disability for which termination of pregnancy is justified.
C: Abnormalities for which *in utero* treatment reduces morbidity.
D: Abnormalities for which immediate postnatal treatment reduces morbidity.

CONCLUSION

Ultrasound scanning is effective in the diagnosis of congenital abnormalities. Although not considered in our paper, it is well recognized that such scanning can also cause avoidable worry and unnecessary medical intervention, principally further scans with no definitive action in many cases.

Many studies on the value of routine screening in pregnancy have been unsatisfactory. Some studies reported negative conclusions in spite of evidence of efficacy both from the study itself and from other work. The main reason for studies yielding such false-negative conclusions is that the objective of scanning was not precisely defined in terms of the specific abnormalities that would be detected and for which action would be taken, so that general outcome categories, such as perinatal mortality, were used; this diluted the results. Another reason for reaching apparent false-negative conclusions is the loss of statistical power by using an inappropriate study design, for example, a randomized trial when this was not needed for some of the key end points. Other studies have led to false-positive conclusions largely on the basis of assumptions—the assumption that detection of an abnormality per se is worthwhile, as well as the assumption that planned postnatal care is better than routine care. The underlying conceptual problem stems from an inappropriate definition of a true-positive, that is, any structural abnormality instead of abnormalities for which an effective intervention would be offered.

In future practice we believe the aim should be to identify and report only those disorders for which an effective intervention exists. We also believe that there is a need to specify the disorders and their intervention to the women before the scan is performed. In this way genuine consent can be obtained. This will require a process of discussion and examination of data so that the specified disorders command a reasonable measure of agreement. Having specified what will be sought and reported, there would no longer be a need to report abnormalities for which there is no effective intervention. Indeed, to do so is unjustified because it causes needless distress and the temptation to carry out further unnecessary medical investigations. We acknowledge that there maybe a reluctance to withhold apparently positive findings for which there is no effective remedy, but the new approach aims to improve the benefit of the fetal abnormality scan, simplify the examination by only seeking specified abnormalities instead of all possible abnormalities, and to better quantify its value.

REFERENCES

1. RCOG/RCR SURVEY on the use of obstetric ultrasound in the UK, 1996. Cited in the Report of the RCOG Working Party on Ultrasound Screening for Fetal Abnormalities—Consultation document. Submitted.

2. CRANE, J.P., M.L. LeFEVRE, R.C. WINBORN, J.K. EVANS, B.G. EWIGMAN, R.P. BAIN, F.D. FRIGOLETTO, D. McNELLIS & THE RADIUS STUDY GROUP. 1994. A randomised trial of prenatal ultrasonographic screening: Impact on the detection, management and outcome of anomalous fetuses. Am. J. Obstet. Gynecol. **171**: 392–399.

3. CHITTY, L.S., G.H. HUNT, J. MOORE & M.O. LOBB. 1991. Effectiveness of routine ultrasonography in detecting fetal structural abnormalities in a low risk population. Br. Med. J. **393**: 1165–1169.

4. CONSTANTINE, G. & J. McCORMACK. 1991. Comparative audit of booking and mid-trimester ultrasound scans in the prenatal diagnosis of congenital anomalies. Prenatal Diagn. **11**: 909–914.

5. GONCALVES, L.F., P. JEANTY & J.M. PIPER. 1994. The accuracy of prenatal ultrasonography in detecting congenital anomalies. Am. J. Obstet. Gynecol. **171**: 1606–1612.

6. LEVI, S., J.P. SCHAAAPS, P. DE HAVAY, R. COULON & P. DEFOOR. 1995. End-result of routine ultrasound screening for congenital anomalies: The Belgian Multicentric Study 1984–92. Ultrasound Obstet. Gynecol. **5**: 366–371.

7. LUCK, C.A. 1992. Value of routine ultrasound scanning at 19 weeks: A four year study of 8849 deliveries. Br. Med. J. **304**: 1474–1478.

8. PAPP, Z., E. TÓTH-PÁL, CS. PAPP, Z. TÓTH, M. SZABÓ, L. VERESS & O. TÖRÖK. 1995. Impact of prenatal mid-trimester screening on the prevalence of fetal structure anomalies: A prospective epidemiological study. Ultrasound Obstet. Gynecol. **6**: 320–326.

9. ROBERTS, A.B., E. HAMPTON & N. WILSON. 1993. Ultrasound detection of fetal structural abnormalities in Auckland 1988–9. N. Z. Med. J. **106**: 441–443.

10. SHIRLEY, I.M., F. BOTTOMLEY & V.P. ROBINSON. 1992. Routine radiographer screening for fetal abnormalities by ultrasound in an unselected low risk population. Br. J. Radiol. **65**: 564–569.

11. STOLL, C., B. DOTT, Y. ALEMBIK & M.P. ROTH. 1995. Evaluation of routine prenatal diagnosis by a registry of congenital anomalies. Prenatal Diagn. **15**: 791–800.

Managed Care and Ultrasound for the Diagnosis of Fetal Anomalies

ELIZABETH J. BUECHLER

Harvard Vanguard Medical Associates, 133 Brookline Avenue, Boston, Massachusetts 02215, USA

ABSTRACT: Managed care organizations and their affiliated group practices approach technology evaluation in a methodical way. This paper reviews the factors used in analysis of ultrasound for the diagnosis of fetal anomalies. It includes one group practice's strategies for ultrasound management while supporting the use of the second trimester fetal survey.

Managed care organizations should, and often do, evaluate technologies as they determine payment issues. This evaluation allows premium dollars to be spent on services that improve care or outcomes. The intent is to decrease waste, while providing coverage for beneficial care. There are a variety of factors that go into an evaluation of ultrasound for the diagnosis of fetal congenital anomalies. This paper will review usual areas for evaluation and provide information about how managed care organizations in general, and our own practice in particular, have resolved this dilemma. The following factors are included in such an evaluation.

Standard of Care in the Community

For the use of ultrasound in pregnancy, the statement from the American College of Obstetricians and Gynecologists may be considered to determine the standard of care in the obstetrical community. The Technical Bulletin from December 1993 states ". . . the routine use of ultrasonography cannot be supported from a cost-benefit standpoint."[1]

Effectiveness of the Technology

A detailed evaluation of the value of ultrasound technology has occurred elsewhere in this conference and is beyond the level of analysis performed by most managed care organizations. Most organizations review the literature, using published studies such as the Helsinki Ultrasound Trial[2] or the RADIUS study.[3] The Helsinki study suggests that there is a decrease in perinatal mortality in the screened population (4.6/1000) compared to the mortality rate for the control group (9.0/1000). This is presumed to be due to an increase in the abortion rate for the screened group. No data show that screening ultrasound improves outcome of the pregnancy other than by allowing termination of pregnancy in selected cases.

Specificity and Sensitivity of the Technology

The specificity of ultrasound in diagnosing fetal anomalies is approximately 99%, but the sensitivity is only 34–53%. False positives can cause considerable anguish to the couple and can be associated with unnecessary testing with its attendant risks and costs. This distressing event is well described in a recent newspaper article from the New York Times.[4] False negatives, on the other hand, provide false reassurance. The parents lose the opportunity to terminate, intervene or prepare as appropriate.

Quality and Availability

An important consideration for any managed care organization is the availability of quality scans. In our region, in and around Boston, Massachusetts, there is easy access to high-quality ultrasound services. This is not the case for all areas of the country. Recently, US Health Care began credentialing physicians for the performance of complete ultrasounds in pregnancy. It is notable that only 16% of the obstetricians who applied passed the criteria.[5]

Benefits for the Patient

A variety of benefits to the patient must be considered in making a decision about coverage of ultrasound services. Identification of a congenital anomaly early in gestation allows the parents to consider opportunities for termination of the pregnancy, intervention in the pregnancy in some circumstances, and the ability to prepare appropriately for the birth. A negative scan, on the other hand, may provide considerable psychological benefit and reassurance.

Costs

The cost to the managed care company can range from a low of $100 for a fetal survey to a high of $662. Cost-effectiveness is mostly conjecture. We presume that there can be savings from routine ultrasound scanning when the parents elect termination of a pregnancy, which would otherwise result in expensive neonatal care for an anomalous newborn. Because of the variation in selection of termination of pregnancy, calculations become complex. Our best calculations have suggested that our group practice will spend approximately $40,000 in routine scanning to identify one fetus with lethal anomalies.

Patient Expectations

Most women speak to their friends, families and co-workers, and many presume that ultrasound is a part of routine prenatal care. Our group practice was averaging one to two complaints per month on this topic until we began offering fetal survey to all pregnant women. Since then, the complaint rate has dropped virtually to zero.

Medicolegal Risk

There have been lawsuits about failure to detect fetal anomalies during obstetrical ultrasound. Lawsuits are also reported for failure to order an ultrasound.[6] For one large malpractice carrier, 7% of their obstetrical claims relate to ultrasound.

After a full evaluation of all of these factors, each managed care organization is required to make a decision about the provision of this service to their patients. A survey of 13 major managed care organizations revealed that they all cover ultrasound when it is determined to be medically necessary by the ordering provider.

Our organization has recommended that obstetrical ultrasound be discussed with every patient at the time of the initial prenatal visit. This discussion should include the potential benefits, particularly in the diagnosis of fetal anomalies, as well as the limitations. We know that many patients believe that a normal ultrasound means a normal baby, and it is important that each woman understand that this is not true. Furthermore, women should be informed that there may be confusing or concerning findings that may cause anxiety for the couple, but that turn out to be insignificant. With this approach, we find that almost all women do opt for a screening fetal survey.

We have also worked on reducing unnecessary use of ultrasound. In particular, we have encouraged providers to obtain dating scans at their best estimate of 18 weeks, so that the dating scan can be done concurrently with a fetal survey. We have written guidelines that help clinicians plan when to repeat scans for reevaluating identified problems, such as fetal hydronephrosis. These guidelines have helped reduce variation, so that some providers are ordering more ultrasounds and others fewer. As noted in FIGURE 1, six of our nine sites moved closer to the mean over time. With this approach, our managed care organization has held steady the number of total ultrasounds ordered, while increasing the number of women who had fetal survey ultrasounds done in the second trimester. In 1993, we averaged 2.25 ultrasounds per pregnancy; in 1996 the average was 2.24 per pregnancy.

Managed care organizations and their affiliated practices are in the business of providing care, not denying it. In making a decision about technology, including ultrasound, we must analyze a variety of factors, some scientific and some not. We are ultimately responsible for the health care of the individual and therefore must weigh highly individual desires and benefits. In the case of ultrasound for the identification of fetus anomalies, the sum of the analysis leads to the conclusion that managed care plans must provide coverage for the routine screening fetal ultrasound, if desired by the patient. It is also essential for the managed care organization to attempt to manage care

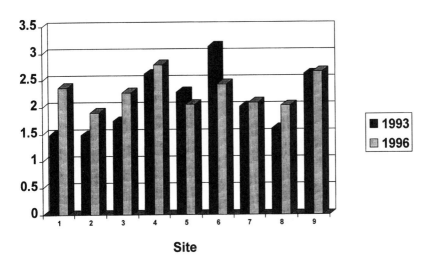

Site

FIGURE 1. Average number of ultrasounds per patient.

Ethical Dimensions of Ultrasound Screening for Fetal Anomalies

FRANK A. CHERVENAK[a,c] AND LAURENCE B. McCULLOUGH[b]

[a]Division of Maternal-Fetal Medicine, The New York Hospital—Cornell Medical Center, New York, New York, USA
[b]Baylor College of Medicine, Center for Ethics, Medicine, and Public Issues, Houston, Texas, USA

ABSTRACT: The ethical dimensions of the debate on routine ultrasound are analyzed. The central role of the informed consent process, based on a respect for the autonomy of the pregnant woman, is presented. Failure to offer quality ultrasound in clinical settings where it is available restricts access to pregnant women to the diagnosis of fetal anomalies and therefore restricts access to the options of abortion and fetal therapy. We show that beneficence- and justice-based considerations do not supersede respect for autonomy.

INTRODUCTION

Whether all pregnant women have an ultrasound examination has become a major issue in contemporary obstetric ultrasound. Debate on this topic has been framed in terms of lack of benefit and excessive cost and objections made to routine obstetric ultrasound on both grounds.[1-3] This framing of the issues has failed to address adequately the implications of the ethical principle of respect for autonomy. The purpose of this article is to identify the ethical implications of respect for autonomy in the debate on routine ultrasound and on this basis to criticize, as clinically and ethically deficient, objections to routine ultrasound based on lack of benefit and excessive cost.

IMPLICATIONS OF RESPECT FOR AUTONOMY

Respect for autonomy is a central principle of both medical ethics and obstetric ethics. Respect for autonomy obliges the physician to acknowledge and respect the patient's values, to elicit the patient's preferences, and in the absence of overriding constraints to implement these preferences.[4] Providing patients with information about diagnostic and therapeutic alternatives is essential for implementing respect of the patient's autonomy in the informed consent process.[5] The formation of preferences by the patient requires, as its necessary condition, such information. Failing to provide the patient information of which the patient is ignorant undermines her autonomy by depriving her of the opportunity to consider alternatives about the management of her pregnancy that she may value highly.

Routinely offering obstetric ultrasound respects the autonomy of pregnant women, whereas not routinely offering obstetric ultrasound systematically disrespects the autonomy of pregnant women,[6] because nondisclosure creates restriction of access to the diagnosis of serious anomalies and, therefore, restriction of access to abortion and

---

[c] Address correspondence to Frank A. Chervenak, M.D., Dept. of Obstetrics and Gynecology, 525 East 68th Street, Room J-130, New York, NY 10021.

therapy for serious fetal anomalies.[7] On no construct of respect for the autonomy of pregnant women and no construct of modern obstetric ethics are such matters ethically and clinically trivial.

The routine offering of obstetric ultrasound means that every pregnant woman should be informed of the availability of this diagnostic modality at the physician's initiative.[6] A practice of discussing ultrasound only when women initiate inquiries makes a sham of respect for autonomy because many women are ignorant of this modality and its ability to detect at least three times the background detection rate of fetal anomalies.[1,2] Respect for autonomy implemented in the consent process creates an affirmative obligation to disclose relevant information.

Prenatal informed consent for sonogram (PICS)[6] should be undertaken in several stages.

1. Shortly after the pregnancy is diagnosed, every pregnant woman should be provided with information about the actual and theoretical benefits and harms of obstetric ultrasound.
2. The pregnant woman should evaluate this information in terms of her own values, something every autonomous patient is qualified to do. At this point in the process, it may be helpful to some women to consider the physician's scientific evaluation of the clinical data that have been reported in the literature.
3. The pregnant woman articulates her preference regarding the use of ultrasound in the management of her pregnancy.
4. The physician provides the pregnant woman with the physician's own recommendation, if he or she has one.
5. There should be a thoughtful and sensitive discussion of any disagreement that may emerge.
6. The woman makes her final decision. This decision should then determine the use of obstetric ultrasound for that pregnant woman.

This process provides a significant role for the physician's clinical judgment and experience, as well as any recommendation the physician thinks is in the patient's interest. Professional integrity requires current, well-informed knowledge of the literature as the basis for any such recommendation. Thus, respect for the pregnant woman's autonomy does not devalue the physician's role; rather, that role is enhanced.

PICS is dependent on the needs of patients, which can vary. What is important is that the physician responds knowledgeably and meaningfully to each patient's needs. Respect for autonomy does not create unreasonable burdens on the conscientious physician.

PICS prevents a dangerous situation in which the physician attempts to manipulate the patient's decision, particularly to promote the possible financial interest of the physician in performing the examination. Because the informed consent process described above emphasizes eliciting the patient's preference before the physician makes a recommendation, only a deliberate distortion of this process creates a slippery slope of manipulating the patient. Doing so, however, would involve a violation of the virtue of professional integrity, a virtue that enjoins the physician never to act primarily on the basis of self-interest, such as monetary reward, in making clinical judgments about the patient's interest. That a well-defined process of informed consent could be undermined is not an unavoidable risk of that process but an avoidable moral failure on the part of the physician.

Routinely offering obstetric ultrasound also creates a bulwark against a clinically much more important slippery slope. Doctors who have strong personal convictions against abortion are disinclined to offer ultrasound because abortion of an anomalous fetus may result from doing so. PICS should be understood as a powerful antidote to this situation by preventing physicians from cloaking personal convictions in the guise of professional judgment. In other words, PICS empowers women to "opt in" for routine ultrasound in centers where this practice is not advocated. PICS also empowers women to "opt out" of routine ultrasound in centers that favor the practice. PICS is thus a powerful antipaternalistic check on physician preference, as is informed consent generally.

LIMITATIONS ON RESPECT FOR AUTONOMY

The authors caution that respect for autonomy should not be regarded as an absolute ethical principle. Instead, as a prima facie ethical principle,[8] respect for autonomy holds only when there are no overriding considerations to the contrary. Two such considerations have been advanced against routine ultrasound: lack of benefit and excessive cost. We will show how each of these objections fails.

Lack of Benefit

An objection to routine obstetric ultrasound based on lack of benefit of routine obstetric ultrasound asserts that beneficence-based considerations override autonomy-based considerations. The RADIUS investigators reported that screening ultrasound did not significantly improve outcome in terms of perinatal morbidity or mortality or maternal morbidity.[1] However, there was significant improvement in detection of fetal anomalies, detection of twin pregnancies, diminished usage of tocolysis, and reduction of the occurrence of postdatism. The RADIUS investigators assumed that these possible benefits would be truly clinical benefits only if they had a documented improvement in perinatal morbidity and mortality. Romero, however, has shown that the RADIUS trial lacked the statistical power to detect the effect of routine obstetric ultrasound on perinatal morbidity and mortality for these four important subsets of patients.[9] Thus, the beneficence-based conclusion of the RADIUS investigators that routine ultrasound lacks clinical benefit is called into question.

There is a further problem with the RADIUS argument: beneficence-based clinical judgment should *not* narrow itself to consideration only of such end points as perinatal morbidity and mortality. Instead, well-formed clinical-ethical judgment must also include the prevention of harm in small but important subsets of patients. We can now see that the RADIUS trial and its interpretation were limited by an unjustifiably narrow concept of beneficence, because it ignored other clinical realities (prevention of unnecessary tocolysis, prevention of undiagnosed twin gestations, ignorance of the presence of fetal anomalies, and inappropriate assignment of postdatism) that are also significant *in and of themselves* in any adequate beneficence-based clinical judgment.

The corrective here is to expand beneficence-based clinical judgment to its proper scope. In well-formed beneficence-based clinical judgment, the physician justifiably offers obstetric ultrasound as a matter of prudence to avoid rare adverse outcomes such as unnecessary tocolysis, provided that such benefits outweigh the possibility of harm from erroneous ultrasound diagnoses. Prudential calculations in well-formed beneficence-based clinical judgment emphasize the seriousness of the outcome, not just the low incidence of the outcome. With respect to seriousness of outcome, the risks of not performing ultrasound are significant even though they are of very low incidence. Therefore, given the seriousness of the outcomes of undetected clinical complications, such as unexpected twins at the time of delivery, it is justifiably risk averse to attempt to prevent those outcomes when in beneficence-based clinical judgment the risks of not performing the ultrasound outweigh the risks of performing it. In the authors' view, *high-quality* ultrasound, which is required as a matter of professional integrity,[7] reduces the risk of harm from erroneous ultrasound and, therefore, tips the balance in favor of this prudential judgment.

Possible bioeffects do not alter this argument, because there are no documented reproducible ill effects of obstetric ultrasound.[10] Moreover, no credible study has documented a serious bioeffect. In prudential clinical judgment, outcomes that remain theoretical have far less weight than serious outcomes that are documented.

The preceding ethical analysis of routine ultrasound based on beneficence reaches two conclusions: (1) End points of overall perinatal morbidity and mortality are not equivalent to well-formed beneficence-based clinical judgment, but only part of it; and (2) prudential beneficence-based clinical judgment supports offering high-quality ultrasound. The first is neutral in the beneficence-based judgment of PICS; the second supports PICS in beneficence-based clinical judgment. Thus, an objection to PICS based on the claim that it provides no benefit fails. Moreover, given the significance to the pregnant woman of the benefits of PICS, namely, to make an informed choice about the management of her pregnancy, central matters of respect for autonomy are at stake.[11] On balance, autonomy-based obligations should clearly be the physician's primary guide in response to objections based on lack of benefit.

Excessive Cost

An objection to routine obstetric ultrasound based on its excessive cost asserts that justice-based considerations override autonomy-based considerations. A central justice-based consideration, cost-effectiveness, concerns identifying the least expensive means to achieve an agreed upon goal. An important goal of obstetric ultrasound is to detect fetal anomalies. DeVore has shown that the cost per detected case of an anomaly in the RADIUS trial is similar to the cost per detected anomaly in the California maternal serum alpha fetoprotein (MSAFP) screening program.[12] Given the improved detection rate in tertiary centers, DeVore has shown that the cost per anomaly detected with quality ultrasound is much less.[12] If the California MSAFP screening program is a reliable touchstone for cost-effectiveness, then routine obstetric ultrasound is surely cost-effective.

A second justice-based consideration, cost-benefit, concerns whether the cost of an intervention in the present saves a greater cost in the future. We interpret DeVore's analysis[12] to suggest that routine ultrasound is cost-beneficial because the cost per anomaly detected with quality ultrasound is far below the neonatal and lifetime costs of those anomalies, assuming that for many pregnancies in which serious anomalies are detected women will elect abortion.

To continue our response to the cost-based objections, let us suppose that routine obstetric ultrasound were not cost-beneficial. The ethical question becomes whether this consideration should automatically override respect for autonomy? Those who answer in the affirmative confront a very daunting burden of proof. First, most theories of justice in Western philosophy give paramount consideration to personal autonomy and freedom, including theories of justice based on utilitarianism. Indeed, John Stuart Mill, the most famous proponent of utilitarianism in the history of Western philosophy, argues for the justice-based centrality of liberty.[13] For the principle of justice to automatically override the principle of respect for autonomy would mark a radical departure from this centuries-long history. Justice-based considerations may justifiably override autonomy-based considerations in those uncommon circumstances in which costs are enormous, even when some benefit results. This was not the case before, and is not the case after, the RADIUS study.

Second, in Western democracies, it is already well understood that respect for autonomy is very costly. As a consequence, that fact, by itself, does not override the importance of autonomy. Such matters as universal suffrage, protection of the rights of citizens accused of crimes, and the public education of children with learning disabilities are very expensive. No credible argument based only on excessive cost has been advanced to conclude that such government rules are ethically unjustified. Similarly, no credible argument can be advanced against PICS, a far less costly form of respect for autonomy exercised about a central individual and social concern, namely, human reproductive freedom.

To be successful against PICS, cost-based arguments would have to show that the cost per detected anomaly is so excessive as to establish conclusively that this excessive cost violates accepted theories of justice. Simply subordinating respect for autonomy to ill-defined considerations of cost, as some have done,[1-3] falls far below this demanding intellectual and policy standard.

CONCLUSION

PICS, the routine offering of obstetric ultrasound, is central to the issue of whether all pregnant women have an ultrasound examination. This is because of the decisive role that the exercise of the pregnant woman's autonomy plays in judgments about the relative benefits and harms of routine ultrasound and the worth to her of the information yielded by high-quality ultrasound. The authors of the RADIUS trial explicitly oppose PICS because most pregnant women will accept ultrasound when it is routinely offered, claiming that this would drive cost and expectations up unrealistically.[2] In effect, they and those who agree with them propose paternalistic denial of important information to pregnant women without any convincing ethical or scientific justification. This makes a mockery of obstetric ethics and thereby the clinical practice of obstetrics. Moreover, it invites the obstetrician to abandon the ethical obligation to serve as an advocate for the pregnant woman.

REFERENCES

1. EWIGMAN, B.G., J.P. CRANE, F.D. FRIGOLETTO, et al. 1993. Effect of prenatal ultrasound screening on perinatal outcome. N. Engl. J. Med. **329:** 821–827.
2. EWIGMAN, B.G., M. LE FEVRE, R.P. BAIN, et al. 1990. Ethics and routine ultrasonography in pregnancy (Letter). Am. J. Obstet. Gynecol. **163:** 256–257.
3. BERKOWITZ, R.A. 1993. Should every pregnant woman undergo ultrasonography? N. Engl. J. Med. **329:** 874–875.
4. McCULLOUGH, L.B. & F.C. CHERVENAK. 1994. Ethics in Obstetrics and Gynecology. Oxford University Press. New York.
5. FADEN, R.R. & T.L. BEAUCHAMP. 1986. A History and Theory of Informed Consent. Oxford University Press. New York.
6. CHERVENAK, F.A., L.B. McCULLOUGH & J.L. CHERVENAK. 1989. Prenatal informed consent for sonogram: An indication for obstetric ultrasonography. Am. J. Obstet. Gynecol. **161:** 857–860.
7. CHERVENAK, F.A. & L.B. McCULLOUGH. 1991. Ethics, an emerging subdiscipline of obstetric ultrasound, and its relevance to the routine obstetric scan. Ultrasound Obstet. Gynecol. **1:** 18–20.
8. BEAUCHAMP, T.L. & J.F. CHILDRESS. 1989. Principles of Biomedical Ethics. 3rd edit. Oxford University Press. New York.

9. ROMERO, R. 1993. Routine obstetric ultrasound. Ultrasound Obstet. Gynecol. **3:** 303–307.
10. AMERICAN INSTITUTE OF ULTRASOUND IN MEDICINE BIOEFFECTS COMMITTEE. 1988. Bioeffects considerations for the safety of diagnostic ultrasound. J. Ultrasound Med. **7:** 10.
11. CHERVENAK, F.A. & L.B. McCULLOUGH. 1995. The threat of the new managed practice of medicine to patient autonomy. J. Clin. Ethics **6:** 320–323.
12. DE VORE, G. 1994. The routine antenatal diagnostic imaging with ultrasound study: Another perspective. Obstet. Gynecol. **84:** 622–626.
13. MILL, J.S. 1982. On Liberty. G. Himmelfarb, Ed. Penguin Books. New York.

Detection of Anomalies: Alternatives to Ultrasound

MARK I. EVANS,[a] JOSEPH E. O'BRIEN,[b] AND GREGORY CRITCHFIELD[b]

[a]Departments of Obstetrics and Gynecology, Molecular Medicine & Genetics, and Pathology, Wayne State University, Detroit, Michigan, USA
[b]Quest Diagnostic Laboratories, Teterboro, New Jersey, USA

ABSTRACT: Ultrasound and biochemical screening are complementary screening tests that each have limitations and advantages. The next several years will see variable progress in the evolution of these techniques, which, it is hoped, will result in an appropriate role for each to achieve a cost-effective, highly sensitive and specific screening approach that will allow couples the most comfort in detecting problems during pregnancy, as well as a high degree of confidence that normal results are accurate.

INTRODUCTION

The premise of this conference and its resultant proceedings is that ultrasound can be used to identify a substantial proportion of fetal anomalies. There is considerable debate about the cost-effectiveness of such screening, particularly when reports have demonstrated wide variability in outcomes that are principally operator dependent. In reality, biochemical screening—first with alpha fetoprotein (AFP) and then with multiple markers—has been the original screening mechanism and ultrasound is the "alternative." Thus, measurements of the effectiveness of ultrasound should be judged against biochemical screening, which is the original gold standard.

We believe that ultrasound and biochemistry are complementary and not competitors. They have overlap, i.e., aneuploidy, and some structural abnormalities, such as neural tube defects. Differences include ultrasound for certain physiologic functions, e.g., cardiac, and biochemical for Mendelian disorders, e.g., Tay-Sachs disease. One major advantage of biochemistry is that its services are readily available nearly everywhere inasmuch as blood specimens can be shipped much more readily and cheaper than people for ultrasound.

One of the major tidal waves overhauling medicine in the 1990s is the emphasis to reduce the cost of medical care while supposedly not reducing the quality of the care received. Such debates have been flourishing, particularly in the United States, where they have been caught up in the current medical-political process, and the shift of health care financing to control by corporate and for-profit sectors. Without the rhetoric, the same process has been occurring throughout the Western world.

The past few years have seen continued advancement in attempts to refine the sensitivity and specificity of chromosomal screening, and to reduce the overall costs of the screening programs per se.[1,2] The idea is to reduce the need for expensive costs of invasive testing that follow a positive screening and also, although not commonly mentioned, to reduce the cost of the care of abnormal newborns who might as a result of screening be detected and terminated.[3,4] Work surrounding such screening and reducing the incidence of birth defects falls into essentially four categories:

1. Use of preconceptual and early pregnancy folic acid to reduce the incidence of neural tube defects (not discussed here)

2. Use of biochemical and ultrasound markers in the second trimester to increase the detection of Down syndrome
3. Expansion of biochemical markers into the first trimester to allow for screening at earlier gestational ages
4. Development of biophysical-ultrasonic characteristics of fetal structure in both the first and second trimesters

SCREENING FOR CHROMOSOMAL ABNORMALITIES

In 1984, Merkatz et al.[5] were the first to publish the association of low maternal serum AFP with an increased risk of chromosomal abnormalities, particularly Down syndrome. In the subsequent years there has been gradual acceptance of the association, as well as an understanding that Down syndrome is not the only aneuploid condition associated with low maternal serum AFP. For example, trisomy 18 has even lower AFP values.[6]

The adoption of wide-scale screening with maternal serum AFP effectively doubled the potential detection of chromosomal abnormalities in the population. Only 20% of Down syndrome babies are born to women over age 35. The addition of a well-coordinated maternal serum AFP screening program can detect approximately 30% of the 80% of cases that are born to women under age 35. The mechanics of biochemical screening, that is, with adjustments for gestational age, race, diabetic status, multiple gestation status, maternal weight, and adjustments via a different database or correction factors for maternal race, have been published previously and will not be repeated here.[7]

In 1988, Wald et al.[8] suggested that a combination of parameters including AFP, beta human chorionic gonadotrophin (β-hCG), and unconjugated estriol (uE$_3$) could significantly increase the detection frequency of Down syndrome to approximately 60% of the total. In their original series they included all women, including those over age 35. Of importance, however, and of much more concern on the western side of the Atlantic, was the fact that approximately 15% of Down syndrome cases in women over age 35 would be missed by the incorporation of such screening. In the United States at least, missed cases that would have otherwise been detected by amniocentesis or chorionic villus sampling (CVS) done for advanced maternal age could pose serious medicolegal risks. In the intervening years, multiple studies have corroborated the increased efficacy of multiple marker screening as opposed to AFP alone in detecting chromosomal abnormalities, particularly Down syndrome.[9–14] There is essentially universal agreement that among the three parameters—AFP, β-hCG, and uE$_3$—if one could choose only one, β-hCG is by far the best. There is a virtual tie for second place in efficacy between AFP and uE$_3$. However, because AFP is already used in America and much of western Europe for the detection of neural tube defects, the only real remaining question is whether adding uE$_3$ as a third parameter is cost-beneficial.

The debate over the use of uE$_3$—i.e., double screening versus triple screening—has become very intense and very emotional with staunch, almost "religious" proponents on both sides. We believe that the studies as a whole suggest that there is no real advantage to adding the third marker. The literature is divided between several studies that say the third marker helps, and others that say it doesn't. Furthermore, since 1991 when Crossley et al.[15] first proposed the β-hCG to AFP ratio be used as a marker, the question of how the data are interpreted has been added into the overall equation of sensitivity and specificity.

A number of papers in the past several years have looked at the various constituents in the marker regimen, with the most important touted being the use in the second trimester of free β-hCG as opposed to the intact β-hCG. Wald and Hackshaw[16] reported in 1993 that the use of free β-hCG as compared to total β-hCG would increase the detection frequency by about 4% for a given false-positive rate used in conjunction with maternal age, AFP, and uE$_3$. Other studies have suggested that, particularly at earlier gestational ages,[14,15] free beta may have both better sensitivity and specificity than the intact molecule.

Several other markers have been investigated over the past few years. Cole *et al.* have proposed "nicked" beta, which is a structurally abnormal form.[17] They found increased effectiveness, but the molecule is relatively labile. In order for the research assay to be usable as a clinical screening test, stability has to be increased. The urea-resistant fraction of neutrophil alkaline phosphatase has also shown promising results.[18] Its manual assay first proposed by Cuckle is too cumbersome for practical use, but automated methods have been developed which should make it practical.[19]

Another promising marker has been the search for fetal cells in maternal circulation. Studies throughout the mid-1990s have suggested that isolation and analysis of fetal cells may, in fact, become practical and useful as a screening test.[20-22] The current state follows essentially two decades of various starts and stops that have alternatively looked promising and very frustrating since Hertzenberg *et al.* first demonstrated detection and enrichment by fluorescent activated cell sorting.[23] Much of the past two decades has focused on ways to improve the efficacy of detection methods primarily centered on the need to increase the enrichment of fetal cells from the maternal blood circulation whose prevalence has been estimated to be approximately 1 in 10,000,000 cells.[24-26]

Three types of fetal cells have been sought extensively in the past several years—trophoblasts, lymphocytes, and nucleated fetal red cells. Trophoblasts, although the most obvious candidates because they are purely fetal, have proven to be very frustrating, in that huge variability is found in their passage through the maternal circulation; most antibodies used that were trophoblast specific have been disappointing.[20] Lymphoblasts have the advantage of being much more stable; in fact, they are commonly too stable. Documentation exists of lymphocytes persisting in the maternal circulation literally decades after a woman's last pregnancy. It certainly could persist from pregnancy to pregnancy if there were a recent miscarriage followed by another pregnancy.

The cell type most likely to be successful is felt to be nucleated red blood cells. Bianchi *et al.*[24] were the first to use slow sorting to isolate nucleated fetal erythrocytes using an antibody to the transfer interceptor. More recent studies have focused on two general approaches—one that uses fluorescent activated cell sorting and another that uses magnetic activated cell sorting.[20,26] Trisomic conceptus is subsequently confirmed by invasive testing and has been found by both methods.[26-28] Although the results are encouraging, further work needs to be done before the screening test becomes practical.

Another area of potential applicability of fetal cells in maternal blood is for the isolation of molecular diagnosis of Mendelian disorders. Lo *et al.*[29] were able to determine fetal Rh status in women known to be sensitized and married to heterozygous men. Geifman-Holtzman *et al.* also determined fetal Rh status using PCR fetal nucleated red cells sorted from maternal blood.[30] The next several years will ultimately determine how successful fetal cell sorting is as a screening test. It was originally hoped that it could be a diagnostic test and replace the need for invasive testing; however, as of this writing, fetal karyotypes cannot be obtained from cells that are isolated, and therefore only FISH-related results are possible. Although FISH is very good as a screening test for aneuploidy, our experiences show that approximately one-third of abnormal karyotypes seen in prenatal diagnosis programs are, in fact, not ones that would be detected by the standard probes for chromosomes 13, 18, 21, X, and Y.[31] Until and unless complete karyotypes can be obtained, fetal cells will not replace invasive testing, but may potentially be an important addition to the armamentarium of screening technologies.

TRISOMY 18

Although screening has generally focused on trisomy 21, our data and those of others have always shown a varied pattern of anomalies detected by screening.[32] A different pattern of analyte levels has been observed in trisomy 18. The values of AFP, hCG, and uE_3 appear to be very low.[33] This suggests a different pathophysiology than for Down syndrome. In Down syndrome, the low levels of AFP and uE_3 and high hCG can be explained as reflecting immaturity of the fetus, that is, all values are consistent with a younger gestational age. In trisomy 18, therefore, that explanation does not work. We have previously shown that there are different patterns of genomically directed intrauterine growth retardation in different aneuploides, but how this translates into serum markers is unclear.[33] Nevertheless, Palomaki et al. have shown that an algorithm can be used to identify the majority of trisomy 18 cases while adding about 0.75% to the population being offered amniocentesis.[34]

FIRST TRIMESTER MARKERS

Since the development of CVS and patient awareness about the availability of first trimester diagnosis, there has been continued pressure both from the public and from the medical community to attempt to move most diagnoses into the first trimester. With women's rights to abortion coming under significant challenge around the world, there has been even further added pressure to achieve this shift. It has become apparent from the results of several preliminary studies that screening for chromosomal abnormalities in the first trimester is probably possible, but that the parameters used will be different from those seen in the second trimester. The most promising parameters in the first trimester appear to be pregnancy-associated plasma protein A (PAPP-A) and free β-hCG.[35–37] Both of these parameters appear to work significantly better than do AFP, total β-hCG, or uE_3. Van Lith et al.[38] showed in a study of 1,348 pregnancies with 53 chromosomally abnormal fetuses that maternal serum β-hCG distributions did not differ significantly from normal, and that only 25% of Down syndrome pregnancies would be detected using the 90th percentile. Brambati et al.[35] showed that the median value of PAPP-A was 0.27 multiples of the median in trisomy 21 at 7 to 11 weeks' gestation, prior to undergoing CVS. Using PAPP-A alone, 60% of Down syndrome cases would be identified for a false-positive rate of 5%. Cuckle and Lilford[39] have shown that using free β-hCG, the detection rate at gestational ages down to 13 weeks remains high, whereas with total β-hCG, it becomes unusable. Spencer et al.[40] showed that the use of free β-hCG would, by their calculations, give an 8–10% improvement compared to the use of intact or total β-hCG. Their conclusions, although hotly disputed by Wald and Hackshaw,[16] do suggest an improvement, particularly at younger gestational ages.

As detailed above, recently a number of studies have looked at parameters such as PAPP-A, free β-hCG, nicked β, urinary gonadotropin protein, SP1, dimeric inhibin, and ultrasound.[1,2,13,17,18,35,40,41–44] This has resulted in a state of confusion as to the most likely best combination of parameters. Ultimately, we believe that with sufficient data, there will be no one best combination or algorithm. The physician will order chromosome screening and, by specifying the demographics the patient's age, ethnic background, and maternal age, a particular cocktail of parameters may be run. Only by potentially tailoring the particular set of biochemical, and perhaps biophysical parameters, can maximal sensitivity and specificity be obtained.

ALGORITHMIC QUESTIONS

The equation used to generate the Gaussian curves has for many years been fundamentally a black box. Analysis of the equations suggests that they are needlessly complex[1,2] and that considerable simplification would produce equal results. Our group has analyzed the mathematical bases upon which these equations were generated, and has several concerns, relating in part to the normalcy of the distribution curves and assumptions made thereof. Logarithmic transformations of the data do not completely satisfy these concerns. We have tried several approaches in large studies to reanalyze the act of mathematical alterations upon screening efficacy, and have shown in publications that the use of discriminant function analysis and/or logistic regression analysis can potentially improve the sensitivity and specificity. Furthermore, analyses of actual outcomes in large series of data, both those of patient populations predominantly in the New York metropolitan area (Quest Diagnostics) and at Romford England (Kevin Spencer), have shown that new equations can be generated that fit the data curves far better than those published and used in most algorithmic equations. The impact of altered equations is such that the likelihood ratios magnify the errors in the curves, so that a substantial variance exists between computed risk rates that are quoted on reports and what experience suggests the real risks are. We believe that quoting patients' risk of considerably under 1 in 2,000 is fraught with inaccuracies, and that the high end of the risk spectrum that averages risks quoted to patients is probably half that of reality. It has long been known that for patients who had amniocentesis because of a low AFP, per se, an abnormality was detected in approximately 1 in every 85 taps, and for double and triple screening the number was about 1 in 45. In a published series of 25,000 patients, we found that for triple screening, the threshold risk was approximately 1 in 180, the mean risk was approximately 1 in 10, the median risk was approximately 1 in 75, and the observed risk was 1 in 147.[1,2] No wonder everybody was confused. We hope we are gradually evolving into a reengineered mathematics of biochemical screening that can give more accurate results, and ultimately reduce the cost of such screening.

PUBLIC POLICY AND ETHICAL ISSUES

The demonstration that multiple marker biochemical screening will detect the majority of fetuses with chromosomal abnormalities such as Down syndrome has set off both policy and ethical debates on both sides of the Atlantic. Haddow *et al.*[45] have shown that in women over age 35, nearly 90% of Down syndrome fetuses can be detected while reducing the number of amniocenteses by perhaps half or more. From purely public health and mathematical perspectives, denying access to women over age 35[46] whose biochemical screens do not meet a risk level sufficiently high enough to warrant expenditure of resources might seem appropriate. However, that would require a reorientation of philosophy and a removal of patient autonomy over such issues. When autonomy and public dollars come into conflict, however, it is not unreasonable to expect disagreements over the appropriate utilization of these resources. Elkins and Brown[47] have argued that the cost of choice for both younger and older women is too high, and that Down syndrome per se is not enough of a problem to warrant screening in the first place. In a pluralistic society, there clearly are a variety of opinions, none of which will suit everyone. Likewise, Marteau[48] has called for increased study of the psychological sequelae of screening, believing that this important characteristic has been studied far too little. Stratham and Green[49] have concluded that the way in which serum screening is being implemented does not always meet the needs of women with positive results. They recommend that appropriate support measures be available for all patients. Connor[50] has argued for biochemical screening to be available for all pregnant women who want it, and that it is cost justified on the basis that the majority of women who have abnormal fetuses will choose to terminate, with subsequent savings to health care expenditures. Waldron and Williams[51] have emphasized that informed consent for screening is still necessary, still a very much overlooked point.

Czeizel et al.[52] summarized the data on what proportion of congenital abnormalities could be detected and prevented. They believe that approximately 51 of 73 congenital abnormality types (70%) could be evaluated. The birth prevalence of all congenital anomalies could, therefore, be reduced from about 65 to 26 per 1,000. Thus, 39 per 1,000 or 60% are preventable. The authors caution, however, that although many congenital abnormalities can be prevented, they do not represent a single pathological category, and there is no single strategy for their prevention that is appropriate.

Macnaughton and MacNaughton Dunn[53] have argued that although termination of pregnancy following the diagnosis of a congenital abnormality should be available, patients should be counseled against termination of pregnancy in minor anomalies.

REFERENCES

1. EVANS, M.I., L. CHIK, J.E. O'BRIEN, B. CHEN, E. DVORIN, M. AYOUB, E.L. KRIVCHENIA, J.W. AGER, M.P. JOHNSON & R.J. SOKOL. 1995. MOMs and DADs: Improved specificity and cost effectiveness of biochemical screening for aneuploidy with DADs. Am. J. Obstet. Gynecol. **172:** 1138–1147.
2. EVANS, M.I., L. CHIK, J.E. O'BRIEN, E. DVORIN, M.P. JOHNSON, E. KRIVCHENIA & R.J. SOKOL. 1996. Logistic regression generated probability estimates for trisomy 21 outcomes from serum AFP and bHCG: Simplification with increased specificity. J. Maternal Fetal Med. **5:** 1–6.
3. EVANS, M.I., M.A. SOBECKI, E.L. KRIVCHENIA, D.A. DUQUETTE, M.P. JOHNSON, A. DRUGAN & R.F. HUME. 1996. Parental decisions to terminate/continue following abnormal cytogenetic prenatal diagnosis: "What" is still more important than "when." Am. J. Med. Genet. **61:** 353–355.
4. PRYDE, P.G., A.E. ODGERS, N.B. ISADA, M.P. JOHNSON & M.I. EVANS. 1992. Determinants of parental decision to abort (DTA) or continue for non-aneuploid ultrasound detected abnormalities. Obstet. Gynecol. **80:** 52–56.
5. MERKATZ, I.R., H.M. NITOWSKY, J.N. MACRI & W.E. JOHNSON. 1984. An association between low maternal serum alpha-fetoprotein and fetal chromosome abnormalities. Am. J. Obstet. Gynecol. **148:** 886–894.
6. NYBERG, D.A., D. KRAMER, R.G. RESTA, R. KAPUR, B.S. MAHONY, D.A. LUTHY & D. HICKOK. 1993. Prenatal sonographic findings of trisomy 18: Review of 47 cases. J. Ultrasound Med. **2:** 103–113.
7. EVANS, M.I., E. DVORIN, J.E. O'BRIEN, J.L. MOODY & A. DRUGAN. 1992. Alpha-fetoprotein and biochemical screening. In Reproductive Risks and Prenatal Diagnosis. M.I. Evans, Ed.: 223–235. Appleton & Lange. Norwalk, CT.
8. WALD, N.J., H.S. CUCKLE, J.W. DENSEM, K. NANCHAHAL, P. ROYSTON, T. CHARD, J.E. HADDOW, G.J. KNIGHT, G.E. PALOMAKI & J.A. CANICK. 1988. Maternal serum screening for Down syndrome in early pregnancy. Br. Med. J. **297:** 883–887.
9. CHENG, E.Y., D.A. LUTHY, A.M. ZEBELMAN, M.A. WILLIAMS, R.E. LIEPPMAN & D.E. HICKOK. 1993. A prospective evaluation of a second-trimester screening test for fetal Down syndrome using maternal serum alpha-fetoprotein, hCG, and unconjugated estriol. Obstet. Gynecol. **81:** 72–77.
10. AITKEN, D.A., G. McCAW, J.A. CROSSLEY, E. BERRY, J.M. CONNOR, K. SPENCER & J. MACRI.

1993. First-trimester biochemical screening for fetal chromosome abnormalities and neural tube defects. Prenatal Diagn. **13:** 681–683.

11. RODRIGUEZ, L., R. SANCHEZ, J. HERNANDEZ, L. CARRILLO, J. OLIVA & L. HEREDERO. 1997. Results of 12 years' combined maternal serum alpha-fetoprotein screening and ultrasound fetal monitoring for prenatal detection of fetal malformations in Havana City, Cuba. Prenatal Diagn. **17:** 301–304.

12. WALD, N., J. DENSEM, R. STONE & R. CHENG. 1993. The use of free b-hCG in antenatal screening for Down's syndrome. Br. J. Obstet. Gynaecol. **100:** 550–557.

13. GOODBURN, S.F., J.R.W. YATES, P.R. RAGGATT, C. CARR, M.E. FERGUSON-SMITH, A.J. KERSHAW, P.J.D. MILTON & M.A. FERGUSON-SMITH. 1994. Second-trimester maternal serum screening using alpha-fetoprotein, human chorionic gonadotrophin, and unconjugated oestriol: Experience of a regional programme. Prenatal Diagn. **14:** 391–402.

14. GARDOSI, J. & M. MONGELLI. 1993. Risk assessment adjusted for gestational age in maternal serum screening for Down's syndrome. Br. Med. J., **306:** 1509–1511.

15. CROSSLEY, J.A., D.A. AITKEN & J.M. CONNOR. 1991. Prenatal screening for chromosome abnormalities using maternal serum chorionic gonadotrophin, alpha-fetoprotein, and age. Prenatal Diagn. **11:** 83–101.

16. WALD, N.J. & A. HACKSHAW. 1993. Antenatal screening for down's syndrome. Br. Med. J. **306:** 1198–1199.

17. COLE, L.A., A. KARDANA, S.Y. PARK & G.D. BRAUNSTEIN. 1993. The deactivation of hCG by nicking and disociation. J. Clin. Endocrinol. Metab. **76:** 704–710.

18. CUCKLE, H.S., R.K. ILES & T. CHARD. 1994. Urinary b-core human chorionic gonadotrophin: A new approach to Down's syndrome screening. Prenatal Diagn. **14:** 953–958.

19. TAFAS, T., M.I. EVANS, H.S. CUCKLE, E.L. KRIVCHENIA, E. RESVANI, S. NASR & P. TSIPOURAS. 1996. An automated image analysis method for the measurement of neutrophil alkaline phosphatase in the prenatal screening of Down syndrome. Fetal Diagn. Ther. **11:** 254–260.

20. ELIAS, S. & J.L. SIMPSON. 1997. Prenatal diagnosis. *In* Emery and Rimoin's Principles and Practice of Medical Genetics, 3rd edit. D.L. Rimoin, J.M. Connor & P.E. Pyeritz, Eds. Churchill Livingstone. New York.

21. ELIAS, S. & J.L. SIMPSON. 1995. Prospects for prenatal diagnosis by isolating fetal cells from maternal blood. Contemp. Rev. Obstet. Gynecol. **7:** 135–139.

22. LEWIS, D.E., W. SCHOBER, S. MURRELL, *et al.* 1996. Rare event selection of fetal nucleated erythrocytes in maternal blood by flow cytometry. Cytometry **23:** 218–227.

23. HERZENBERG, L.A., D.W. BIANCHI & J. SCHRODER. 1979. Fetal cells in the blood of pregnant women: Detection and enrichment by fluorescence-activated cell sorting. Proc. Natl. Acad. Sci. USA **76:** 1453–1455.

24. BIANCHI, D.W., A.F. FLINT, M.F. PIZZIMENTI. *et al.* 1990. Isolation of fetal DNA from nucleated erythrocytes in maternal blood. Proc. Natl. Acad. Sci. USA **87:** 3279–3283.

25. BIANCHI, D.W. & K.W. KLINGER. 1992. Prenatal diagnosis through the analysis of fetal cells in the maternal circulation. *In* Genetic Disorders and the Fetus. 3rd edit. A. Milunsky, Ed.: 759. Johns Hopkins University Press. Baltimore, MD.

26. GANSHIRT-AHLERT, D., R. BORJESSON-STOLL, M. BURSCHYK, *et al.* 1994. Detection of fetal trisomies 21 and 18 from maternal blood using triple gradient and magnetic cell sorting. Am. J. Reprod. Immunol. **30:** 194–201.

27. ELIAS, S., J. PRICE, M. DOCKTER, *et al.* 1992. First trimester prenatal diagnosis of trisomy 21 in fetal cells from maternal blood. Lancet **34:** 1033.

28. GANSHIRT, D., R. BORJESSON-STOLL, M. BURSCHYK, *et al.* 1994. Noninvasive prenatal diagnosis: Isolation of fetal cells from maternal circulation. *In* Seventh International Conference on Early Prenatal Diagnosis. H. Zakuk, Ed.: 19. Monduzzi Editore. Bologna.

29. LO, Y.M.D., P.J. BOWELL, M. SELINGER, *et al.* 1993. Prenatal determination of fetal RhD status by analysis of peripheral blood f rhesus negative mothers. Lancet **341:** 1147–1148.

30. GEIFMAN-HOLTZMAN, O., I.M. BERNSTEIN, BERRY, S.M. *et al.* 1996. Fetal RhD genotyping in fetal cells flow sorted from maternal blood. Am. J. Obstet. Gynecol. **174:** 818–822.

31. EVANS, M.I., G.P. HENRY, W.A. MILLER, T.H. BUI, R.J. SNIDJERS, R.J. WAPNER, P. MINY, M.P. JOHNSON, D. PEAKMAN, A. JOHNSON, K. NICOLAIDES, W. HOLZGREVE, S.A.D. EBRAHIM & L. JACKSON. International, collaborative assessment of limitations of

chromosome-specific probes and fluorescent in situ hybridization: Analysis of expected detections in 73,000 prenatal cases. American Society of Human Genetics, October 18–22, 1994, Montréal.

32. DRUGAN, A., E. DVORIN, F.C. KOPPITCH, A. GREB, E.L. KRIVCHENIA & M.I. EVANS. 1989. Counseling for low maternal serum alpha-fetoprotein should emphasize all chromosome anomalies, not just Down syndrome! Obstet. Gynecol. **73:** 271–274.

33. JOHNSON, M.P., M. BARR, JR., F. QURESHI, A. DRUGAN & M.I. EVANS. 1989. Symmetrical intrauterine growth retardation is not symmetrical: The ontogeny of organ specific gravimetric deficits in midtrimester and neonatal trisomy 18. Fetal Diagn. Ther. **4:** 110–119.

34. PALOMAKI, G.E., J.E. HADDOW, G.J. KNIGHT, N.J. WALD, A. KENNARD, J.A. CANICK, D.N. SALLER, M.G. BLITZER, L.H. DICKERMAN, R. FISHER, D. HANSMANN, M. HANSMANN, D.A. LUTHY, A.M. SUMMERS & P. WYATT. 1995. Risk-based prenatal screening for trisomy 18 using alpha-fetoprotein, unconjugated oestriol, and human chorionic gonadotropin. Prenatal Diagn. **15:** 713–723.

35. BRAMBATI, B., M.C.M. MACINTOSH, B. TEISNER, S. MAGUINESS, K. SHRIMANKER, A. LANZANI, I. BONACCHI, L. TULUI, T. CHARD & J.G. GRUDZINSKAS. 1993. Low maternal serum levels of pregnancy associated plasma protein A (PAPP-A) in the first trimester in association with abnormal fetal karyotype. Br. J. Obstet. Gynaecol. **100:** 324–326.

36. MACINTOSH, M.C.M., R. ILES, B. TEISNER, K. SHARMA, T. CHARD, J.G. GRUDZINSKAS, R.H.T. WARD & F. MULLER. 1994. Maternal serum human chorionic gonadotrophin and pregnancy-associated plasma protein A, markers for fetal Down syndrome at 8–14 weeks. Prenatal Diagn. **14:** 203–208.

37. MACRI, J.N., R.V. KASTURI, D.A. KRANTZ, E.J. COOK, N.D. MOORE, J.A. YOUNG, K. ROMERO & J.W. LARSEN. 1990. Maternal serum Down syndrome screening: Free b-protein is a more effective marker than human chorionic gonadotropin. Am. J. Obstet. Gynecol. **163:** 1248–1253.

38. VAN LITH, J.M.M. FOR THE DUTCH WORKING PARTY ON PRENATAL DIAGNOSIS. 1992. First-trimester maternal serum human chorionic gonadotrophin as a marker for fetal chromosomal disorders. Prenatal Diagn. **12:** 495–504.

39. CUCKLE, H. & R. LILFORD. 1992. Antenatal screening for Down's syndrome. Br. Med. J. **305:** 1017–1018.

40. SPENCER, K. 1993. Antenatal screening for Down's syndrome. Br. Med. J. **306:** 1616.

41. MACINTOSH, M.C.M., R. ILES, B. TEISNER, K. SHARMA, T. CHARD, J.G. GRUDZINSKAS, R.H.T. WARD & F. MULLER. 1994. Maternal serum human chorionic gonadotrophin and pregnancy-associated plasma protein A, markers for fetal Down syndrome at 8–14 weeks. Prenatal Diagn. **14:** 203–208.

42. MACRI, J.N., R.V. KASTURI, D.A. KRANTZ, E.J. COOK, N.D. MOORE, J.A. YOUNG, K. ROMERO & J.W. LARSEN. 1990. Maternal serum Down syndrome screening: Free b-protein is a more effective marker than human chorionic gonadotropin. Am. J. Obstet. Gynecol. **163:** 1248–1253.

43. CUCKLE, H.S., R.K. ILES & T. CHARD. 1994. Urinary B-core human chorionic gonadotrophin: A new approach to Down's syndrome screening. Prenatal Diagn. **14:** 953–958.

44. WARD, N.J., J.W. DENSEM, L. GEORGE, S. MUTTUKRISHNA & P.G. KNIGHT. 1996. Prenatal screening for Down's syndrome using inhibin-A as a serum marker. Prenatal Diagn. **16:** 143–153.

45. HADDOW, J.E., G.E. PALOMAKI, G.J. KNIGHT, G.C. CUNNINGHAM, L.S. LUSTIG & P.A. BOYD. 1994. Reducing the need for amniocentesis in women 35 years of age or older with serum markers for screening. N. Engl. J. Med. **330:** 1114–1118.

46. CUCKLE, H.S. 1992. Maternal serum screening policy for Down's syndrome. Lancet **340:** 799.

47. ELKINS, T.E. & D. BROWN. 1993. The cost of choice: A price too high in the triple screen for Down syndrome. Clin. Obstet. Gynecol. **36:** 532–540.

48. MARTEAU, T.M. 1993. Psychological consequences of screening for Down's syndrome. Br. Med. J. **307:** 146–147.

49. STATHAM, H. & J. GREEN. 1993. Serum screening for Down's syndrome: Some women's experiences. Br. Med. J. **307:** 174–176.

50. CONNOR, M. 1993. Biochemical screening for Down's syndrome: The NHS should provide it for all pregnant women who want it. Br. Med. J. **306:** 1705.

51. WALDRON, G. & E.S. WILLIAMS. 1993. Serum screening for Down's syndrome: Informed consent is vital. Br. Med. J. **307:** 500–502.
52. CZEIZEL, A.E., Z. INTÔDY & B. MODELL. 1993. What proportion of congenital abnormalities can be prevented? Br. Med. J. **306:** 499–502.
53. MACNAUGHTON, M. & P. MACNAUGHTON DUNN. 1992. Ethical aspects of termination of pregnancy following prenatal diagnosis. Int. J. Gynecol. Obstet. **39:** 1–2.

Comparison of First and Second Trimester Screening for Fetal Anomalies

GIUSEPPINA D'OTTAVIO, GIAMPAOLO MANDRUZZATO,
YORAM J. MEIR, MARIA ANGELA RUSTICO, LEO FISCHER-TAMARO,
GIANCARLO CONOSCENTI, AND ROBERTA NATALE

Department of Obstetrics and Gynecology, Istituto per l'Infanzia "Burlo Garofolo", Trieste, Italy

ABSTRACT: Four thousand fifty unselected pregnant women bearing a total of 4,078 fetuses were examined by transvaginal sonography (TVS) at 14 weeks of gestational age and rescreened via transabdominal sonography (TAS) at 21 weeks. Fifty-four of 88 anomalies were correctly identified at first scan whereas 34 were not; of these, 24 were discovered at second trimester rescreening, and the remaining 10 were observed later in pregnancy or after birth. The sensitivity of TVS screening with respect to final outcome was 61.4% (54 of 88 malformations in total) and 69.2% in comparison to TAS screening results (54 malformations detected among 78 recognized within 21 weeks). The association between fetal malformation and chromosomal aberrations was also investigated: in our study population there were 21 aneuploides, 14 of which were recognized because of abnormal findings at the 14 weeks' TVS, 5 at the TAS rescreening, and 2 after birth in neonates free of structural abnormalities.

INTRODUCTION

Prenatal ultrasonography is increasingly used in surveillance of pregnancy, above all for the identification of fetal malformations which still represent one of the principal causes of perinatal mortality and morbidity.[1] Early detection of fetal abnormalities is desirable in order either to avoid late termination of pregnancy in case of severe fetal malformations or to introduce more effective therapeutic strategies for treatable conditions.

Visualization of detailed fetal anatomy in the first trimester has improved as a result of technological progress in ultrasound machines and the introduction of transvaginal sonography (TVS). Transvaginal sonography has deeply modified our knowledge of the physiology and pathology of early stages of pregnancy. We have learned that a strict correlation exists between embryologic events and their sonographic appearance;[2] however, as far as early detection of fetal malformations is concerned, a delay still exists between what is happening *in utero* and what we can image on the screen. It depends not only on technical problems of machine resolution and fetal position, but mainly on our incomplete knowledge of the natural history of several malformations and our tendency to look for "signs" of abnormal conditions which we usually find in later stages of pregnancy.

One of the principal aims of studying structural defects in the first or early second trimester is to elucidate such a history, in order to improve our ability in modifying this history.[3] Thus far several studies concerning the diagnostic potential of TVS have been

[a] Address correspondence to Dr. Giuseppina D'Ottavio, Dept. Obst. Gyn., Istituto per l'Infanzia "Burlo Garofolo," Via dell'Istria 65/1, Trieste, Italy.

published; their results seem to be encouraging, although they were obtained by highly specialized operators and mostly in highly selected pregnancies.[4–7] There is still a paucity of data available on the use of TVS in screening the low-risk population for congenital malformations.[8] Our study aims to evaluate the accuracy of TVS as a screening tool for detecting fetal malformations in a nonselected population of pregnant women. For this purpose we compared the results obtained by using second trimester TA scanning with those obtained using TVS at 13–15 weeks' gestation.

MATERIAL AND METHODS

From March 1991 to December 1996, 4,050 unselected consecutive pregnant women, bearing a total of 4,078 fetuses, were recruited at their initial visit at our institution and offered a TVS scan at the average gestational age of 14 weeks in addition to the TA screening usually performed between 20 and 22 weeks.

To fulfill the technical requirements of a screening test[9] (comfort, speed, and affordability), ultrasonographic examinations were performed by several operators with different degrees of experience, using adequate instruments (ACUSON 128 XP10 and XP4 provided with either a 5.0 MHz TV probe or a 3.5–5.0 multifrequency TA probe) in a fixed scanning time of maximum 30 min, generally considered sufficient for a complete fetal anatomic survey. All women underwent both examinations with the exception of 30 who chose termination of pregnancy on the basis of the first screening results. The outcome is known for all pregnancies.

We considered as target conditions of our screening all the structural malformations that had been already recognized by ultrasound screening programs, independent from their seriousness or gestational age of previous detection. We excluded only isolated cases of choroid plexus cyst (CPC), partial reduction of fingers, pyelectasis in which the proportion of renal pelvis to kidney width was less than 50%, small septal defects or mild valve stenoses of no clinical relevance and which didn't require surgical repair. Moreover, we considered as markers of fetal aneuploidy all structural malformations including any abnormality of nuchal region (NRA): septated and nonseptated cystic hygromas and nuchal edema consisting of thickening of the nuchal fold of at least 4 mm at 13–14 weeks and of 6 mm at 20–22 weeks.

All cases of CPC and bilateral pyelectasis were recorded, but they were considered neither as malformations nor as markers of chromosomal abnormalities, if isolated. The evaluation of fetal karyotype was suggested only in the case of association with other signs and also if they were detected later in pregnancy. Gestational age was confirmed by measuring biparietal diameter (BPD) and femur length.

RESULTS

During the study period we found in our unselected population an overall prevalence of target abnormalities of 2.1% (88 malformed fetuses out of 4,080 screened). In the fetuses examined by TVS, 54 abnormalities were detected whereas 34 were not; of these, 24 were detected at transabdominal rescreening and the remaining 10 were observed later in pregnancy or after birth (FIG. 1). No false positive results were recorded at first screening, because any doubt in interpretation of unclear findings of the TVS approach was resolved within the subsequent two weeks. A partial agenesis of corpus callosum and a large atrial septal defect were found at TA rescreening and were not confirmed after birth.

The sensitivity of TVS screening with respect to the final outcome was 61.4% (54 of

TABLE 1. Results of Transvaginal Sonographic Screening for Fetal Anomalies

Area	Detection Rate	True Positive	False Negative vs. TAS	False Negative vs. Birth
Nuchal Region	30 / 30	6 Septated c. hygroma 9 N. septated c. hygroma 15 Nuchal edema		
Skeleton	8 / 16	O. imperfecta Hypophosphatasia 2 Clubfoot 3 Cleft lip and palate Multiple hemivertebrae	Radial agenesis Clubfoot 3 Cleft lip and palate Agenesis of sacrum	Heterozygous Achondrondroplasia Clubfoot
Urinary tract	6 / 12	Megacystis 3 Megacystis + other 2 Hydronephrosis	Pelvic kidney 3 Hydronephrosis	Bladder extrophy Hydronephrosis
CNS	4 / 7	Exencephaly Iniencephaly Dandy-Walker Spina bifida	Holoprosencephaly Dandy-Walker var. Spina bifida	
Cardiovascular	4 / 15	TOF EFE+ Ao stenosis Dilated RV + ASD(+CLP) HLHS (+NSCH)	TOF Ao Stenosis 4 AVC (1 incomplete) HLHS VSD (+CPC+CH)	Ao stenosis Ao coarctation TAPVR
Abdominal wall Gastrointestinal	2 / 6	Gastroschisis Omphalocele	Rt. diaphragmatic hernia	 2 Esophageal atresia Anorectal atresia
Miscellaneous			CAML Epignathus	
Total	54 / 88	54	24	10

TOF, tetralogy of Fallot; EFE, endocardial fibroelastosis; Ao, aortic RV, right ventricle; ASD, atrial septal defect; CLP, cleft lip and palate; AVC, atrioventricular canal; HLHS, hypoplastic left heart syndrome; NSCH, nonseptated cystic hygroma; VSD, ventricular septal defect; CPC, choroid plexus cyst; CH, clenched hand; TAPVR, total anomalous pulmonary venous return; CAML, cystic adenomatoid malformation of the lung.

88 malformations in total) and 69.2% in comparison to TA screening results (54 malformations detected among 78 recognized within 21 weeks).

A nuchal region abnormality was the most frequent type of malformation detected in the early scan, including six cases of septated cystic hygroma, nine cases of nonseptated cystic hygroma, and 15 cases of focal edema. The other detected anomalies were eight skeletal malformations, six urinary tract anomalies (mainly low obstructions associated in different ways with abnormalities of other organs), four major defects of the central nervous system, four congenital heart diseases, and two abdominal wall defects. The two missed abnormalities—classified as other—were a case of epignathus and one of cystic-adenomatoid malformation of lung, respectively (FIG. 1).

The correlation of fetal malformations with chromosomal abnormality was investigated in 73 cases by performing fetal karyotype; 12 neonates were evaluated after birth. In four cases results are unknown due to cell culture failure. We found prenatally 19 aneuploides and 52 normal karyotypes: the most frequent association between a structural defect and karyotype aberration was found among the fetuses with a nuchal region abnormality (FIG. 2).

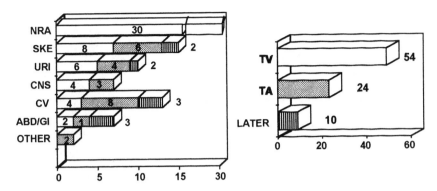

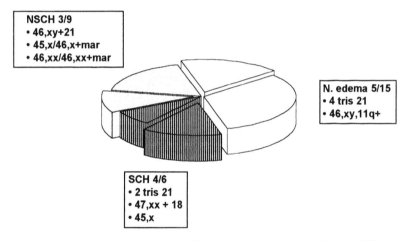

FIGURE 1. Malformations detected at 14 weeks by transvaginal sonography, at 21 weeks by transabdominal sonography or later (*n* = 88).

FIGURE 2. Nuchal region abnormalities and chromosomal aberrations (*n* = 30).

DISCUSSION

In TABLE 1 the results of TVS screening are reported in detail; they are compared with those obtained by the midtrimester TAS rescreening or later. Two cases of severe skeletal dysplasia, namely, one of the earliest reported diagnosis of osteogenesis imperfecta[10] and a case of hypophosphatasia (FIG. 3), were correctly identified, whereas a case of heterozygous achondroplasia was missed, also at TA screening. It is well known that this pathology is not usually apparent until advanced midtrimester, expecially in nonrecurrent cases.

We diagnosed only two cases of talipes at first screening; clubfoot however, can be minimal at early stages of pregnancy. Cleft lip and palate can be clearly defined at 14 weeks[11] as our three early diagnoses also demonstrate, only if a convenient plane is cor-

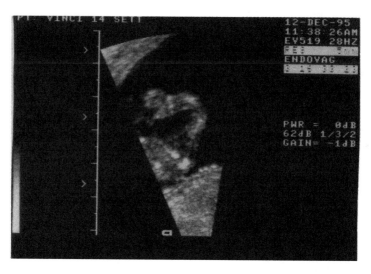

FIGURE 3. Extremely shortened and hypomineralized upper limb in a 14-week fetus affected by congenital hypophosphatasia.

rectly achieved. Probably more time or a higher probe frequency could have improved the detection rate, and with more experience the radial aplasia and the agenesis of the sacrum could have been detected.

As for urinary tract abnormalities, all cases of bladder outlet obstruction, resulting in megacystis (isolated in one case and associated with other malformations in the remaining three), were correctly identified, whereas we missed four cases of hydronephrosis (three detected at TA rescreening and one later in pregnancy), of which the progressive nature is well known.

With respect to central nervous system malformation, a case of holoprosencephaly was missed at the very beginning of the study, a Dandy-Walker malformation was detected, while the isolated hypoplasia of cerebellar vermis, or Dandy-Walker variant, was recognized only by means of TA screening. We missed a case of spina bifida in a twin pregnancy in the fetus farthest from the probe because of a poor visualization of the spine. We suspected the anomaly in the other fetus at 14 weeks on the basis of the intracranial findings (FIG. 4A and B) but we were not able to detect the small vertebral defect without meningocele until two weeks later.

Both abdominal wall defects, a large omphalocele and a small gastroschisis (FIG. 5), were detected at first screening while a right diaphragmatic hernia was missed; its recognition, however, was difficult also at TA rescreening. All cases of gastrointestinal tract obstruction were missed at both screenings because of their progressive nature.

Fetal cardiac anatomy can be assessed at early midtrimester,[12] and defects grossly altering the four-chamber view can be detected (as in the case of endocardial fibroelastosis shown in the FIG. 6). However, alteration in chamber size (i.e., less severe forms of hypoplastic left heart), and difference in size between great vessels (i.e., tetralogy of Fallot, aortic stenoses or coarctation) may not be apparent until later in the pregnancy.[13] As far as the missed atrioventricular canal malformations are concerned, in one case the defect was incomplete, and in two of the remaining cases the visualization of the cardiac structures was defined as unsatisfactory by the operators. It is possible that a longer scanning time would have led to a better detection rate.

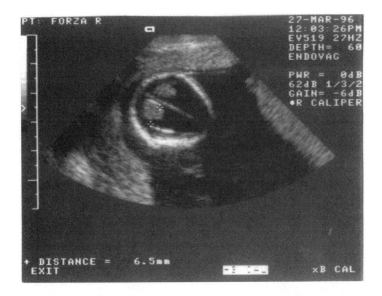

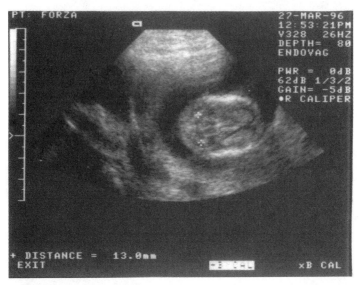

FIGURE 4. Cranial findings associated with spina bifida at 14 weeks: (*upper scan*) transverse sonogram of the cranium demonstrates moderate dilation of lateral ventricle and (*lower scan*) transcerebellar scan shows obliteration of the cisterna magna and the cerebellar hemispheres wrapped around the brain stem (banana sign).

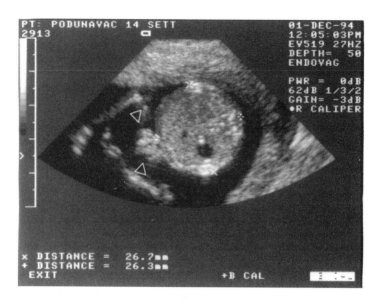

FIGURE 5. Gastroschisis. Transverse scan at 14 weeks' gestational age shows a relatively small amount of bowel eviscerated through an anterior abdominal wall defect.

An extremely important observation that arises from our data concerns the high rate of aneuploides correlated with nuchal region abnormalities. This high correlation was found not only in large septated cystic hygromas, but also in cases of less severe or transient abnormalities, such as nuchal edema or nonseptated hygroma (TABLE 2).

The correlation of fetal malformations with chromosomal abnormalities is also re-

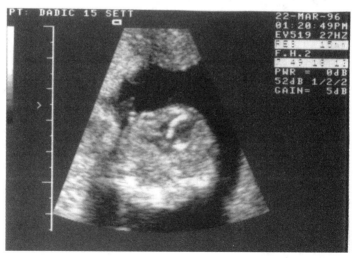

FIGURE 6. Endocardial fibroelastosis. Transverse scan on fetal torax demonstrating an abnormally echogenic endocardium at 15 weeks' gestational age.

TABLE 2. Fetal Malformations and Chromosomal Aberrations

Area	TVS Diagnosis	Aneuploidy/ Available Karyotype	Chromosomal Abnormality	TAS Diagnosis	Aneuploidy/ Available Karyotype	Chromosomal Abnormality
Nuchal Region						
Septated c. hygroma	6	4/5	2 Trisomy 21 47,xx + 18 45,x			
N. septated c. hygroma	9	3/9	46,xy + 21 45,x / 46,x + mar 46,xx/46,x + mar			
Nuchal edema	15	5/15	4 Trisomy 21 46,xy,11q+			
Skeleton	8	0/6		6	1/6 Agenesis of sacrum	69,xxx
Renal	6	1/4 Megacystis +*	46,xy/47,xy+18	4	1/4 Bil hydronephrosis	46,xx20q+
CNS	4	0/4		3	0/3	
Cardiovascular	4	1/3 Dilated RV+ ASD**	46,xx-14+ t(13;14)	8	2/8 2 CHD + cpc	2 Trisomy 18
P. Abdominal	2	0/2		1	0/1	
Other				3	1/3 Pyel + short limb	47,xy + 21
Total	54	14/48 (29.2%)		25	5/25 (20.0%)	

TVS, transvaginal sonography; TAS, transabdominal sonography; AVC, atrioventricular canal; RV, right ventricle; ASD, atrial septal defect; CHD, congenital heart defect; cpc, choroid plexus cyst; *= clubfoot+clenched hand; **=cleft lip and palate. None of the 9 malformations detected after the 22nd week gestational age or later was associated with chromosomal anomalies.

ported in TABLE 2. Out of 21 aneuploides that were present in our study population, 14 were detected on the basis of first screening ultrasonographic abnormal findings, five on that of TA screening, whereas two babies with Down syndrome were born, free of any structural abnormality. And this high detection rate reflects the substantial advantage of early transvaginal sonography in comparison with transabdominal scan.

In planning an early sonographic screening for fetal malformations three kinds of problems should be taken into consideration. Among the technical problems are the small size of the structures and the restriction of imaging plans, which lead to a variable rate of organ visualization. It may be improved by using multifrequency probes for a better organ-targeted evaluation and prolonging the scanning time until a complete evaluation of fetal anatomy has been achieved, but this could be in contrast with a screening policy. The operator's experience has a determining role, as shown also in our experience, looking at the trend of true positive and false negative results in three subsequent periods of 20 months each in our study, by using the same instruments in the same scanning time (FIG. 7). Therefore, better-trained operators will obtain, without any doubt, better results. Finally, the biological problem concerning the natural history of fetal malformations may be reduced with collaborative studies, but presently there are still some significant structural anomalies which cannot be ruled out by transvaginal sonography. This means TVS cannot yet replace midtrimester TA screening; how-

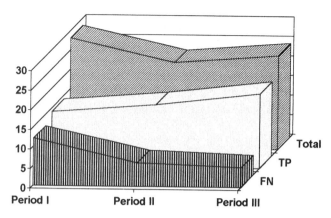

FIGURE 7. True positive (TP) and false negative (FN) trend in three subsequent periods of the study.

ever, it should be recommended as an additional technique, also in low-risk pregnancies, because more than one-half of malformations can be recognized, and a higher proportion of chromosomal aberrations can be suspected mainly on the basis of transient markers that have been proved to disappear at more advanced stages of pregnancy.[14]

REFERENCES

1. CHUNG, C. S. & C. MYRIANTHOPULOS. 1987. Congenital anomalies: Mortality and morbidity, burden and classification. Am. J. Med. Genet. **27:** 505–510.
2. TIMOR-TRITSH, I.E., D.B. PEISNER & S. RAJU. 1990. Sonoembryology: An organ-oriented approach using a high-frequency vaginal probe. J. Clin. Ultrasound **18:** 286–298.
3. ROTTEM, S. 1995. IRONFAN—A sonographic window into the natural history of fetal anomalies. Ultrasound Obstet. Gynecol. **5:** 361–363.
4. CULLEN, M. T., J. GREEN, J. WHETHAM, et al. 1990. Transvaginal ultrasonographic detection of congenital anomalies in the first trimester. Am. J. Obstet. Gynecol. **163:** 466–476.
5. ACHIRON, R. & O. TADMOR. 1991. Screening for fetal anomalies during the first trimester of pregnancy: Transvaginal versus transabdominal sonography. Ultrasound Obstet. Gynecol. **1:** 186–190.
6. BONILLA-MUSOLES, F. M., F. RAGA, M. J. BALLESTER, et al. 1994. Early detection of embryonic malformations by transvaginal and color Doppler sonography. J. Ultrasound Med. **13:** 347–355.
7. YAGEL, S., R. ACHIRON, M. RON, et al. 1995. Transvaginal ultrasonography at early pregnancy cannot be used alone for targeted organ ultrasonographic examination in a high-risk population. Am. J. Obstet. Gynecol. **172:** 971–975.
8. D'OTTAVIO, G., Y. J. MEIR, M. A. RUSTICO, et al. 1995. Pilot screening for fetal malformations: Possibilities and limits of transvaginal sonography. J. Ultrasound Med. **14:** 575–580.
9. HANNIGAN, V. L. 1991. The periodic health examination. In Prevention and Screening in Office Practice: Contemporary Management in Internal Medicine. A. K. Diehl, Ed.: 3–26. Churchill Livingstone. New York.
10. D'OTTAVIO, G., L. FISCHER-TAMARO & G. P. MANDRUZZATO. 1993. Early prenatal ultrasonographic diagnosis of osteogenesis imperfecta: A case report. Am. J. Obstet. Gynecol. **169:** 384–385.

11. BRONSHTEIN, M., I. BLUMENFELD, J. KOHN, *et al.* 1994. Detection of cleft lip by early second-trimester transvaginal sonography. Obstet. Gynecol. **84:** 73–76.

12. ALLAN, L. D., R. SANTOS & T. PEXIEDER. 1997. Anatomical and echocardiographic correlates of normal cardiac morphology in the late first trimester fetus. Heart **77:** 68–72.

13. JOHNSON, P., G. SHARLAND, D. MAXWELL, *et al.* 1992. The role of transvaginal sonography in the early detection of congenital heart disease. Ultrasound Obstet. Gynecol. **2:** 248–251.

14. NADEL, A., B. BROMLEY & B. R. BENACERRAF. 1993. Nuchal thickening or cystic hygromas in first- and early second-trimester fetuses: Prognosis and outcome. Obstet. Gynecol. **82:** 43–48.

Psychological Impact of the Announcement of a Fetal Abnormality on Pregnant Women and on Professionals

J.-J. DETRAUX, FR. GILLOT-DE VRIES, S. VANDEN EYNDE, A. COURTOIS, AND A. DESMET

Center for Study and Training in Special Education, and Department for Developmental Psychology, Université Libre de Bruxelles, Brussels, Belgium

ABSTRACT: The psychological impact of the announcement of a fetal abnormality after ultrasound examinations is examined in relation to the building up of the mother-child attachment. It represents the "psychological cost" of such techniques. Understanding the subjective experience of the patients could increase the effectiveness of clinical practice. We have assumed that the relationship between parents and professionals is a critical element that contributes to the establishment of an emotional link between the mother and her child. Pregnant women, mothers, and professionals were approached for interviews and by questionnaires including anamnestic data, opinions, and projective methods. The results showed that the women with fetopathy were less centered on themselves during the pregnancy. Long-term effects were found to be important. In pregnant women, ultrasound examination was experienced with satisfaction even if some ambivalence remained. In mothers with an impaired child, ultrasound examination was viewed as a technique with low reliability. Professionals reported not having preparation in making such an announcement. We concluded that a need exists for better management of the modalities of ultrasound examinations. Many parents have expressed their need for psychological support.

INTRODUCTION

Many studies have shown that the announcement of an impairment in the newborn child creates emotional disturbance in the parents. Some authors refer to an "emotional traumatism" to qualify this severe disturbance. Various feelings such as anxiety, prostration, depression, and loneliness are generally found in mothers. Reality is denied and parents always express a sudden loss of reference. Further, their self-image is severely altered.

Similar emotional traumatism has been reported in professionals who have to announce bad news to parents. In particular, for the gynecologist-obstetrician, the feeling of having failed in his or her mission—that is, to deliver a healthy child—as well as difficulty in communicating with parents about this failure, is present.[1]

As techniques of prenatal screening for fetal abnormalities continue to develop, the announcement of a birth defect is now made more frequently during pregnancy. The question of the psychological impact of such an announcement at this stage arises, especially in relation to the building of bonds between mother and child. Various studies suggest that ultrasound examinations give parents the opportunity to visualize their future child and thereby facilitate the process of attachment.[2–6]

However, even if the ultrasound examination is considered by most pregnant women as a desired examination, one offering reassurance and visualization of the fetus, a certain number of women do not. Fellous[7] considers three categories of women:

1. Those who experience this examination positively: they are often primiparous and they have undergone a first examination by ultrasound; the screening announces more symbolically the pregnancy.
2. Those who are quite indifferent: either they have other privileged ways to communicate with their child, or the image of the child is deceptive.
3. Those who experience negatively the examination because the ultrasonography breaks the phantasmic image of the child to be born by giving them a "reality" too quickly. Soulé[8] refers to a "voluntary interruption of phantasm."

Other studies[9] consider ultrasound examination as the opportunity for the woman to interpret and reinterpret continuously what they can see on the screen.

In every case, the importance of an adequate relationship between the future mother (and the future father, who is more and more present during ultrasound examination sessions) and the specialist is noted. For example, the silence of the professional during the examination, although necessary for concentration, is experienced by women as the signal that something could be wrong.

When prenatal screening leads to the announcement of a fetal abnormality, anxiety increases. When the abnormality is confirmed, feelings of guilt arise and are reinforced by the ambivalence found in every pregnancy—the normal desire to have a child in good health and the intense desire "to harm the child."[10] When the fetus is impaired, parents feel that they are being punished for their bad thoughts. Further, the parents' abilities are questioned—they have not succeeded in making a "normal" child; they have not been able to do as other parents and as their own parents have done. Those feelings increase their pain and create a narcissistic wound. The contrast between the "real" child and the imagined child will be accentuated suddenly. Parents will not be able to fantasize about the imagined child any more unless they deny the diagnosed abnormality. The announcement of the abnormality obliges the parents to mourn the imagined child.

Ayers and Pickering[11] pointed out that "there is a big difference between routine ultrasound examinations in which no fetal abnormalities are found and ultrasound examinations in which fetal abnormalities are suspected or diagnosed, especially if this results in termination of the pregnancy or later perinatal loss" (p76). After a short review of the literature on this topic, they concluded that the potentially negative psychological effects of ultrasound examinations are greater among women with a fetal abnormality and that the benefits of those examinations are less apparent in those patients.

However, even if they know that the ultrasound examination of the second trimester of pregnancy aims at detecting possible malformation or abnormality, women (and men) experience a positive event and receive sufficient information. The exception to this was found in women who had experienced problems in a previous pregnancy.[12]

In a study on long-term psychological responses of women after pregnancy termination due to fetal abnormalities, Salvesen *et al.*[13] concluded that the long-term psychological stress responses in women to pregnancy termination following ultrasonographic detection of fetal abnormalities do not differ from the stress responses found in women experiencing a perinatal loss.

We can conclude from those studies that the understanding of what the subjective experience of the patients is could increase the effectiveness of clinical practice. Further, we assume that the ultrasound examinations are an interactive process between the parents and a professional. Therefore, the professional's feelings are to be taken into account in the analysis of the situations.

In our study, we have assumed that

- pregnancy is a period of psychological change which interacts with the experience of maternity; therefore, the announcement of a fetal abnormality creates a traumatism and a real "crisis" in life.

- the announcement of the abnormality creates a narcissistic wound: the intensity of this wound decreases over time as parents become able to face the real child.
- the experience of parents is influenced by the modalities of the announcement of such abnormalities and, in particular, the context of the relationship between the parents and the professionals, which is an important element that contributes to the establishment of an emotional link between the mother and her child; in addition, technical information and adequate psychological preparation allow the mother to manage the pain that follows the announcement.

MATERIALS AND METHODS

The research is divided into three parts. In part 1, four samples of women were approached:

- women with a normal pregnancy and without previous medical problems (control group 1)
- women with a diagnosed fetal abnormality but no decision regarding pregnancy termination (target group 1)
- mothers with children born without any problem (control group 2)
- mothers with a child having a perinatal malformation detected before or after the birth (target group 2)

In part 2, a sample of professionals (gynecologists and some pedatricians) were questioned. In part 3, a follow-up was conducted of mothers who had a child with a cardiopathy that was detected before birth.

Four maternity centers (two in Brussels and two in Liège), as well as a children's hospital, were involved in this research.

Part 1

One hundred three women (74 were between 20 and 29 years of age and 29 were older than 30) were contacted. TABLE 1 shows mean age, nationality, and level of education of the women. The distribution of the diagnosed abnormalities for the target samples "women with fetopathy" and "mothers with an impaired child" is shown in TABLE 2. The "women with fetopathy" were met after the announcement, but before a decision regarding termination of the pregnancy was made.

Questionnaires included (1) anamnestic data on both mother and father, on the follow-up of the pregnancy, the examinations, health of the woman, the circumstances of the announcement, and so on, (2) feelings about experiencing pregnancy, delivery, suspicion and eventual announcement of an abnormality, and medical follow-up. Various questionnaires were used such as semantic differential classifications of items and satisfaction ratio scales. All questionnaires were completed during interviews with the women.

Results

Pregnant Women

Although all subjects had the same number of living children, target women had more pregnancies than did control women. For 53% of target women, abnormality was

TABLE 1. Characteristics of Subjects (*n* = 103)

	Pregnant Women		Mothers	
	Control 1	Target 2	Control 2	Target 2
Age Range				
< 20	—	1	—	1
20–24	7	7	—	6
25–29	13	3	22	14
> 30	6	6	8	9
Nationality				
Belgian	19	15	27	27
UE	3	2	2	2
Others	4	—	1	1
Level of studies				
< Elementary school	2	—	—	2
Junior high school	2	3	5	7
High school	9	5	8	13
Non University Sup. school	4	5	9	5
College	9	4	8	3

TABLE 2. Diagnosed Abnormalities

	Pregnant Women	Mothers with a Handicapped Child
Cardiopathy	5	4
Central nervous system	2	4
Urogenital tract defects	2	4
Gastrointestinal tract defects	4	6
Hereditary abnormalities	1	4
Others	3	8

diagnosed between the seventh and ninth month of pregnancy; for 29%, the diagnosis was made between the fourth and sixth month.

The desire for a child was present in both groups. However, the control subjects wanted to have other children, whereas only 60% of the target women wanted to have more. In both groups, more than 50% of the subjects experienced an enriching pregnancy. In the target group, however, women made a clear distinction between the period previous to and the period after the announcement. A certain ambivalence seemed to exist in target women, especially regarding their own body image. The body was reported as "destroyed" more frequently in this group than in the control group. In general, the experience of the pregnancy was significantly less satisfactory in the target group than in the control group (Fisher test, $p < .048$) Regarding anxiety, no differences were found between the groups. Pregnant women were generally afraid for the child's development. However, clinical interviews revealed that target women were more able to manage their anxiety. Although efforts to control anxiety were considerable, those efforts seemed to be a condition of pursuing their pregnancy.

Surprisingly, target women were less fearful about the delivery. The results showed that those women presented a tendency to deny the difficulties and were less centered on themselves or the pregnancy. All their thoughts were centered on the child to be born, without permitting themselves to experience their own body narcissistically.

With respect to the medical follow-up and especially the use of ultrasound screening, all the subjects agreed that the antenatal examination was not dangerous for the fetus. However, target women were more informed about the technical aspects of the examinations. We observed a significant difference (Fisher test, $p < .015$) regarding the level of satisfaction: controls were more satisfied than were target subjects. The function of reassurance was less effective in the target group. Further, the wish for more ultrasound examinations was significantly greater in the control group than in the target group (Fisher test, $p < .036$). The target subjects used nurses more frequently as confidants than did the control subjects (Fisher test, $p <.022$) (TABLE 3).

Regarding the detection of an abnormality, all the women reported that, if detected, the abnormality must be immediately told to the parents. Information about the viability of the fetus and concrete solutions was also expected. Only a very few women wanted to delay obtaining that information. Further, the pregnant women reported that the announcement of the abnormality should be done by the couple's "regular gynecologist/specialist." If termination of the pregnancy was decided, they felt that pediatricians should be associated during the follow-up.

Mothers

Fifty percent of the mothers of both the target and control groups were primiparous. For target mothers, the abnormality was detected at birth or a few months after the birth. The desire for a child was equal and high in both groups, but target mothers expressed significantly more often that they did not want another child (Fisher test, $p < .01$). The pregnancy was enriching for all women, and the best moment was the confirmation of the pregnancy.

We also observed that target mothers were more inclined to mention more frequently that their own body was "destroyed" by the pregnancy. No difference was found regarding the level of anxiety during pregnancy. The delivery was experienced positively in both groups. The knowledge about the ultrasound examination was similar in both groups. The image obtained by ultrasonography allowed a majority of women to be aware that the baby could have a malformation. Ultrasound examination was generally experienced as useful and as one mean among others to detect abnormalities. However, control subjects reported more often that ultrasound examination was too expensive (Fisher test, $p < .04$). Target subjects said that they would agree to pay more if necessary and found that ultrasound examinations remained absolutely necessary despite the fact that this technique was not able to detect the abnormality of their own newborn (TABLE 4).

TABLE 3. Attitudes of Pregnant Women

	Target (%)	Control (%)
Experience of Pregnancy		
Pregnancy does not contribute to personal enrichment	36	8
Pregnancy is enriching	64	92
Negative experience of pregnancy	33	8
Experience of Ultrasound Examinations		
Level of satisfaction for ultrasound	64	96
Wish for further examinations	57	100
Use of nurses as confidants	100	46

TABLE 4. Attitudes of Mothers

	Target (%)	Control (%)
Desire for another child		
No desire	62	30
Experience of ultrasound examination		
Anxiety associated with ultrasound examination	67	10
Dissatisfaction	17	0
Too expensive	19	50

Finally, the confidence attached to the relationship with the specialist who detected the abnormality and the target mother was not broken.

Part 2

One hundred twenty gynecologists were contacted and 40% agreed to answer the questionnaire. Forty-five percent of the gynecologists worked in private practice or in a hospital, but all of them followed pregnancies until delivery. Only 42% could be considered specialized in ultrasound examinations. The practitioners were not familiar with the situation of effective suspicion or detection of an abnormality because only 50% of them had met five cases during the last two years. As a consequence, almost 50% of the gynecologists estimated that it was not necessary to have further training in ultrasonography. Generally, the subjects thought that if the ultrasound examination were more expensive for the women, they would no longer request this kind of examination. This result is clearly in contradiction with the parents' expectations.

The answers to the questionnaires showed that the practitioners preferred to do routine ultrasound examinations themselves rather than to refer patients to a specialized center. If a specific examination were to be performed by a more competent colleague, they expected to maintain a privileged relationship with the patient during the whole pregnancy.

It seems that a certain ambivalence exists in gynecologists regarding the perception of ultrasound examination because of the difficulty in managing adequately the human relationship along with with the technical aspects of this kind of examination. The practitioners experienced the suspicion or the detection of an abnormality as a critical moment, and 50% of them felt that they were not prepared for this situation. Sadness, doubt, and uneasy feelings were found. By giving a diagnosis of abnormality, they experienced a feeling of failure, powerlessness or even personal incapacity. They also expressed their difficulties in coping with the parents' pain. Communication with them was therefore experienced as very difficult, and this was especially true when the whole family was present during the announcement. Further, reactions of the fathers were perceived as more aggressive than reactions of the mothers. Finally, all the practitioners estimated that the more serious the abnormality the more difficult the announcement was to make. Therefore, and unsurprisingly, a majority of gynecologists were quite undecided as how to act and what to say.

However, the gynecologists agreed that they themselves had to manage the announcement—even if inadequately—as opposed to leaving it to another specialist. Clearly, parents and professionals agreed that a privileged relationship had to be maintained in all cases.

Part 3

Eleven mothers who had a child with a cardiopathy diagnosed before birth (age range: 1 to 6 years) were submitted to a clinical investigation. Anamnestic questionnaires, projective techniques (adapted pictures from Thematic Apperception Test of Murray), and nondirective interviews were used. Seven dimensions were approached: the experience of the pregnancy, impact of medical examinations, the announcement of the abnormality, delivery, anxiety just after birth, parents–child relationships, and continuous questioning regarding the present situation of handicap.

TABLE 5 shows the general characteristics of mothers, fathers, and children. In all cases, the arrival of the child was expected. TABLE 6 shows the given diagnosis, the moment during the pregnancy at which the announcement was made, the modalities of delivery, the presence or not of operations after birth, and familial antecedents.

Results

In the majority of women, the pregnancy was experienced negatively, filled with anxiety and culpability.

The announcement of a cardiopathy in the fetus created a narcissistic wound. It did not allow the woman to focus on her own body. The relationship between the couple was generally reinforced as the father tried to keep his role of protector.

Medical examinations during pregnancy were associated with anxiety, but the privileged relationship with the gynecologist allowed the parents to cope with anxious feelings. Ultrasound examination appeared at first as a method to visualize the future child, meet a certain reality and follow the pregnancy, but second it created anxiety. The examination was then considered as "having the power" to reveal the abnormality.

The delivery was experienced as a happy moment and created reassurance. It seemed that the painful aspects were forgotten. However, the pain, which had sometimes been restrained over many weeks, expressed itself suddenly with intensity. The pain seemed to be magnified by being face-to-face with the real child. Fantasies linked to the loss of the child were numerous especially when the mothers were separated from their new-

TABLE 5. Characteristics of Eleven Mothers and Fathers with a Child with a Cardiopathy

	Mother		Father		Child			
No.	Age (years)	Occupation	Age (years)	Occupation	Age (years)	Sex	Siblings (n)	Order
1	32	Restaurant worker	28	Restaurant worker	3.3	M	1	Twin
2	38	At home	38	Advocate	5.5	M	2	1
3	30	Educator	30	Butcher	2	M	1	2
4	34	Teacher	39	Administration	5	M	0	—
5	33	At home	36	Teacher	1.5	F	1	2
6	21	Housemaid	28	Printer	1	M	0	—
7	31	Artist	37	Writer	5.6	F	1	1
8	34	At home	28	Mason	2.4	F	1	2
9	31	Teacher	31	Optician	5.6	F	1	2
10	29	Administration	30	Administration	2	M	1	2
11	27	At home	33	Technician	4	M	0	—

TABLE 6. Characteristics Surrounding Eleven Children with a Cardiopathy

	Mother's Desire for Child	Diagnosis	Period When Diagnosed	Delivery Mode	Surgery	Familial Antecedents
1	++	Transposition of great vessels	7th month	Cesarean 8th month	No	No
2	+	Transposition of great vessels	30th week	Normal	Yes	No
3	+	Intraventricular communication	6th month	Cesarean 7th month	Yes	No
4	+	Tetralogy of Fallot	7th month	Cesarean	Yes	No
5	+	Dysrhythmia	7th month	Cesarean	No	Yes
6	+	Tetralogy of Fallot	6th month	Normal 8th month	Yes	No
7	++	Tetralogy of Fallot	4th month	Normal	Yes	No
8	+	Tetralogy of Fallot	7th month	Normal 8th month	Expected	No
9	++	Multiple diagnosis	6th month	Normal	Yes	Yes
10	+	Multiple diagnosis	Suspected 7th month	Normal	Yes	No
11	++	Multiple diagnosis	7th month	Normal	Yes	No

born. This separation was experienced as evidence that the child was sick and that they were not able to give birth to a normal child. In some mothers, feelings of guilt and child deprivation induced hyperactive behavior, which may have an adaptive role. Indeed, to be active corresponded clearly to the possibility of being a "good" mother again, of feeling useful, and of restraining to a certain degree the anxiety with which they had to cope.

Medical care increased the difficulties that the mothers had in interacting with their child; they were continuously fearful of a fatal condition. We observed the same feelings in mothers carrying an abnormal fetus, i.e., those of an anticipated mourning. Some mothers tended to overprotect their child and to make the process of separation-individuation difficult.

Mothers did not formulate plans for the future and tended to live day by day with the risk of withdrawing within themselves. Finally, we found that the intensity of the pain maintained itself over time, as was shown by the mothers with an older child.

CONCLUSIONS

Our study has indicated that in pregnant women psychological consequences of a fetal abnormality seemed mainly related to a difficulty in experiencing their own body narcissistically. Long-term effects were observed, which could increase the mother's overprotective behavior. Those women, however, were able to cope with their feelings of anxiety, especially if the relationship between their gynecologist and the specialist to whom they were referred when a suspicion of abnormality occurred was adequately managed.

The potentially negative psychological effects of ultrasound examinations found by Ayers and Pickering[11] are probably related to the absence of such management. In other words, we can assume that women are able to cope with anxiety and benefit further from information given by the practitioner, but only under certain conditions. In particular, the possibility given to pregnant women to express their own feelings allows them to contain their pain. A structure is then established and acts in a positive way for the future.

As our subjects pointed out, their gynecologists are probably the best persons with whom to dialogue. The gynecologists have to prepare their patients to cope with more specialized examinations and possible outcomes. When a pathology is detected, information must be delivered as quickly as possible. Ideally, at least one interview with the couple, the gynecologist, and the specialist in ultrasonography would be the best way to make the parents feel secure. The presence of a pediatrician would be also helpful.

Further, providing parents with the opportunity to meet other parents who have experienced the same problem may be beneficial. Groups of parents, led by a competent professional and/or a psychologist not involved in the medical decision to be made about the future child, probably provide considerable help for a certain number of parents.

Both pregnant women and mothers with an abnormal child make considerable efforts to act just like other pregnant women and mothers. At birth, anxiety is at least partly linked to the early separation between the mother and the child. We therefore assume that it is important to leave time to the mother to discover her baby before he or she is transferred to a specialized unit. During the stay in maternity, the staff must be available to answer questions and facilitate contacts with colleagues of the specialized unit. It reflects a staff that is well prepared.

The hyperactive behavior shown by the mothers can have an adaptive role. We think that it is important to involve the mothers in nursing in order to reinforce their feelings of being a "good mother."

The mothers who discover the abnormality of the child at or just after birth experience ultrasound examinations as very useful and, if necessary, would agree to pay more for them. As recent studies have shown, a follow-up with the mother and the father after the announcement will give them the opportunity to gradually meet their child, with her or his characteristics and competencies. Perceptions that the professionals have about the future development of the child directly influence the parents' capacity to cope with their handicapped child as well as to establish a partnership with the professionals.[1,14] Again, adequate training of the staff is necessary.

There is probably no ideal way to announce bad news to parents. Therefore, the professionals have to be conscious that their own difficulties in coping with the birth defect will directly interact with the anxiety of the women. A systemic approach is thus necessary to understand how the attitude of the practitioner could magnify reactions of inadequacy by parents.

Finally, ethical considerations must be taken into account. Antenatal diagnosis, made with more and more sophisticated techniques and competencies, is desirable. It allows not only better psychological preparation in making a decision regarding termination of pregnancy, but also in taking care of the future impaired child. It should be stressed, however, that any detection is ethically correct only if consequences are correctly assumed. Women are able to cope with a birth defect, but need professionals who are responsive to their psychological difficulties.

REFERENCES

1. DETRAUX, J.-J., CH. DEBRUYNE & K. FRAITURE. 1989. L'annonce du handicap en milieu hospitalier. *In* La révélation du handicap. Actes du Vème colloque AIR, Macon. pp. 13–18.
2. STEWART, N. 1986. Women's views of ultrasonography in obstetrics. Birth **13:** 39–43.

3. LUMLEY, J. 1990. Through a glass darkly ultrasound and prenatal bonding. Birth **17.4:** 214–217.

4. HYDE, B. 1986. An interview study of pregnant women's attitudes to ultrasound screening. Soc. Sci. Med. **22:** 587–592.

5. GILLOT-DE VRIES, FR. 1988. Social and psychological research methods in the evaluation of prenatal screening procedures. Eur. J. Obstet. Gynecol. Reprod. Biol. **28:** 93–103.

6. LERUM, L. & G. LABIONDO. 1989. The relationship of maternal age, quickening and physical symptoms of pregnancy to the development of maternal-fetal attachment. Birth **16.1:** 13–16.

7. FELLOUS, M. 1991. La Première Image: Enquête sur l'Échographie Obstétricale. Nathan. Paris.

8. SOULE, M. 1985. Enfant imaginaire, enfant dans la tête. *In* G. Delaisi de Parseval, Ed. Objectif Bébé, une Nouvelle Science de la Bébélogie. Ed. Autrement. Paris.

9. BOYER, J.-P. & P. PORRET. 1988. Impact imaginaire de l'échographie obstétricale sur les parturientes à partir de la possibilité de connaître le sexe de l'enfant à naître. Dossiers Obstétrique **157:** 3–9.

10. PASINI, W., M. BYDLOWSKI, E. PAPIERNIK & E. BEGIN. 1984. Relations Précoces Parents-Enfant. Simel. Paris.

11. AYERS, S. & A. D. PICKERING. 1997. Psychological factors and ultrasound: Differences between routine and high-risk scans. Ultrasound Obstet. Gynecol. **9:** 76–79.

12. EURENIUS, K., O. AXELSSON, I. GALLSTEDT-FRANSSON & P.-O. SJODEN. 1997. Perception of information, expectations and experiences among women and their partners attending a second-trimester routine ultrasound scan. Ultrasound Obstet. Gynecol. **9:** 86–90.

13. SALVESEN, K. A., L. OYEN, N. SCHMIDT, U. F. MALT & S. H. EIK-NES. 1997. Comparison of long-term psychological responses of women after pregnancy termination due to fetal anomalies and after perinatal loss. Ultrasound Obstet. Gynecol. **9:** 80–85.

14. VAN CUTSEM, V. 1993. Naissance d'un Enfant Porteur d'un Handicap: Quand les Parents et les Professionnels se Découvrent Partenaires. Ed. AP³, Bruxelles.

15. DETRAUX, J.-J., FR. GILLOT-DE VRIES, A. COURTOIS, A. DESMET & S. VANDEN EYNDE. 1994. Impact de l'examen anténatal par échographie pour la détection précoce d'anomalies chez le foetus: Aspects psychologique et sociaux. Unpublished report. ULB, Brussels.

16. GILLOT-DE VRIES, FR., J.-J. DETRAUX & S. VANDEN EYNDE. 1997. Approche du vécu maternel suite à l'annonce d'une anomalie foetale. *In* Actes du Colloque de Psychiatrie Périnatale, Monaco, 1996, PUF. In press.

Legal Problems Related to Obstetrical Ultrasound

ROGER C. SANDERS

Ultrasound Institute of Baltimore, 20 Crossroads Drive, Suite 211, Owings Mills, Maryland 21117

ABSTRACT: Malpractice suits related to fetal anomalies are now the most common type of litigation involving ultrasound, surpassing ectopic pregnancy. Missing an anomaly on a sonogram performed for a standard indication, such as dating, is the most frequent type of litigation. Other causes of litigation include invented anomalies and unrecognized anomalies that are visible in retrospect on the ultrasonic images. Rarer causes of malpractice problems relate to failure to communicate the results of a sonogram in a timely fashion, failure to inform the patient of the findings about the sonogram at the time the patient is seen, and failure to perform ultrasound studies for anomalies when there is clinical indication to do so, such as elevated alpha-fetoprotein or polyhydramnios. The level of protection given by the obstetrical guidelines are discussed. Particular areas of concern relate to litigation involving missed fetal heart malformations, spina bifida, absent distal limbs, and twins.

Over the past 16 years, I have collected legal cases related to ultrasound from a variety of different sources. Earlier on, two surveys of ACOG and AIUM members gave details of a number of cases. Since that time, new cases have been accumulated either from contact with expert witnesses, from the physician being sued, or from a monthly review of settled cases.

This survey shows that obstetrical ultrasound is responsible for 75% of recorded cases, with gynecological ultrasound responsible for 10% and abdominal ultrasound responsible for another 10%. Miscellaneous smaller areas, such as breast ultrasound, account for another 5% (TABLE 1). The various categories of obstetrical malpractice will be considered in the sections that follow.

INVENTED LESIONS

Invented lesions are unusual with today's equipment (TABLE 2). Two cases of invented fetal death were reported. These were cases in which fetal death was diagnosed on a real-time sonogram; a subsequent induced delivery resulted in the delivery of a live infant. Both of these cases were performed with relatively early real-time systems and occurred in obese patients. These cases are at least 10 years old. In addition, there were three examples of fetuses that were diagnosed as anencephalic by ultrasound, but which proved to be normal at birth or termination. Two of these cases also are old ones, dating back at least 15 years; one, however, is of more recent origin. In two cases of renal agenesis in which the fetus was said to have no kidneys, at termination or early delivery, kidneys were found. Both of these cases were examples of premature rupture of membranes, so there was severe oligohydramnios which made the kidney area difficult to examine. In one instance, a fairly large pocket of amniotic fluid was present and, in retrospect, at least one kidney could be seen. In a case of supposed amniotic band syndrome, reexamination of the images suggest that the correct diagnosis was unfused

TABLE 1. Legal Cases Related to Ultrasound

	n	%
Obstetrical	318	(75)
Gynecological	45	(11)
Abdominal	29	(7)
Neurological	1	(.2)
Eye	4	(1)
Breast	2	(.5)
Miscellaneous	28	(6)
Total	427	

TABLE 2. Type and Number of Invented Lesions

Carcinoma of the pancreas	1
Intrauterine devices in the uterus	3
Fetal death	2
Anencephalic	3
Renal agenesis	2
Mole	2
Ectopic	2
Gallstones	4
IUGR	1
Amniotic bands	1
Hydrocephalus	2
Abnormal abdominal wall	1
Retained products	1

amniotic membranes rather than amniotic band syndrome. There were two cases of invented hydrocephalus. In these cases, the echopenic insula was mistaken for a dilated lateral ventricle. Further, there were two cases in which ectopic pregnancy was diagnosed when a ruptured or intact corpus luteum cyst was present. In another case—one of invented retained products—only blood was found at a dilation and curettage.

MISREPORTED CASES

Among the group of 31 misreported lesions (TABLE 3), 18 were misdated fetuses. In these cases, either a third trimester sonogram was confidently reported as being consistent with a 36 weeks' or later gestational age, and the fetus was dated by the third trimester sonogram or an earlier sonogram had been performed; a sonogram in the third trimester, however, was thought to be more consistent with the clinical examination and the fetus was redated. Both of these are well-known errors which should not occur today. First or second trimester dating is much more accurate than any attempt to date in the third trimester, when standard ultrasonic dating can be 4–5 weeks off the mark.

Ten fetal anomalies could be diagnosed in retrospect, although they were not recognized at the time of the study. One example of hydrocephalus was missed at 15 weeks. The subtle dilated lateral ventricle is visible in retrospect. In another example, with posterior urethral valve syndrome, the bladder was said to be large, but the keyhole distention of the inferior aspect was not recognized. Bilateral hydronephrosis was diagnosed, but there was no comment on the visible dilated ureters.

TABLE 3. Type and Number of Misreported Cases

Misdated fetus	18
Fetal anomaly	10
Hydrocephalus	2
Posterior urethral valves	1
Decidual cast	9
Size underestimated	3
Early pregnancy called mole > radiotherapy	1
Spina bifida	2
Intrauterine device not seen	1
Bladder called ovarian cyst	3
Bladder called mass in child; surgery and death	1
Miscalled ovarian cancer	6
Appendiceal abscess called bicornuate uterus	1
Buttock sarcoma called abscess	1
Wrong side of double uterus identified	1
Tampax called pelvic mass	1

Two cases of spina bifida could be seen in retrospect. In one instance, a videotape created by the sonographer showed the spina bifida, but none of the images that were permanently recorded and reported on by the radiologist showed the spina bifida or any of the secondary cranial changes. This sonogram was performed in 1993, prior to the requirement that the cerebellar view be included under the obstetrical guidelines.

Size was underestimated in three macrosomic cases. A suboptimal measurement technique was used in these patients. A common problem was that the abdominal circumference was not measured along the outer edge of the abdomen, but rather along the inner edge, resulting in an underestimate of abdominal size. In a second group, the crucial abdominal circumference measurement was derived from an oblique or squashed abdominal circumference view. No comment was made on the poor quality of the abdominal circumference measurement.

In an early case from 1979, a 9-week pregnancy was called a mole. By contrast injection within the apparent mole, the placenta was actually made to confirm the diagnosis of mole, and the patient was given radiotherapy. In fact, a viable normal intrauterine pregnancy was present.

MISSED DIAGNOSIS

Missed diagnoses are the most sizable group with 156 reported cases (TABLE 4). By far, the largest subgroup is missed fetal anomalies with spina bifida as the most common problem. For most of the time during which this survey was performed, the view of the cranium that shows the cerebellum and cisterna magna was not a required part of the obstetrical guidelines. The recent incorporation of the cerebellar view into the guidelines in 1995 should decrease the frequency with which spina bifida is missed. In some instances, the diagnosis could be suspected by a partial lemon deformity of the skull. In almost all instances, limited and/or suboptimal views of the lumbosacral spine were obtained.

The next most common type of missed diagnosis is ectopic pregnancy. Most of these cases occurred before the introduction of the endovaginal probe. Since that time, this type of litigation has become much less common although it still occurs. In some

TABLE 4. Type and Number of Missed Diagnoses

Ectopic pregnancy	45
Twins	22
Monoamniotic twins	1
Fetal anomalies	61
Spina bifida	23
Hydrocephalus	6
Missing limbs	12
Posterior urethral valves	1
Microcephaly	1
IUGR	4
Abruptio	2
Macrosomia	1
Hypoplastic heart	1
Rhythm problems	1
Trisomy 13	2
Trisomy 21—Nuchal thickening	1
Placenta previa	13
Placenta percreta	1
Abruptio—No images	2
Appendix abscess	2
Gallstones	2
Hepatic abscess	1
Ovarian cancer	3
Pancreatic abscess	1
Transplant tumor	1
Trophoblastic disease	1

cases, particularly with interstitial pregnancy, the pregnancy may be thought to be an intrauterine pregnancy. In others, the diagnosis was missed, although a large mass was found at the time of surgery shortly after the sonogram. In a number of instances, an ectopic pregnancy was missed because a decidual cast was considered to be a normal early gestational sac rather than a decidual cast.

A second large subgroup is missing limbs. Since the obstetrical guidelines do not require visualization of the arms, distal legs, and feet, a competent study with all of the views that correspond with the obstetrical guidelines can be performed, and yet the absence of the distal limbs will not be observed by the reporting physician. It is difficult for the average layman to understand how this seemingly obvious mistake can be made. Yet, all of us who practice ultrasound on a daily basis know that observation of all four limbs is not that easy.

Four cases of intrauterine growth retardation were missed because an earlier sonogram was overlooked, and no comparison with the dates of the new sonogram was made. In some instances, even though the earlier scan was performed within the same institution, no comparison was made between the dates of the new sonogram and those obtained from the old one.

In the three cases of holoprosencephaly, two with trisomy 13, the fetus was born with gross facial anomalies and lobar holoprosencephaly. In reviewing the ultrasound studies, the face was not shown; it is not a required component of the obstetrical guidelines. The views of the cranium were surprisingly normal, which is not surprising because the cranial changes of lobar holoprosencephaly may be very subtle.

In the 13 examples of missed placenta previa, no midline longitudinal view of the lower segment of the uterus was obtained. This is a view that is required by the obstetrical guidelines. The missed placenta percreta and abruptio were very subtle cases that were understandably missed.

OBSTETRICAL PROCEDURES

Procedures accounted for a surprisingly low number of the law suits; 14 were related to problems with amniocentesis (TABLE 5). In six, all old cases, amniocentesis was performed without a concomitant sonogram and problems arose. The absence of the sonogram was blamed for the poor outcome. In eight, ultrasound was used, but was said to be used in a suboptimal fashion or not used for the actual needle placement. In three exchange transfusions, a poor outcome was blamed on a combination of poor puncture technique and poor sonogram performance.

FRAUD

Fraud related to obstetrical sonograms was seen four times in this series. In one instance, obstetrical sonograms were performed by a radiologist who billed for the sonogram, and then bills were also submitted by the obstetrician. In two instances, clinics in large cities performed a number of unnecessary sonograms on a group of indigent patients. The indigent patients were offered money or drugs in exchange for the fabrication of a story that would justify the performance of the sonogram for Medicaid or Medicare.

An infertility specialist invented a novel method of allegedly increasing fertility. He injected patients with weekly doses of HCG. The patients felt pregnant and developed enlarged breasts and other changes of pregnancy related to the HCG dose. Weekly sonograms were then performed to document the alleged pregnancy. The HCG was discontinued at 12 weeks and the patients were told that they had resorbed the fetus. Ultrasound charges of approximately $2,000 per pregnancy were generated. Hundreds of "pregnancies" were treated in this fashion.

FAILURE TO PERFORM ULTRASOUND

Failure to perform ultrasound for an accepted indication is an increasingly common category (TABLE 6). A number of recognized indications for ultrasound exist which were identified by the National Institutes of Health consensus panel in March 1984. This conference laid out 26 accepted indications for obstetrical ultrasound. Routine ultrasound was not among those indications considered standard care. Two suits for routine obstetrical care did not succeed. The four cases in which ultrasound was unavailable for emergencies were related to ectopic pregnancy, placenta previa or abruptio. In one case, ultrasound was not performed prior to a second trimester abortion; after the

TABLE 5. Procedures

No sonogram for amniocentesis	6
Misperformed sonogram for amniocentesis	8
No sonogram for abscess drainage	1
Liver mass—Bloody pleural effusion	1
Poor outcome for exchange transfusion for hydrops	3

abortion had been performed, a much larger fetus than expected was delivered which was clinically viable. In a number of instances, the fetus was "large for dates" and no ultrasound was performed; in many, a multiple pregnancy was eventually shown to be present. Because twins were unexpected, complications at delivery occurred with the second twin. In a number of cases, macrosomia was unexpectedly present, and complications at delivery, such as Erb's palsy, occurred.

"Small for dates" was also cited as a common indication for failure to perform ultrasound. These were cases in which intrauterine growth retardation (IUGR) was undiagnosed, and the fetus either died or suffered complications related to the IUGR. In four instances, an increased alpha-fetoprotein was not followed by further investigation, whether by ultrasound or amniocentesis. In one instance, ultrasound was not performed when there had been a previous case of spina bifida and the next pregnancy also had a spina bifida. In five instances, the patient presented with a very similar story to that of a previous ectopic pregnancy, yet no ultrasound study was performed.

MISCELLANEOUS

Among the miscellaneous group, several cases related to obstetrical ultrasound (TABLE 7). In one, an abortion occurred after the sonogram, and the plaintiff alleged that the transducer pressure induced the abortion. In another case, 14 sonograms were performed with a small fetus, the mother thought that the small size of the fetus was related to the effects of ultrasound, when in fact, the concern was to track IUGR accurately. In yet another case, a lawyer claimed he could interpret a normal obstetrical

TABLE 6. Situations in Which There Was Failure to Perform Ultrasound

For routine obstetrical care	2
Ultrasound unavailable for emergencies	4
Prior to second trimester abortion	1
Biophysical profile	1
Breast ultrasound	1
Neonatal intracranial	1
Uncertain dates	1
Twins—Failure to do biophysical profile	1
Large for dates	15
Multiple pregnancy	9
Macrosomia complications	4
Hydrocephalus	2
Breech vs. cephalic	1
Increased AFP	4
IUGR	7
In diabetes	1
Possible congenital heart defect	1
Oligohydramnios	1
Postmature	3
Premature	1
Previous anomaly	1
Previous ectopic	5
Failure to follow up previously diagnosed previa	1
Earlier scans raised question of anomaly	2
With ovarian cancer	1
With vaginal bleeding and abruptio	1
With pelvic mass—24-week twins	1

sonogram after a sonographer told him that the diagnosis was normal. He refused to pay the professional fee for the radiologist. In another instance, a sonographer released the information that twins were present in a patient who was up for a promotion. She alleged that she failed to get the promotion because her employer learned from the sonographer that she was about to have twins.

DISCUSSION

Although the series has been accumulated over many years, new cases are being added at a rate of 35–40 cases per year with the large majority being of obstetrical origin. The obstetrical guidelines have, on the whole, been helpful. If a quality sonographic series that corresponds to the guidelines is available, this is often an adequate defense if a finding is missed. However, there are some vague areas in the guidelines, e.g., the region of the spine. The absence of the cerebellar view in the initial set of guidelines meant that many spina bifida cases were misdiagnosed. It has become clear that the American College of Obstetricians and Gynecologists' approach that advocates visualizing but not documenting ultrasonic findings does not stand up in court. Absence of documentation is considered equivalent to missing a lesion.

Several new trends came to light from this review. It is increasingly expected that all structural defects in a fetus will be found, and a missed hand or foot can provoke a legal suit. Particularly dangerous areas include missed multiple pregnancy, missed placenta previa, missed ectopic pregnancy, and missed spina bifida. Although the obstetrical guidelines do provide considerable protection against lawsuits, additional views which help protect one are (1) detailed views of the lower lumbar spine and sacral region with sagittal, coronal, and transverse projections; (2) documentation that all limbs are present, if possible with views of both feet and both hands; (3) views that show the orbits, face, and mouth are very helpful in excluding conditions such as trisomy 13; (4) concerning several suits related to the heart, it is possible that if outflow tract views had been taken, as well as the four-chamber view that is now mandated by the guidelines, these suits might have been avoided. (Since the obstetrical guidelines were first published in 1986, two additional views have been included in the performance of a standard survey: the four-chamber view of the heart, as well as the view that shows the cerebellum and nuchal thickening.)

Why is litigation so common in obstetrical ultrasound? As already mentioned, the long life expectancy of the infant means that the expected award is very large, and it is not uncommon to hear of structured settlements as high as $25–27 million. These

TABLE 7. Miscellaneous Cases

Gallbladder study mixed with another
Transducer pressure induced abortion
14 sonograms for IUGR
Eye ultrasound burst parasitic bleb
Lawyer claims he could interpret sonogram
Loss of sexual desire
Breech of security—twins
Mistyping there was "no" intrauterine device
Doctor failed to read the report of liver stones
Condyloma due to vaginal probe condom loss
Wrong sex diagnosed

awards sound enormous, but are in practice less expensive. Such awards are structured so that $250,000–300,000 per year is given out. An insurance policy may be bought for approximately $2 million to generate these annual payments. (The insurance company makes the assumption that the deformed infant will not live until age 72.) The lawyer's share of the $2 million is approximately 40% (i.e., $800,000). A second important reason why litigation related to obstetrical ultrasound is common is that predictions about normality are being made *in utero,* and it is all too evident when the baby emerges if the predictions are wrong. Such immediate and obvious evidence of a mistake is not nearly as common as in other aspects of medicine. Some of the plaintiffs in cases of deformed babies are indigent and live within the center of large cities. A significant factor in large awards is the difference between the likelihood of a verdict for the plaintiff when one compares inner-city neighborhoods with suburban courts. Inner-city courts are much more likely to award large amounts to plaintiffs than suburban courts. Inner-city juries are greatly influenced by seeing misshapen and deformed children in court whether or not the deformity relates to the negligence.

According to standard legal teaching, there are four aspects to negligence which is the basis of almost all suits in obstetrical ultrasound: (1) There should be negligence; (2) negligence should be the responsibility of the care provider; (3) negligence should have an assessable monetary value; and (4) negligence should be responsible for the problems that the fetus has. In many instances, there is negligence, but it is not the cause of the child's disability. The presence of disability induces a favorable mental climate in the jury so that a sizable award is given.

Performing diagnostic ultrasound requires competent sonographic technique and up-to-date interpretation. Misdiagnosis and/or mismanagement, as in any other part of obstetrics, has the potential for a sizable obstetrical malpractice award.

Teaching Sonography in Obstetrics and Gynecology

G.C. DI RENZO AND G. CLERICI

Center of Perinatal Medicine, Institute of Obstetrics and Gynecology, University of
Perugia, Italy

*The ultrasound examinations in the area of obstetrics and
gynecology should preferably be in the hands of
obstetricians/gynecologists. If for logistic reasons, technicians
and/or midwives are involved, they should be adequately
trained by a medical expert, preferably an
obstetrician/gynecologist and have continuous supervision.
Clinical follow-up should be an essential part of every
routine ultrasound examination.*
(FIGO [1])

More than 35 years ago, Ian Donald first showed ultrasound images in his historical
paper published in Lancet. In a relatively short period of time ultrasound proved to be
the most important diagnostic breakthrough in the practice of obstetrics and gynecology in this century.

Three significant advances have revolutionized the scope of diagnostic ultrasound:
gray-scale imaging, real-time scanning, and Doppler technology. Technical improvements in ultrasonic instrumentation opened up new ways in the visualization and evaluation of normal and abnormal fetal anatomy and normal and pathological conditions
of the female pelvis. Three-dimensional sonography, high-resolution surface sonography (12 to 40 MHz), angiosonography with the new power-color technology, and so on,
are opening new frontiers in finding solutions to obstetrical and gynecological problems.

To understand and to use this high technology is one of the biggest ventures in
modern obstetrics and gynecology. The only way to achieve this goal is a "revolution"
in teaching the subject and an adequate and controlled diffusion of this complex diagnostic tool. In fact, the rapid diffusion of sonography was not accompanied by appropriate teaching of the operators. Many practitioners were tempted to enter the business of obstetrical and gynecological sonography because, unfortunately, in many
countries no credentials were required.[2-4] Only a medical degree (and sometimes not
even that) and enough money to buy an ultrasound machine were required and, often,
the preparation of sonographers was entrusted to chance.[5]

Today, only in a few countries have scientific societies formulated guidelines for obstetrical and gynecological sonographic examinations (TABLE 1).[6, 7] We, however, do not
know whether these are followed in teaching programs or still remain "on paper."
Problems related to the inadequate use of this diagnostic tool are frequent with serious
medico-legal and social consequences such as mistakes in the detection of fetal anomalies. Nevertheless, the severity of this situation has induced only a few scientific societies to promote the regulation of this diagnostic methodology.

We believe that the most effective way to solve such a problem is to recognize the obstetrical and gynecological sonographer as a specific person configured by a precise
teaching formulation.[8] The main questions to ask are, What titles are needed for access
to the training programs? and what should the structure of these programs be?

For the first question, we have to point out how obstetrical and gynecological sonog-

TABLE 1. Countries With and Those Without Guidelines for Sonographic Screening

Yes	No
Italy	Belgium
Spain	Croatia
Israel	United Kingdom
United States	Ireland
	Czech Republic
	Romania
	Russia
	Sweden
	Slovenia
	Turkey
	Hungary
	Cyprus
	Germany
	Poland
	Switzerland

raphy is characterized by high specificity. It is not possible or adequate to perform a pre-natal diagnosis of fetal anomalies without the necessary knowledge of embryology, genetics, and teratology. It is also difficult to imagine sonography in monitoring a risk pregnancy without deepening one's knowledge of obstetrical pathophysiology. Therefore, endocrinological gynecological knowledge is fundamental for use of sonography in the correct way and with all its particularities in the solution of problems related to fertility and sterility; moreover, oncological gynecological knowledge is of basic importance for the evaluation of pelvic masses, etc. The interpretation of sonographic data requires not only a specific obstetrical and gynecological background, but also a great integration of clinical, instrumental, and laboratory data. Some examples are the close relationship between the clinic, sonography, and cardiotocography in the evaluation of fetal well-being and the relationship between sonography and laboratory data in the diagnosis and treatment of infertility problems.

The specificity of this methodology currently assumes particular importance because there is an attempt, by radiologists or by other specialists, to isolate obstetrical- and gynecological-specific issues. Structuring suitable training courses for obstetrical and gynecological sonography is the first essential way to face this tendency. We should evaluate two considerations: first, it is evident that different levels of competencies exist and that the validity of sonography, as a diagnostic tool, is strongly related to the sonographer's ability and to the quality of the equipment; and second, sonography is often required in emergency situations. Thus, it is appropriate that every sonographer be able to perform a standard obstetrical and gynecological examination.

Moreover, sonography examinations are presented on two different levels: the first identifies the execution of a routine basal examination; the second identifies examinations performed on patients with particular clinical problems, in specialized centers, by experienced sonographers. It is also commonly accepted that an emergency level of sonography consists of recording elementary data such as fetal heart beat, fetal presentation, etc. The same thing can be said for gynecological sonography.

We believe that the postgraduate schools in obstetrics and gynecology and those in radiology should give a theoretical and a practical basis for emergency exams performed for first aid. On this basis, the specialist should understand the limits and the possibilities of first- and second-level sonography. Training in postgraduate schools should be considered as essential preparation, accessible to interested operators, for theoretical and practical specialist training courses in obstetrical and gynecological sonography which must include the basal competencies for first- and second-level sonography (TABLES 2–4). Different levels of these specialist training courses should be anticipated: the first should guarantee the necessary competencies for the first-level examination and should be open to all obstetrical and gynecological specialists, midwives, and radiologists. Second-level courses should be planned for second-level sonography examinations, accessible therefore only to those who already attended the

TABLE 2. Requirements for Centers of Basic Training

Establish recognized center(s) in each country
FIGO/ISUOG Committee to supervise centers
Requirements for each center, with reevaluation every 3–5 years
- Sufficient number of doctors with experience to act as trainers—need for initial assessment
- Sufficient teaching and training material passing through the department, e.g., relating to fetal anomalies, obstetric medical pathologies, ectopic pregnancies, infertility, gynecologic emergencies, etc.
- Sufficient high-quality equipment available for training
- Good documentation and retrieval of data
- Good pathologic service (for audit)
- Postgraduate meetings (genetics, clinical pathology, etc.)
- Library facilities
- Support of hospital administration (letter of intent, etc.)

TABLE 3. Practical and Theoretical Aspects in Achieving Basic Training

FIGO/ISUOG Committee determines number of trainees

Practical part: delivered only by the recognized centers; according to material, it should last at least 6 months for continuous training or 18 months for part-time training (2 days per week)

Theoretical part
- Regional basic courses
- FIGO/ISUOG members to visit and check
- Standardized designed courses
- Audiovisuals, video, prepared by the FIGO Committee
- 5-day course, possibly after training
- Contents: basic physics, artifacts, bioeffects, instrumentation, organization, maternal-fetal physiology, anatomy of normal female pelvis, clinical applications
- Periodicity: at least one course per year per region. Initially the FIGO/ISUOG Committee organizes the course: 4–5 local speakers + guest speakers; English language

FIGO/ISOUG Committee prepares standard program and requirements; submission for approval by trainers

TABLE 4. Basic Training—Certification and Accreditation

Certification
- MCQ
- Book of cases (at least 10 log books)
- Video tests

The standard of the teaching and training course program is ensured by an accreditation which also serves as an incentive for physicians to attend the course

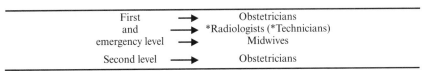

FIGURE 1. Relations between levels of sonography and sonographers. *(*In selected countries)*

first-level courses and who have sufficient background knowledge in the field of obstetrics and gynecology.

Thus, we believe that the first-level and emergency sonography should be performed not only by obstetrical and gynecological specialists, but also by midwives and radiologists—only if they have an accreditation in obstetrical and gynecological sonography, that is, if they have attended the first level of specialistic training courses (FIG. 1). Finally, the sonographic examinations should be performed by a very experienced sonographer with a wide background knowledge in the field of obstetrics and gynecology. Practically, we think that second-level sonography should be performed by obstetricians who have attended advanced-level training courses and therefore have the necessary competencies and credentials.[9-13]

As has been shown, this is a serious situation: many people waste a lot of words about teaching, confirming that this is necessary and basic for the future of gynecology and its improvement; the truth is, however, that nobody intends to put words into practice, nobody decides the right rules to follow, and nobody establishes how young specialists really should learn new methodologies. The reason for this lack is, probably, that old practitioners have no resources or interest in making teaching a reality. The consequences are that new generations of specialists, those who probably would have enthusiasm in their profession and would have the energy to spend improving themselves and increasing their knowledge, do not know how to learn what they are going to practice on patients after postgraduate school.

We think that now is the time to formulate teaching programs and to structure teaching methods. This should be the task of the exponents of the scientific societies, institutions, and all people qualified to teach. They have to dedicate time and resources to train a new generation of sonographers. We hope that these people will be available soon, leading us to ameliorate our diagnostic capabilities.

REFERENCES

1. FIGO NEWS. 1992. Recommendations on the use of ultrasound and Doppler technology in clinical obstetrics and gynecology. Int. J. Gynecol. Obstet. **37:** 221–228.
2. ARDUINI, D. 1994. Teaching ultrasonography in the field of obstetrics and gynecology. Ultrasound Obstet. Gynecol. **4:** 1–3.
3. ISUOG EDUCATION COMMITTEE. 1993. Ultrasound Obstet. Gynecol. **3:** 73–76.
4. ISUOG EDUCATION COMMITTEE. 1996. Ultrasound Obstet. Gynecol. **8:** 363–365.
5. BENACERRAF, B.R. 1993. Who should be performing fetal ultrasound? Ultrasound Obstet. Gynecol. **3:** 1–2.
6. COPEL, J.A. 1996. Obstetrics and gynecology ultrasound laboratory accreditation in the USA. Ultrasound Obstet. Gynecol. **7:** 161–162.
7. WLADIMIROFF, J.W. 1992. ISUOG in a united Europe and beyond. Ultrasound Obstet. Gynecol. **2:** 383–384.
8. FORTUNY. 1997. Prenatal diagnosis: A plea for multidisciplinarity, education and training. Ultrasound Obstet. Gynecol. **9:** 1–3.

9. TRUDINGER, B.J. 1994. The ultrasound examination: Content and cost containment. Ultrasound Obstet. Gynecol. **4:** 89–94.
10. EIK-NES, S.H. 1995. Fetal structural disorders—Large series are emerging. Ultrasound Obstet. Gynecol. **5:** 364–365.
11. EIK-NES, S.H. 1993. The fetal examination. Ultrasound Obstet. Gynecol. **3:** 83–85.
12. MARSAL, K. 1992. Ultrasound—An indispensable diagnostic tool for the obstetrician. Ultrasound Obstet. Gynecol. **2:** 235–237.
13. REED, K.L. 1996. Why (not) do obstetrical ultrasound? An observation on uncertainty. Ultrasound Obstet. Gynecol. **8:** 1–2.

Ultrasound Screening for Fetal Anomalies in Developing Countries: Wish or Reality?

ASIM KURJAK[a] AND MILAN KOS

Ultrasonic Institute, Medical School, University of Zagreb, Sveti Duh 64, 10000 Zagreb, Croatia

ABSTRACT: The main problems related to the screening of fetal anomalies in developing countries do include general ones of limited resources for health care and specific ones related to ultrasonographic practice, education, and instrumentation. The strategy to improve the detection of fetal anomalies is reliable, but has to be targeted to the following cornerstones: maintenance of obligate minimum of quality in perinatal care, establishment of three ultrasonographic examinations as a basic prerequisite of antenatal care, enhanced importance of first trimester screening, and a uniform program of education of sonographers, emphasizing the standardization of basic examination. Because of limited resources for perinatal care, we have to be highly responsible in selection of echographic instrumentation and appropriate education, subject to rigorous cost-benefit analysis.

INTRODUCTION

During the past 15 years, the development of screening for fetal anomalies has profoundly affected perinatal care. This has been due mainly to dramatic advances in imaging and biochemical techniques, along with the relative increase of fetal abnormalities as the cause of perinatal and neonatal mortality and morbidity. Congenital defects are significantly related to death during the perinatal period (25%), in infancy (50%), and in severe mental and physical handicaps in children (50%). They will affect some 3 to 5% of all pregnancies.[1]

For many anomalies, early prenatal diagnosis dramatically increases the chances of recovery. In severe conditions, with currently no existing effective therapy, early detection allows termination of pregnancy.

Prenatal diagnosis of major birth defects results in a lower perinatal mortality rate, which is the result of second trimester termination of pregnancies with severe fetal malformations. It has to be pointed out that such termination results in lower health care costs because of avoidance of long-term care that major malformations require.

For all developing countries, the cost of medical care has become a major concern. Because of limited resources for maternal and child care, we have the responsibility to select carefully which tests and procedures are used and how often.

None of the existing screening tests for congenital anomalies can detect, with a high degree of accuracy, every risk factor or every kind of anomaly. This is because of the extent and variety of anomalies, the potential of every pregnancy to be affected, and the low overall incidence or risk of occurrence. In practice, programs that utilize various screening tests must coexist. Three basic types of programs have been shown to be effective in detecting congenital defects:[1]

1. *Ultrasound* screening programs for the detection of severe malformations and some trisomies
2. Chromosomal screening programs based on the *age* of the mother and the reproductive history

---

[a] Corresponding author.

3. *Biochemical* screening programs that allow selection of risk cases for chromosomal and structural anomalies

ULTRASOUND SCREENING FOR FETAL ANOMALIES

Ultrasonography is the fundamental technique for prenatal diagnosis of malformations. However, the results obtained with this method are significantly influenced by the level of the examination. This is the next major problem of ultrasound screening in developing countries. Sensitivity and specificity of ultrasonography, for the detection of fetal anomalies, depend mainly on the training and expertise of the sonographer, and on the quality of the equipment used.

Following the above statements, inadequate education and worn-out machines are the next problems related to limited resources in developing countries.

First, the strategy of ultrasonographic antenatal care in developing countries has to be directed according to the EAGO recommendation for developing countries (1993): obligatory minimum of three scannings during pregnancy for every pregnant woman.

Second, the diagnostic capacity of ultrasound examinations has to be improved. Progressive improvements in ultrasound equipment have permitted its diagnostic capacity to obtain a high detection rate. Romero, in an excellent review, has analyzed five studies together with the results available from the Helsinki trial.[2-6] He found that of the 52,295 patients screened, ultrasound had an overall sensitivity of 50.9%, a specificity of 99.9%, a positive predictive value of 95.9%, and a negative predictive value of 99.26%.[2,4]

However, these results are only obtainable when three basic prerequisites are present:

1. Sufficient preparation of the sonographer, who should be an expert in fetal dismorphology
2. Use of the appropriate instrumentation
3. Correct management of prenatal diagnosis allowing the sonographer sufficient time, as well as access to acceptable ultrasound tests for all gestations at the appropriate period. Appropriate management must include a system of EAGO-recommended suitable levels of ultrasound expertise.

Level 1: Standard obstetric echography and brief examination, general anatomy examination, elementary biometry. This level is performed by general practitioners, private clinicians, and doctors having relatively little experience in prenatal diagnosis.

Level 2: Particular study of fetal anatomy, detection of minor and major fetal malformations including the sonographically detectable markers of fetal chromosomal abnormalities. This level is performed by experienced clinicians located within a hospital and who belong to a subregional organization.

Level 3: Expertise in special fetal anatomy and functional study, performed by sonographers specially trained in the fields of echocardiography, echoneurography, and blood flow investigations, operating within main regional perinatal centers and collaborating in team work with specialists in other areas.

PROBLEMS RELATED TO ULTRASOUND SCREENING IN DEVELOPING COUNTRIES

The main problems related to the screening of fetal anomalies in developing countries can be subdivided into two groups: (1) General problems of health care and

(2) problems related to ultrasonography. In the first group are issues concerning populations with a lower level of health education, a lower level of complete perinatal care (fewer number of visits per patient, maternal unemployment), lack of management and organization following the principles of subordination and centralization (regarding levels of expertise), and data collection.

Ultrasonography-related problems include inadequate education of sonographers, use of poor-quality equipment, a consistently low detection rate of fetal anomalies, and a lack of authorized supervision.

It is completely utopian to try to solve all of these problems; rather, the strategy of improvement has to be guided by the logic of incurring minimal costs that result in maximal benefit. In developing countries, all equipment must be subjected to rigorous cost-benefit analysis because funds are limited. Expensive equipment without skilled specialists is a waste of money; analogously, the ability to make a complicated diagnosis is often wasted if no clinicians or facilities to treat the patient are available.[7] When used rationally and with appropriate technology, ultrasonography seems certain to become of increasing importance in developing countries where competing, more expensive, imaging modalities such as magnetic resonance imaging or digital radiography cannot replace its widescale use. Therefore, ultrasonography represents a method of choice among imaging techniques in developing countries.[8]

The difficulties in ultrasound screening are such that the purchase of ultrasound equipment without making provision for operator training is contrary to sound health care practice and is unlikely to be cost-effective. No technique is worthwhile without appropriately trained specialized physicians. Training is at least as important as proper choice of equipment. The World Health Organization (WHO) scientific group has stressed in its report the need for appropriate training of general practitioners and specialists meant to use ultrasound. A physician coming from a small hospital should be trained on the same type of unit that he is going to use in practice. Training programs have been developed, tested, and implemented in recognized centers willing to modify their existing programs in line with the needs of WHO. The Ultrasound Institute, University of Zagreb, was the first center of that kind.[7]

STRATEGY TO IMPROVE THE DETECTION OF FETAL ANOMALIES IN DEVELOPING COUNTRIES

- The imperative of lower health care costs is influencing the possibilities for perinatal care, but *the obligate minimum of quality has to be maintained.*
- Organize a national population-health-education program that includes *sonography as a basic part of antenatal care.*
- Enhance efficacy of *first trimester screening* with biochemical and sonographic markers for aneuploides (nuchal fold, omphalocele, plexus chorioideus cyst, hyperechoic bowel). Unfortunately, human and logistic benefit to the patient of first trimester diagnosis is worth adding it to a screening program as long as a second trimester scan is always used as a follow-up.
- Ensure a *minimum of three ultrasound examinations* (at 10, 20, and 30–34 weeks) stressing the importance of the second trimester scan (18–20 weeks) at level 1, for every pregnant woman and proposed by the national health care program. A second trimester scan, even without regard to the quality of equipment, would date pregnancy with very reasonable accuracy. It also would give the best opportunity to identify major anomalies at a time when termination of pregnancy is still available (FIG. 1).

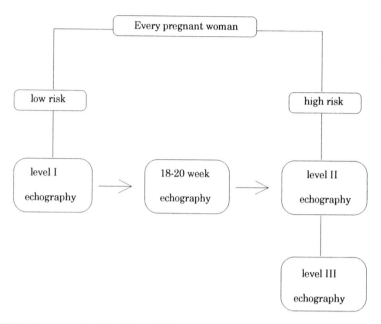

FIGURE 1. Recommended algorithm of ultrasonographic scanning regarding level of expertise, gestational age, and risk factors.

- Form *regional tertiary centers* (integrating echographic levels II and III), which connect with subordinate networks in other hospitals and outlying practices allowing possibilities of adequate supervision and concentration of cases.
- Uniform education of sonographers (residency programs, postgraduate studies, international courses) emphasizing standardization of basic examination and training in recognition of anomalies with the lowest detection rates (congenital cardiac defects, diaphragmatic defects).[7-9]
- Finally, the very serious and important problem in developing countries of *collecting data* from different diagnostic centers and their statistical analysis should addressed, as well as publication of these results.

It is difficult, if not impossible, to determine the incidence of various types of congenital defects that are diagnosed by means of ultrasound and the real incidence of these malformations diagnosed at birth. The main reason for this problem is again the lack of financial resources, first hardware and second, adequate software programs. Even though it is hoped that this problem will be solved in time, the importance of the availability of these data has to be stressed to all those involved in public health service in developing countries.

REFERENCES

1. CARRERA, J.M. & G.C. DI RENZO, Eds. 1993. Recommendations and protocols for prenatal diagnosis. *In* Report of the European Study Group on Prenatal Diagnosis. European Association of Perinatal Medicine.: 13–33.

2. Romero, R. 1993. Routine obstetric ultrasound (Editorial). Ultrasound Obstet. Gynecol. **3:** 303–307.
3. Leivo, T. *et al.* 1996. Cost-effectiveness of one-stage ultrasound screening in pregnancy: A report from the Helsinki ultrasound trial. Ultrasound Obstet. Gynecol. **7:** 309–314.
4. Skupski, D.W. *et al.* 1996. Routine obstetric ultrasound examination: A clinical and ethical evaluation. *In* Fetus as a Patient. F. Chervenak & A. Kurjak, Eds.: 203–212. The Parthenon Publishing Group. New York.
5. Luck, C.A. 1992. Value of routine ultrasound scanning at 19 weeks: A four-year study. Br. Med. J. **304:** 1474–1478.
6. Shirley, I.M., F. Bottomley & V.P. Robinson. 1992. Routine radiographer screening for fetal abnormalities in an unselected low risk population. Br. J. Radiol. **65:** 564–569.
7. Kurjak, A. Ed. 1986. Diagnostic Ultrasound in Developing Countries (Foreword). p. 1. Mladost. Zagreb.
8. Leihtinen, E. 1986. WHO's approach to the use of ultrasound and other diagnostic imaging modalities in developing countries. *In* Diagnostic Ultrasound in Developing Countries. A. Kurjak, Ed.: 11–21. Mladost. Zagreb.
9. Gottesfeld-Hohler Ultrasound Think Tank. 1995. Proceedings. Lake Arrowhead, California, September 1995.

Prevalence of Chromosomal Abnormalities in Low-Risk Pregnancies with Fetal Anomalies

MARIA BELLOTTI,[a] GIULIA ROGNONI, MADDALENA BOZZO, SIMONA FIORE, SERENA RIGANO, MARIA GRAZIA GRIMOLDI, AND MAURO BUSCAGLIA

Department of Obstetrics and Gynecology, Department of Pathology, Citogenetics Laboratory, ISBM San Paolo, University of Milan, Italy

INTRODUCTION

Most fetuses with major chromosomal defects have morphological abnormalities or peculiar morphometric features, which an accurate ultrasonographic examination can identify. On the other hand, chorionic villus sampling (CVS) and amniocentesis for determining fetal karyotype should be avoided when estimated risk for chromosomal defects is lower than the related risk of fetal loss for invasive procedures. The fetal loss rate varies, according to different experiences, from 0.5 to 5.2%[1,2] for amniocentesis and from 0.4 to 14%[3] for CVS, respectively, whereas the estimated prevalence for trisomy 21 at a maternal age >35 years is >1/148 and >1/193 at 10 and 16 weeks of gestation, respectively.

In a population of pregnant women with a maternal age <35 years, not at risk for chromosomal defects, the ultrasound screening performed at 20 weeks of gestation for morphological anomalies and the third trimester screening for growth restriction can identify the fetuses at risk for chromosomal abnormalities. In these cases we could suggest a fetal blood sampling for rapid karyotyping,[5,6] although the related loss ranges from 0.8 to 4%.

The aims of our work are (1) to verify whether the fetal population selected by ultrasound screening for FBS, on the basis of detected morphological or morphometric abnormalities, is really at risk for chromosomal abnormalities; and (2) to analyze the different diagnosed anomalies in order to identify which patterns of morphological anomalies are correlated to chromosomal defects.

MATERIALS AND METHODS

From January 1991 to December 1996, 344 singleton low-risk pregnancies were referred to our prenatal diagnosis unit with evidence or a suspicion of fetal structural anomalies at an ultrasound screening examination performed between 20 and 32 weeks of gestation. A second level ultrasound examination was performed in each patient in order to confirm the presence of the fetal malformation, to define the presence of associated anomalies, and to define the severity of the evidenced defects. Major and minor, isolated and associated malformations were considered. Minor signs included: choroid plexus cysts, single or associated, nuchal edema, olygoidramnios, and single umbilical artery.

---

[a] Address correspondence to Maria Bellotti, M.D., Department of Obstetrics and Gynecology, The San Paolo Biomedical Institute, Via di Rudinì, 8-20142 Milan, Italy.

A fetal blood sampling to obtain a rapid fetal karyotype on lymphocytes was performed in all these patients. Fetal blood sample was obtained with percutaneous, free hand needling, using a G-22 spinal needle, under ultrasound guidance (Ansaldo AU 590 with convex probes 3.5–5 MHz). The target was mainly the placental insertion of the umbilical, but in a few cases the chosen site was a free loop because of the position of the placenta or of the fetus. The mean age of the pregnant women was 30 ± 5 years. The mean gestational age at the cordocentesis was 25 ± 5 weeks.

RESULTS

The overall chromosomal anomalies and their relationship with fetal abnormalities are summarized in TABLES 1 and 2. The prevalence of trisomy 21 was 30% (19 cases), trisomy 18 was 31% (20 cases), and trisomy 13 12% (8 cases).

Other chromosomal anomalies such as translocations, deletions, and triploides were detected in 27%. Among minor signs, isolated single umbilical artery and oligo- or polidramnios are not associated with chromosomal anomalies.

CONCLUSIONS

In a population not at risk for chromosomal defects (maternal age is 30 ± 5 years.) ultrasonographic screening selected a group of fetuses on the basis of morphological or morphometric abnormalities. The prevalence of chromosomal defects in this selected group is high (18%), thus justifying the fetal blood sampling for rapid karyotyping despite the invasive procedure and related risk of fetal loss.

The gestational age at diagnosis reflects both the problems and the peculiarity of ultrasound screening and the developmental shape of fetal morphology. Morphometric alterations (minor signs) are evidenced earlier in gestation because of their specific diagnostic window. Major and more complex malformations (heart and brain) were diagnosed later on, probably for a better ultrasonographic evidence of anomalies.

In our experience, no significant difference exists between isolated versus multiple malformations, except for syndromic fetuses in which more than three major malformations were detected. On the other hand, syndromic fetuses represent a particular

TABLE 1. Relationship between Fetal Abnormalities and Chromosomal Anomalies

Fetal Anomaly	n	Age (years)	Weeks at Diagnosis	Chromosomal Anomalies (n)
Brain	60	28 ± 6	28 ± 5	11 (18)[a]
DTN	10	32 ± 2	26 ± 5	2 (20)
Heart	61	31 ± 4	25 ± 5	12 (20)
Urinary tract	56	30 ± 5	23 ± 5	8 (14)
Gastrointestinal	10	28 ± 10	27 ± 9	2 (20)
Abdominal wall	15	31 ± 5	26 ± 6	3 (20)
Minor signs	40	30 ± 4	23 ± 3	8 (17)
Syndromic fetuses	58	29 ± 4	25 ± 5	16 (28)
Others	34	31 ± 2	27 ± 2	1 (3)
Total	**344**	**30 ± 5**	**25 ± 5**	**63 (18)**

[a] Numbers in parentheses are expressed as percentages.

TABLE 2. Fetal Anomalies and Their Relationship to Chromosomal Anomalies

Fetal Anomalies	n	Chromosomal Anomalies		Isolated Anomalies	Chromosomal Anomalies		Multiple Anomalies	Chromosomal Anomalies	
		n	rate		n	rate		n	rate
Brain	60	11	18	35	7	20	25	4	16
DTN	10	2	20	—	—	—	10	2	20
Heart	61	12	20	17	4	23.5	44	8	18
Urinary tract	56	8	14	22	2	9	34	6	18
Gastrointestinal	10	2	20	3	1	33	7	1	14
Abdominal wall	15	3	20	11	2	18	4	1	25
Minor signs	40	7	17	33	6	18	9	2	22
Syndromic fetuses	58	16	27	—	—	—	58	16	27
Others	34	1	3	—	—	—	34	1	3
Total	**344**	**63**	**18**	**119**	**22**	**18**	**225**	**41**	**18**

NOTE: No significant differences between isolated and multiple malformations were found. In two cases we detected two associated minor signs.

group easily detectable at a routine ultrasonographic examination. Malformations can be related to all the major chromosomal defects. The prevalence of trisomy 21 in this population is 30%; trisomy 18 is 31%; and trisomy 13 is 12%.

REFERENCES

1. TABOR, A., J. PHILIP, M. MADSEN, *et al.* 1986. Randomised controlled trial of genetic amniocentesis in 4,606 low-risk women. Lancet **1:** 1287–1293.
2. BUSCAGLIA, M., L. GHISONI, M. BELLOTTI, *et al.* 1995. Genetic amniocentesis in biamniotic twin pregnancy by a single trans abdominal insertion of the needle. Prenatal Diagn. **15:** 17–19.
3. CAMERON, A.D., K.W. MURPHY, M.B. MCNAY, *et al.* 1994. Midtrimester chorionic villus sampling: An alternative approach? Am. J. Obstet. Gynecol. **171:** 1035.
4. BUSCAGLIA, M., L. GHISONI, M. BELLOTTI, E. FERRAZZI, *et al.* 1995. Percutaneous umbilical blood sampling: Indications, changes, procedures and loss rate in nine years' experience. Fetal Diagn. Ther. **11:** 106–113.
5. ALLAN, L.D., G.K. SHARLAND, S.K. CHITA, *et al.* 1991. Chromosomal anomalies in fetal heart disease. Ultrasound Obstet. Gynecol. **1:** 8–11.
6. NICOLAIDES, K.H., C.H. RODECK, I. LANGE, *et al.* 1986. Rapid karyotyping in non-lethal fetal malformations. Lancet **1:** 283–287.

Placement of Amniotic Bladder Catheter in a Fetus with Low Urinary Obstruction

J. CODESIDO, M. IGLESIAS-DIZ, R. UCIEDA, I. SILVA, E. CABO, C. GONZÁLEZ, AND J. AGUILAR

Department of Obstetrics and Gynecology, General University Hospital of Galicia, Santiago de Compostela, Spain

CLINICAL CASE OF A LIVING NEWBORN AFTER PLACEMENT OF AMNIOTIC BLADDER CATHETER

Ultrasound scanning in a 32-year-old expectant mother revealed a cystic mass in fetal pelvis and abdomen in week 17 of gestation. The mass was $47 \times 30 \times 32$ mm and occupied the pelvis of a feet-down male fetus (FIG. 1) with a biometry of 16 weeks and scarce amniotic liquid. The diagnostic impression was that of fetal mega-bladder secondary to low urinary obstruction, probably posterior urethral valves. We performed amniocentesis for karyotype (only 10 cc due to the oligoamnios), which revealed a normal 46XY formula; at the same time we pierced and emptied the pelvic formation for analysis, extracting 30 cc of transparent liquid, whose biochemical analysis was compatible with fetal urine and functioning kidneys[1]—sodium (mEq/L): 84; potassium (mEq/L): 3.1; creatinine (mg/dL): 1.1; osmolarity (mOsm/kg): 178.

When the patient was 20 weeks and 4 days from amenorrhea, the fetal bladder measured $69 \times 51 \times 56$ mm and acute oligoamnios was present, we decided to insert an amniotic bladder catheter. Although not a fail-safe method because of a high incidence of obstructions of the shunt, displacements, and fetal damages, possibilities of success at that age of gestation are very high.[2,3]

The operation took place under general anesthesia using a scanner-guided trocar; uterus inhibitors and antibiotics were administered prophylactically to the mother. Twenty-four hours later ultrasound scanning revealed amniotic liquid in normal quantities, an abdomen of 61×54 mm and fetal bladder of 18×12 mm with the catheter in its interior (FIG. 2). We carried out successive ultrasound scanning, with the amniotic liquid remaining at normal quantities and the fetus placing itself head-down a week after the operation; we also found more acute renal hypoplasia in the left kidney from week 29 onward.

We decided to do a cesarean section at week 35 and 3 days, after a period of maturing with corticoids and a large decrease in amniotic liquid. The patient gave birth to a male baby of 2.675 grams who breathed spontaneously, with an Apgar score of 9-10-10.

Although the results of the method are uncertain,[4,5] in this particular case it has been decisive for the patient, in restoring an adequate amniotic fluid, allowing pulmonary development, and decreasing the effects of a continual renal obstruction.[6,7]

The placement of the catheter in the bladder was examined and found to be well positioned, with urine flowing through it. The catheter was kept functioning during the first three days of life until we managed to introduce, with difficulty, a urinary catheter. We found renal hypoplasia, with a moderate degree of renal insufficiency of uncertain prognosis.

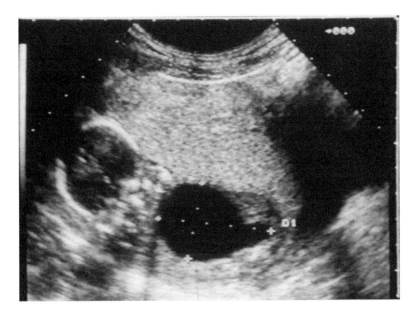

FIGURE 1. Ultrasound scanning revealed cystic mass in fetal pelvis and abdomen in week 17 of gestation.

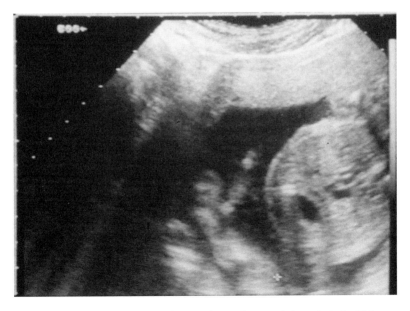

FIGURE 2. Twenty-four hours later ultrasound scanning revealed amniotic liquid in normal quantities and fetal bladder with the catheter in its interior.

The Importance of Rehabilitation on Detection of Congenital Limb Reduction Defects by Prenatal Ultrasound Screening

A.K. DASGUPTA

Disablement Services Centre, St. Mary's Hospital, Milton Road, Portsmouth PO3 6BR, England, United Kingdom

OBJECTIVE

The study was undertaken to find out the impact of prenatal ultrasound screening in determining the prior-to-birth rehabilitation consultation.

METHODS

Between 1992 and 1997, 140 (86.96%) cases of reduction defects were identified from the records of 161 congenital limb deformity cases. Only 54 (33.54%)—31 males, 23 females—fulfilled the selection criteria of age below 20 years (mean age 9.98; range 0.4–19.1 years) because 20 years ago prenatal ultrasound screening was not a routine phenomenon. Retrospective information on limb defects, prenatal ultrasound screening, the input of a rehabilitation team, the cost of prosthetic rehabilitation were collected from the records of those 54 cases and analyzed.

RESULTS

Forty-two cases (24 males, 18 females) were of transverse reduction defects, 8 (6 males, 2 females) had longitudinal defects, and 4 (1 male, 3 females) had both transverse and longitudinal defects (FIG. 1a). Single or multiple anomalies are shown in FIGURE 1b. Forty cases (23 males, 17 females) were of upper limb defects (26 left arms, 14 right arms) and FIGURE 1c shows the level of deficiency. Eight cases (6 males, 2 females) had lower limb reduction defects (4 in right legs, 3 in left legs, bilateral in 1) (FIG. 1d). The average cost of prostheses including maintenance of 52 out of 54 limb wearers in a year was £74,741.42 because two children did not require prostheses. The departmental expenditures for prostheses per person per year were £3259.41 for lower limbs, £1590.14 for upper with lower limbs, and £1029.61 for upper limbs. Cases with reduction defects (16.67%) were identified in prenatal ultrasound screening (TABLE 1). Rehabilitation physicians, prosthetists, occupational therapists, and physiotherapists were mostly involved in after-birth consultations. Early consultations were with the rehabilitation physicians but delayed consultations were with occupational/physiotherapists.

DISCUSSION

The prevalence at birth of congenital limb reduction defects is about 5 per 10,000 births (range, 3 to 8 per 10,000).[1] The notified live-born limb reduction deformity ba-

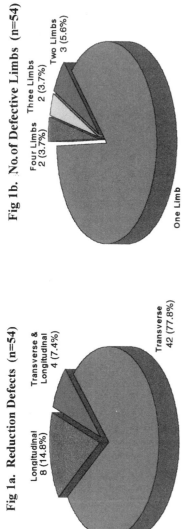

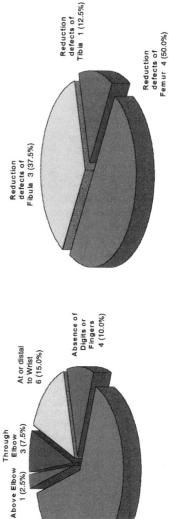

FIGURE 1. Congenital limb reduction defects.

TABLE 1. Prenatal Ultrasound Screening and Prebirth Rehabilitation Consultation

	Ultrasound Screening with Reduction Defects	
Results (*n*=54)	*n*	%
Positive	9	16.67
Negative/Not done/Not known	45	83.33
Prebirth consultation	2	3.70

bies[2] were 194, of which 4 (2.06%) had multiple anomalies. In the Portsmouth center during 5 years, 140 cases (old and new) of reduction defects were found, of which 54 (40.30%) were selected below the age of 20 years. Of the 54, 7 (12.96%) had more than two anomalies. Transverse reduction defects were more common than the longitudinal reduction defects. Lower limbs involvement was low, and the majority was upper limb deficiency. The ratio was 1:4. Nine cases (16.67%) of reduction defects were identified on ultrasound prenatal screening and 83.55% were not. The prenatal ultrasound screening is therefore of limited value in determining the prevalence of reduction defects. The findings from Glasgow, United Kingdom,[3] also supported this, because only 18 (13.43%) cases were prenatally diagnosed from the data of 134 cases of limb reduction defects for the period of 1980–1991. If, on prenatal screening, the limb reduction defect is discovered, the decision to terminate the pregnancy sometimes arises. Prebirth rehabilitation consultation will be beneficial to the mother if the parents accept the deformity and the mother wishes to continue the pregnancy. This is preferable in comparison to the child being born with a deformity after a normal pregnancy, without knowledge of the abnormality during prenatal period even having had a routine ultrasound screening. In this center, only two cases (3.70%, that is, 22.22% of the ultrasound positive cases) were referred for prebirth consultations, but all 54 cases had afterbirth consultation. During consultation, particular attention is given to attitude, motivation, and mental state of the parents regarding the acceptance of the deformity and the prosthetic rehabilitation of the child. Sometimes counseling is necessary for the parents. Here, the parents of 27.78% of the children had difficulty in accepting the after-birth deformity and the future outcome. During prebirth consultation, reassurance, some idea of prosthetic management, and introduction to other team members are necessary. Early postdelivery consultation is required to confirm the type of congenital anomaly. Initially, parents are usually introduced to other children with a similar deformity and their parents. The concept of various types of prostheses and its outcome are usually explained. Use of arms and training in walking are usually given by occupational therapists and physiotherapists. More training and the cost of prostheses will depend upon the type of training and technological advances. The involvement of social workers will depend upon the home circumstances. Prostheses, especially the upper limbs, are usually given within 5–6 months (previously as late as 3–4 years). Here, 11 (20.37%) children were prosthetically rehabilitated within six months, and the majority (18.52%) were with upper limbs. Early rehabilitation is, however, important because there will be less chance of delayed acceptance or rejection of prostheses.

CONCLUSION

Low detection and low referral rate during the prenatal period suggest that prenatal ultrasound screening has limited value in detecting limb deficiency. Early detection with improved technology in ultrasound during prenatal screening will definitely help in decision making and also increases the chances of effective rehabilitation of both the child and its parents, involving a multidisciplinary team.

REFERENCES

1. BROWN, N., J. LUMLEY, C. TICKLE & J. KEENE. 1996. Congenital Limb Reduction Defects. The Stationery Office. London.
2. OFFICE OF THE NATIONAL STATISTICS. Congenital Anomaly statistics notification, England and Wales, 1994. The Stationery Office. MB3, 10. London.
3. LE-HA CHI, D.H. STONE & W.H. GILMOUR. 1995. Impact of prenatal screening and diagnosis on the epidemiology of structural congenital anomalies. J. Med. Screening **2:** 67–70.

Impact of Ultrasound Screening for Facial Cleft on Mother-Child Relationships

S. MAES,[a,d] A. DEMEY,[b] AND J. APPELBOOM-FONDU[c]

Hôpital des Enfants Reine Fabiola, Université Libre de Bruxelles, Departments of Child Psychiatry,[a] Plastic Surgery,[b] and Child and Adolescent Psychopathology,[c] 15, av. J.J. Crocq, B-1020 Brussels, Belgium

INTRODUCTION

The cleft lip and/or palate is one of the most common congenital malformations. In Belgium, if this defect is detected during an echography in the course of a routine checkup, parents are not systematically told for fear of provoking a psychological strain which could be damaging for a pregnancy that is normal in all other respects. The doctor withholds the information until birth, thus jeopardizing this key stage of the parents' early bonding with the child.

When the mother is told of the malformation during a routine prenatal echography, she is, naturally, traumatized. Subsequently, the psychological defense mechanisms are put into play, leading to the acceptance of the diagnosis. She will have started the mourning process for the imagined child before birth and will be prepared to welcome it into the world. A prenatal announcement, however, also presents some risks. If the mother's imagination runs away with herself when she is told of the diagnosis, whether due to a maternal psychological fragility or an imprecise medical explanation, she is in danger of turning her imagined child into a monstrous image. She will fear the moment of giving birth and finally the pregnancy will become a painful time for her. In order to achieve a more precise awareness of the psychological impact of a prenatal diagnosis on the mother-child relationship, we carried out a prenatal study on mothers of children suffering from a cleft lip-palate.

METHOD AND POPULATION

Fifty-nine mothers of children between the ages of 6 and 18 months, who had received surgical treatment at the Hôpital Universitaire des Enfants Reine Fabiola (HUDERF) for the surgical closure of a cleft lip or lip-palate, received a written, semidescriptive questionnaire. Twenty-two questionnaires were returned to us fully completed. Using these questionnaires, the mothers involved in this study were asked questions about their personal experiences and relationships. They gave their opinion on the most appropriate time to be told about the diagnosis.

Among the 22 newborn children taking part in the study, 16 suffered from a cleft lip-palate and 6 suffered only a cleft lip. The average age of the babies when the questionnaires were disseminated was 11.5 months with a standard deviation of 4.5 months.

---

[d] Corresponding author.

RESULTS

- Eight mothers were given a prenatal diagnosis. Seven of these mothers said, with hindsight, they preferred this method of announcing the anomaly. The eighth did not underline any of the choices, wishing to qualify her answer according to "the capacity of the parents to be told the news."
- Among the 14 mothers who only became aware of the defect at birth, 9 would have preferred a prenatal diagnosis.
- Of the total of 22 women questioned, 16 (72.7%) were in favor of a prenatal diagnosis, whereas in fact only 8 mothers (36.3%) were actually told in this way.

DISCUSSION

Except for the mother who did not provide an answer, the mothers who received a prenatal diagnosis advocate this type of procedure. Being told of the defect is a traumatic moment, but each time parents were told, they were provided with descriptive, etiologic, and therapeutic information and support and were given very encouraging prognoses. This made it easier for them to bond with their child at an early stage.

Fourteen mothers were told of the anomaly at birth. Most of these mothers, that is, 9 (64.3%), would have preferred a prenatal diagnosis in order to take advantage of the support offered when the announcement is made. Among the 14 mothers told of the anomaly at birth, 5 (37.5%) preferred prenatal diagnosis in hindsight. One of them said that the joy of the birth helped her to overcome her trauma, but that the trauma continues within the family. The four others suffered a psychologically difficult pregnancy and considered that they were too fragile to face up to the shock of a prenatal diagnosis.

It should be noted that several mothers spontaneously said that the most appropriate moment to be told was between the seventh and eighth month of the pregnancy. The following reasons were given: they were not in a position to make the difficult choice of whether or not to have an abortion; the parents would have enough time to get over the initial shock; the waiting time is sufficiently short to allow them to keep their imagination and anxieties under control until the birth of their child.

The first results of this study need to be confirmed by a broader sample in order to obtain data which are statistically representative.

CONCLUSION

Despite being a traumatic experience, a prenatal diagnosis of a cleft lip, carried out under suitable conditions[1,2] during an echography,[3] has a positive impact on the future mother-child relationship. All the parents who took part in the study said that they were helped considerably by the information given to them,[4,5] especially by meeting the pediatric surgeon before the birth. The fact that the child is surrounded by a cohesive multidisciplinary team reassures these parents. On the other hand, any doubt expressed by the providers of care and felt by the parents can give rise to considerable anxiety. A prenatal detection also allows the medical team at the birth to prepare themselves to welcome this newborn baby and its family. A mother who was psychologically fragile during pregnancy, will clearly be as fragile—and possibly more so—when she is giving birth. If the doctor considers that it is necessary to postpone the announcement of the diagnosis, then psychological assistance must be available at birth. At all times, this type of support may prove to be necessary for some parents.

The psychological approach toward these children must be integrated within a multidisciplinary team, which is responsible for the subsequent therapeutic follow-up. The well-being of these children and of their family begins before the actual birth, and it is important to take this into consideration during the obstetric procedures.

REFERENCES

1. DECANT, D. 1985. L'annonce du handicap. Le point de vue du psychanalyste. L'Enfance **6:** 28–34.
2. ROY, J. & H. HUGUET-PECH. 1987. The physician and the disclosure of a handicap in a neonate: A review of the literature. Early Child Dev. Care **27:** 73–89.
3. MOLENAT, F. *et al.* 1984. La révélation anténatale par échographie d'une anomalie faciale et ses effets sur la place de l'enfant à naître. Sem. Hôp. Paris **60:** 1941–1944.
4. CLIFFORD, E. & E.C. CROCKER. 1971. Maternal responses: The birth of a normal child as compared to the birth of a child with cleft. Cleft Palate J. **Jul.:** 298–306.
5. FAUFMAN, F. 1991. Managing the cleft lip and palate patient. Pediatr. Clin. North Am. **38:** 1127–1147.

Ongoing Surveillance for Neural Tube Defects and Down Syndrome in a Large Urban Maternal Newborn Hospital

P.R. WYATT,[a] A.M. SUMMERS, G. DIMNIK, B. POLLARD, AND N. SHILLETTO

Department of Genetics and Prenatal Diagnosis Unit, North York General Hospital, 4001 Leslie Street, Toronto, Ontario, Canada M2K 1E1

INTRODUCTION

North York General Hospital is a large general hospital in Ontario's biggest urban center—the Greater Toronto area (population 4,500,000). The hospital serves as a base for a large regional genetic center with over 2,500 invasive procedures per year and processing 16,000 maternal sera for triple screens per year. The hospital has a large maternal newborn program with about 4,000 deliveries per year. The number of births at the hospital represents about 3% of all the births in the province. As a result of the regional genetic center being based in a large maternal newborn hospital, a large accessible newborn and prenatal service can be followed to evaluate the impact of prenatal diagnostic care.

In Ontario, all medical services are paid by a single tax-based system. Once a medical service is recognized as an insured service, it is available to all. The patient has no direct medical costs to pay individually for services such as amniocentesis, ultrasound, maternal serum screening, or abortion. Maternal serum screening (by triple marker) was approved in Ontario as a provincial service in 1993. Thus, there are no major individual financial restrictions to assess to any prenatal diagnostic service.

However, in Ontario, because currently no provincial birth defects registry exists, only local surveillance can occur regarding impact or trends of prenatal services. We have prospectively, since 1982, been following all pregnancies where births occurred in the hospital. Virtually all patients registered with the hospital prior to 20 weeks and received their prenatal care at the regional center. We have been able to evaluate all cytogenetic records, birth records, prenatal diagnosis records, and autopsy reports.

Using an estimate prevalence of 1 in 500 in pregnancies at the second trimester for trisomy 21 and 1 in 1,200 births for neural tube defects (NTDs), the anticipated number of cases of trisomy 21/NTDs was identified for each year. This was then considered to be the expected number of cases per year.

All cases of chromosomal disease and/or NTD were then reviewed from the birthing population (birth, stillbirths, medical abortion) and any recognizable syndromes excluded (trisomy 18 with NTD, Meckel-Gruber, etc.); these became the actual cases identified for the population. The primary referral reason by which the case was originally identified—for example, cases with a positive maternal serum screen (+MSS) who were also over 35 were counted as detected by + MSS—was also recorded.

FIGURE 1 shows the expected versus actual cases identified in the 54,191 births followed. FIGURE 2 shows the actual cases sorted by detection method (+ MSS, ultra-

[a] E-mail: pwyatt@nygh.on.ca

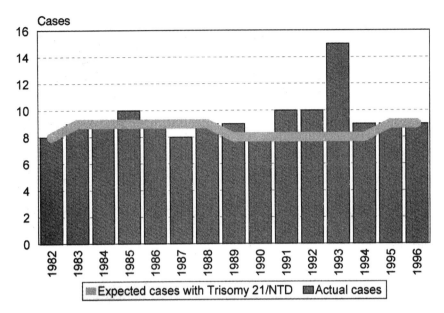

FIGURE 1. Expected and actual cases of trisomy 21 and/or neural tube defects (NTDs) in birthing population at North York General Hospital (based on newborn occurrence of 1 NTD per 1,200 births and trisomy 21 at 1 per 500 pregnancies at 16 weeks).

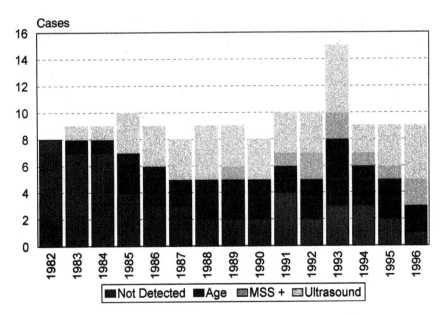

FIGURE 2. Primary method of detection of trisomy 21 and/or neural tube defects in birthing population at North York General Hospital (maternal age 35 or older at delivery, ultrasound abnormality detected, or positive maternal serum screen).

sound, age, or not detected). Although cases of trisomy 21/NTD may be prenatally detected, the information may be used to improve the treatment available to the child at birth rather than pregnancy termination.

RESULTS AND CONCLUSIONS

In a local population, monitoring of birth outcomes and prenatal services can confirm utilization rates of prenatal services and the impact of prenatal care on pregnancies outcome. There is a direct correlation between the availability of all modalities of prenatal diagnostic services and the newborn occurrence of trisomy 21 and NTDs. Small local population surveillance, however, does not provide significant numbers of cases for evaluation of the impact of new (or existing) prenatal diagnostic services for fetal disease.

Consideration should be given by all those involved in prenatal diagnostic services for large-scale population information linkage to assess and evaluate the impact of prenatal care. Some issues that should be addressed by the international cooperation include:

- Standardization of data collection through international cooperation for prenatal diagnosis
- Linkage of prenatal diagnosis information to national census records for country-to-country comparison
- Development of international standards for data collection relating to ultrasound (standardization of fetal measurement, international quality assurance programs for MSS, cytogenetics, ultrasound).

Index of Contributors

TM8414-1

7